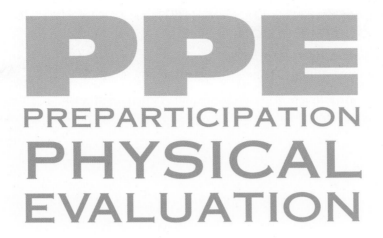

PPE
PREPARTICIPATION
PHYSICAL
EVALUATION

Fourth Edition

AMERICAN ACADEMY OF FAMILY PHYSICIANS

AMERICAN ACADEMY OF PEDIATRICS

AMERICAN COLLEGE OF SPORTS MEDICINE

AMERICAN MEDICAL SOCIETY FOR SPORTS MEDICINE

AMERICAN ORTHOPAEDIC SOCIETY FOR SPORTS MEDICINE

AMERICAN OSTEOPATHIC ACADEMY OF SPORTS MEDICINE

EDITORS
DAVID T. BERNHARDT, MD
WILLIAM O. ROBERTS, MD, MS

PUBLISHED BY

American Academy of Pediatrics
DEDICATED TO THE HEALTH OF ALL CHILDREN™

National endorsements of *Preparticipation Physical Evaluation*, Fourth Edition

- Endorsed by the American Heart Association
- Endorsed by the National Athletic Trainers' Association

Additional materials, including post-publication endorsements or statements of support, will be available at the *Preparticipation Physical Evaluation* Web site, accessible via www.ppesportevaluation.org.

Library of Congress Control Number: 2009911351

ISBN: 978-1-58110-376-2

MA0537

PREPARTICIPATION PHYSICAL EVALUATION WORKING GROUP AND AUTHORS

AUTHORING SOCIETIES

American Academy of Family Physicians
American Academy of Pediatrics
American College of Sports Medicine
American Medical Society for Sports Medicine
American Orthopaedic Society for Sports Medicine
American Osteopathic Academy of Sports Medicine

Editors

David T. Bernhardt, MD
William O. Roberts MD, MS

Organization Representatives

Joel S. Brenner, MD, MPH
John D. Campbell, MD
Dennis A. Cardone, DO
Cindy J. Chang, MD
William Dexter, MD
John P. DiFiori, MD
Jonathan A. Drezner, MD
Kimberly G. Harmon, MD
Rob Johnson, MD
Deryk Jones, MD
Amanda Weiss-Kelly, MD

ADDITIONAL CONTRIBUTORS

American Academy of Pediatrics
Anjie Emanuel, MPH
Mark Grimes
Jeanne Christensen Lindros, MPH
Jeff Mahony

American College of Sports Medicine
James R. Whitehead

American Heart Association
Robert M. Campbell, MD

American Medical Society for Sports Medicine
Jody Gold

American Orthopaedic Society for Sports Medicine
Patti Davis, MPH
Lisa Weisenberger

American Osteopathic Academy of Sports Medicine
Susan M. Rees

■ TABLE OF CONTENTS

■ PREFACE

The preparticipation physical evaluation (PPE) is used in a variety of settings from youth sports to high school and college sports; however, there has not been a systematic approach to its implementation or evaluation. Since publication of the first edition of the *Preparticipation Physical Evaluation* monograph in 1992, there continues to be debate surrounding the effectiveness of the PPE as a screening tool for athlete safety and participation clearance. The PPE has not been studied with great rigor to determine its effectiveness in achieving goals of improving safety and health for the athletes participating in sports. Significant criticism and concerns have been raised regarding the ability of the PPE to affect outcomes, such as reducing risk of injury or sudden cardiac death. In particular, the ability of the PPE to detect athletes at risk for potentially catastrophic events, such as sudden cardiac death, has been questioned. There are several "public health" issues embedded within the topic of sports participation screening. If electrocardiogram or other screening tests or procedures are valuable for the select few who participate in organized sports, should they not be essential for all children if we are to promote exercise as a path to long-term health? The decisions to screen should be based on outcomes that truly save lives and then offered across the population, not just to athletes.

Despite these concerns, the author societies (American Academy of Family Physicians, American Academy of Pediatrics, American College of Sports Medicine, American Medical Society for Sports Medicine, American Orthopaedic Society for Sports Medicine, and American Osteopathic Academy of Sports Medicine) recognize the important role the PPE might play, not only for screening athletes, but also in the overall provision of health care by promoting regular exercise, particularly in the adolescent population.

This fourth edition of the PPE monograph reflects a rigorous attempt by the writing team to identify and outline both evidence-based and expert opinion principles and practices in the examination and activity clearance. The process included
- Definition of the issues surrounding the PPE
- An extensive review of the literature
- Use of position, policy, and consensus statements from major organizations
- Review of expert opinion
- Extensive peer review by other experts from all the author societies (assisting in content revisions)

This edition of *Preparticipation Physical Evaluation* has been reviewed extensively, and we greatly appreciate the excellent recommendations of the many professionals from the 6 societies who have reviewed the document. These individuals include experts in primary care and multiple specialties, both private practice and academic settings.

The author societies hope that this guide will serve to enhance the health and safety of athletes and all active people. In addition to facilitating care of the athlete, a standardized approach to the PPE will set the stage for data collection that may lead to future insights and changes based on outcomes.

CHAPTER 1

Introduction

The overarching goal in performing a preparticipation physical evaluation (PPE) is to promote the health and safety of the athlete in training and competition. The PPE has traditionally been considered a screening tool for injuries, illness, or factors that might place the athlete or others at risk for preventable illness or injury. The author societies (American Academy of Family Physicians, American Academy of Pediatrics, American College of Sports Medicine, American Medical Society for Sports Medicine, American Orthopaedic Society for Sports Medicine, and American Osteopathic Academy of Sports Medicine) hope that this monograph will serve to enhance the health and safety of all athletes whether or not they participate in organized sports and will make the PPE an enjoyable, informative, and useful experience for both the examiner and the athlete. A more standardized approach to the PPE will provide a tool to facilitate care of the athlete and set the stage for data collection leading to future changes based on outcome data. Ideally, the examination will uncover conditions that might require further investigation or treatment and identify conditions that would interfere with safe or optimal athletic performance.

For the PPE to be effective as a screening tool, it must identify diseases or processes that will affect the athlete, be sensitive and accurate, and be practical and affordable. Currently, data on the ability of the PPE to meet these criteria are lacking and research demonstrates that the PPE has little effect on the overall morbidity and mortality of athletes.[1] Despite this lack of efficacy data, the examinations are widely performed, with every state requiring some level of PPE for scholastic athletes. Some argue that "the PPE as currently practiced is ineffective and illogical" and "a research agenda that would provide data to more effectively promote adolescent health both on and off the playing field" is sorely needed.[2]

The National Federation of State High School Associations (NFHS) considers the PPE a prerequisite to participation; however, the NFHS has neither the authority to make the PPE a requirement nor the ability to standardize the PPE format across all of its member state associations. Simply adopting a standard format across all 50 states would improve the ability to judge the efficacy of the examination and help develop an evidence base to improve the examination at the high school level. At the collegiate level, the NCAA recommends, and most institutions require, a PPE at least on entrance to the program.[3,4] Outside of scholastic-based competition, programs like Special Olympics require a PPE for its athletes (see Chapter 7).

Youth sports governing bodies do not have uniform or consistent requirements for a PPE. This large group of young athletes participates with little or no formal screening prior to sports activity other than routine well-child examinations. Therefore, many young athletes do not have their first structured PPE until just prior to their first scholastic-based sports activity. In addition, every child should be active for health reasons, and many children and adolescents participate in vigorous exercise or activities that are not organized and never have any formal PPE screening. With the large number of young athletes participating in physical activity outside of the scholastic or organized sports arena, it would make sense to incorporate the PPE into all routine well-child and adolescent care with the implied public health message that all children and adolescents should be active.

Requirements regarding the high school scholastic sport PPE vary widely by state in content, length, and comprehensiveness. This variance is well illustrated by several studies that demonstrated that most PPE forms used in high school, and often in college, do not follow American Heart Association (AHA) guidelines regarding appropriate cardiac screening.[5-7] In a number of states, providers of varying levels of training and expertise are permitted to administer the PPE for high school athletes.[6] Equally wide variation exists in how physicians approach, conduct, and document these examinations.

While acknowledging these concerns, the author societies agree that the PPE, when thoroughly and consistently performed and supervised by qualified and licensed physicians, may be an effective tool in identifying medical and orthopedic conditions that might affect an athlete's ability to participate safely in sports. The PPE also serves as an important component of adolescent health care. For many, if not most, adolescents, the PPE is their only contact with a medical provider in any given year[5,8] and, unfortunately, for some adolescents, PPE screening examinations may be the only contact with the health care system. This limited exposure to the health care system emphasizes the need for the examination to be performed by an athlete's primary care physician in the medical (or health care) home. While the PPE is not intended to substitute for athletes' regular health maintenance examinations, it provides an opportunity to facilitate general health care, update immunizations, and establish a medical home. Ideally, the PPE findings will be used by physicians and ancillary health team members (certified athletic trainers, sports physical therapists, and others) as part of an overall health care program that focuses on the prevention, assessment, treatment, and rehabilitation of athletic injuries.

The purpose of the PPE is to facilitate and encourage safe participation, not to exclude athletes from participation. While a systematic review[9] of the PPE (>20,000 examinations) found only 3 athletes that were excluded, most individual studies report that 0.3% to 1.3% of athletes are denied clearance to participate during the PPE, with 3.2% to 13.9% requiring further evaluation prior to participation.[6,8,10-14]

■ ROUTINE SCREENING TESTS

Routine laboratory, cardiac, and pulmonary screening tests for PPEs remain controversial. However, because evidenced-based studies indicate their utility are lacking, the PPE working group concurs that no routine screening tests are required during the PPE for clearance of asymptomatic athletes.

This judgment hinges on the difference between screening tests and case finding diagnostic tests. The value of a screening test or procedure depends on 2 variables: (1) the predictive value of the proposed screen, which is in turn affected by the prevalence of the condition in the population being screened, and (2) the ability to reduce morbidity and mortality by identifying the condition with the screening method. The screening test must also be acceptable in terms of cost and potential side effects. The value of a case finding diagnostic test, on the other hand, is in its ability to pinpoint a condition for which suspicion already exists by history or physical examination.

When evaluating screening tests with the aforementioned criteria, studies have not supported the use of such tests as urinalysis, complete blood count, chemistry profile, lipid profile, ferritin level, or sickle cell trait in the PPE.[15-19] Similarly, cardiopulmonary screening with electrocardiogram (ECG), echocardiogram, exercise stress testing, or spirometry lacks research to demonstrate that it clearly meets these criteria in asymptomatic athletes.[20-26]

Of particular concern to physicians, parents or guardians, and athletes is the issue of cardiovascular screening. The decision to increase the level of screening for sudden cardiac death prevention is controversial and difficult. The current literature and expert opinion recommendations are addressed in Chapter 6A: Cardiovascular Problems to help with this decision. This will be an area of potentially rapid change over the next few years, and it will be important for all of us to keep abreast of the topic. Key to this decision is the specificity and sensitivity of our current testing when applied to more than 6 million athletes annually. For example, ECG screening in Italy has reduced the incidence of sports-related sudden cardiac death to the level currently reported in the United States, where ECG screening is not recommended by the AHA, in part because of the large number of false-positive examinations.[27,28] While the state of ECG use in US athlete screening is evolving, the current state is well described in a 2008 article by Lawless and Best,[29] "Although the literature is lacking well-controlled prospective trials, the sensitivity in detecting underlying cardiac disease in this population is about 51% to 95%, depending on the type of underlying disease and the population being studied. Since many of the conditions that cause SCD [sudden cardiac death] in athletes demonstrate similar ECG findings as to what is seen in normal athletic adaptation, clinicians need to follow some simple rules in ECG interpretation in athletes, and they need to be prepared for the consequences of both over- and under-interpretation of the ECG in this group."

Findings from the PPE medical history or physical examination may indicate a need to arrange specific case finding diagnostic tests. The examining physician may elect to defer clearance for sports participation while awaiting completion of diagnostic testing, but specific recommendations to test for targeted conditions are not part of the standardized screening examination. For example, a complete hematologic profile may be recommended to check for anemia or nutritional deficiency in an athlete who has fatigue, pallor, performance decline, heavy menstrual bleeding, low calorie intake, or a diet lacking red meat. A lipid profile to test for familial dyslipidemia is recommended in a student-athlete who has a family history of premature atherosclerotic heart disease or dyslipidemia. Urinalysis may be indicated in an athlete with dysuria, hematuria, or a family history of certain types of kidney disease. Urine screening, not as a part of the PPE but as part of a drug testing program for performance-enhancing drugs, is common among elite amateur and professional athletes and is becoming more common for intercollegiate athletes.

Mandatory human immunodeficiency virus (HIV) screening is discouraged because of the low risk of transmission, although certain boxing organizations require it.[30,31] While mandatory testing of athletes for HIV or hepatitis is not recommended,[32,33] voluntary testing should be encouraged for high-risk athletes who have exposure to blood products, symptoms suggestive of disease, or significant risk factors detected during the PPE. The current literature and expert opinion regarding testing for certain blood-borne diseases will be reviewed in Chapter 6C: General Medical.

This monograph is intended to provide a state-of-the-art, practical, and effective screening tool for physicians who perform PPEs for athletes in middle school, high school, and college. It is intended for use as a stand-alone screening examination that can be easily incorporated into routine preventive examinations within the medical home. The process and forms are designed to apply in most settings (office, school, urban, rural) and are easily adaptable to suit individual or institutional needs.

The fourth edition includes descriptions of goals, objectives, timing, setting, and structure of the examination; details the history, physical examination, and clearance considerations; lists return-to-play guidelines; addresses medicolegal and ethical concerns; and explores future research and the use of electronic formats. The text of the monograph reviews the rationale for the primary and secondary history questions as well as the examination maneuvers. While most of the content remains, as in previous editions, based on the expert opinion level of evidence, whenever there is higher-level evidence for the content, it will be noted in the text (see Table 1-1 for evidence rating). Numerous references are provided, including Web

TABLE 1-1. NATIONAL HEART, LUNG, AND BLOOD INSTITUTE EVIDENCE SCALE[a]

Evidence Category	Sources of Evidence	Definition
A	Randomized controlled trials (rich body of data)	Evidence is from endpoints of well-designed RCTs (or trials that depart only minimally from randomization) that provide a consistent pattern of findings in the population for which the recommendation is made. Category A therefore requires substantial numbers of studies involving substantial numbers of participants.
B	Randomized controlled trials (limited body of data)	Evidence is from endpoints of intervention studies that include only a limited number of RCTs, post hoc or subgroup analysis of RCTs, or meta-analysis of RCTs. In general, Category B pertains when few randomized trials exist, they are small in size, and the trial results are somewhat inconsistent, or the trials were undertaken in a population that differs from the target population of the recommendation.
C	Nonrandomized trials, observational studies	Evidence is from outcomes of uncontrolled or nonrandomized trials or from observational studies.
D	Panel consensus judgment	Expert judgment is based on the panel's synthesis of evidence from experimental research described in the literature and/or derived from the consensus of panel members based on clinical experience or knowledge that does not meet the above-listed criteria. This category is used only in cases where the provision of some guidance was deemed valuable but an adequately compelling clinical literature addressing the subject of the recommendation was deemed insufficient to justify placement in one of the other categories (A through C).

Abbreviation: RCT, randomized controlled trial.
[a]National Institutes of Health and National Heart, Lung, and Blood Institute. Clinical guidelines on the identification, evaluation, and treatment of overweight and obesity in adults: the evidence report. NIH Publication 98-4083. 1998:228.

sites, to support the discussion, provide useful resources, and offer a basis for further inquiry. The sections have been reconfigured to make them more user-friendly based on feedback from the previous edition and include system-based history, examination, and clearance sections, particulars for athletes with special needs, administrative concerns, and future directions. Succinct, comprehensive, easily used forms (pages 153–156) are supplied for athletes, parents or guardians, and clinicians.

■ REFERENCES

1. Best TM. The preparticipation evaluation: an opportunity for change and consensus. *Clin J Sport Med.* 2004;14:107–108
2. Bundy DG, Fuedtner C. Preparticipation physical evaluations for high school athletes: time for a new game plan. *Ambul Pediatr.* 2004;4:260–263
3. Montalto NJ. Implementing the guidelines for adolescent preventive services. *Am Fam Physician.* 1998;57(9):2181–2190
4. MacAuley D. Does preseason screening for cardiac disease really work? The British perspective. *Med Sci Sports Exerc.* 1998;30(10 suppl):S345–S350
5. Krowchuk DP, Krowchuk HV, Hunter M, et al. Parents' knowledge of the purposes and content of preparticipation physical examinations. *Arch Pediatr Adolesc Med.* 1995;149(6):653–657

6. Fuller CM. Cost effectiveness analysis of screening of high school athletes for risk of sudden cardiac death. *Med Sci Sports Exerc.* 2000;32(5):887–890

7. Glover DW, Maron BJ. Profile of preparticipation cardiovascular screening for high school athletes. *JAMA.* 1998;279(22):1817–1819

8. Carek PJ, Futrell M. Athletes' view of the preparticipation physical examination. *Arch Fam Med.* 1999;8(4):307–312

9. Stickler GB. Are yearly physical examinations in adolescents necessary? *J Am Board Fam Pract.* 2000;13(3):172–177

10. Klein JD, Slap GB, Elster AB, et al. Access to health care for adolescents: position paper of the Society for Adolescent Medicine. *J Adolesc Health.* 1992;13(2):162–170

11. Rosen DS, Elster A, Hedberg V, et al. Clinical preventive services for adolescents: position paper for the Society for Adolescent Medicine. *J Adolesc Health.* 1997;21(3):203–214

12. Fuller CM, McNulty CM, Spring DA, et al. Prospective screening of 5,615 high school athletes for risk of sudden cardiac death. *Med Sci Sports Exerc.* 1997;29(9):1131–1138

13. Lyznicki JM, Nielsen NH. Cardiovascular screening of student athletes. *Am Fam Physician.* 2000;62(4):765–774

14. Koester MC, Amundson CL. Preparticipation screening of high school athletes: are recommendations enough? *Phys Sportsmed.* 2003;31(8):35–38

15. Lombardo JA, Robinson JB, Smith DM, et al. *Preparticipation Physical Evaluation.* Kansas City, MO: American Academy of Family Physicians, American Academy of Pediatrics, American Medical Society for Sports Medicine, American Orthopaedic Society for Sports Medicine, American Osteopathic Academy of Sports Medicine; 1992

16. Dodge WF, West EF, Smith EH, et al. Proteinuria and hematuria in school children: epidemiology and early natural history. *J Pediatr.* 1976;88(2):327–347

17. Peggs JF, Reinhardt RW, O'Brien JM. Proteinuria in adolescent sports physical examinations. *J Fam Pract.* 1986;22(1):80–81

18. Taylor WC III, Lombardo JA. Preparticipation screening of college athletes: value of the complete blood cell count. *Phys Sportsmed.* 1990;18(6):106–118

19. Vehaskari VM, Rapola J. Isolated proteinuria: analysis of a school-age population. *J Pediatr.* 1982;101(5):661–668

20. Ades PA. Preventing sudden death: cardiovascular screening of young athletes. *Phys Sportsmed.* 1992;20(9):75–89

21. Epstein SE, Maron BJ. Sudden death and the competitive athlete: perspectives on preparticipation screening studies. *J Am Coll Cardiol.* 1986;7(1):220–230

22. Feinstein RA, Colvin E, Oh MK. Echocardiographic screening as part of a preparticipation examination. *Clin J Sport Med.* 1993;3(3):149–152

23. Lewis JF, Maron BJ, Diggs JA, et al. Preparticipation echocardiographic screening for cardiovascular disease in a large, predominantly black population of collegiate athletes. *Am J Cardiol.* 1989;64(16):1029–1033

24. Maron BJ, Bodison SA, Wesley YE, et al. Results of screening a large group of intercollegiate competitive athletes for cardiovascular disease. *J Am Coll Cardiol.* 1987;10(6):1214–1221

25. Rupp NT, Brudno DS, Guill MF. The value of screening for risk of exercise-induced asthma in high school athletes. *Ann Allergy.* 1993;70(4):339–342

26. Rupp NT, Guill MF, Brudno DS. Unrecognized exercise-induced bronchospasm in adolescent athletes. *Am J Dis Child.* 1992;146(8):941–944

27. Corrado D, Pelliccia A, Bjørnstad HH, et al. Cardiovascular pre-participation screening of young competitive athletes for prevention of sudden death: proposal for a common European protocol. *European Heart J.* 2005;26:516–524

28. Maron BJ, Thompson PD, Ackerman MJ, et al. Recommendations and considerations related to preparticipation screening for cardiovascular abnormalities in competitive athletes: 2007 update. *Circulation.* 2007;115:1643–1655

29. Lawless CE, Best TM. Electrocardiograms in athletes: interpretation and diagnostic accuracy. *Med Sci Sports Exerc.* 2008;40(5):787–798

30. Mast EE, Goodman RA, Bond WW, et al. Transmission of blood-borne pathogens during sports: risk and prevention. *Ann Intern Med.* 1995;122(4):283–285

31. Drotman DP. Professional boxing, bleeding, and HIV testing. *JAMA.* 1996;276(3):193

32. Mitten MJ. HIV-positive athletes: when medicine meets the law. *Phys Sportsmed.* 1994;22(10):63–68

33. American Medical Society for Sports Medicine, American Academy of Sports Medicine. Human immunodeficiency virus and other blood-borne pathogens in sports. *Clin J Sport Med.* 1995;5(3):199–204

CHAPTER 2

Goals and Objectives

The preparticipation physical evaluation (PPE) has been adopted as a standard of care by many organizations and countries. Unfortunately, there is little agreement on the nature, content, and efficacy of these examinations.[1] The most important goal of the PPE is to promote the health and safety of athletes. This goal is facilitated by adhering to the primary objectives (Box 2-1). The secondary objectives take advantage of the athlete's contact with the physician (and health care system) during the PPE (see Box 2-1) to influence health care and prevention. Ultimately, the PPE provides the medical background on which physical activity decisions will be made by the individual athlete's physician or the team physician and associated medical staff. It is well documented that 75% or more of medical and orthopedic conditions are detected by the history alone.[2–4] Accordingly, this monograph focuses on the history as the most relevant aspect of the PPE. Where possible, the forms include validated questions (eg, from the Youth Risk Behavioral Survey) and recommendations from consensus documents by other organizations, such as the American Heart Association and the United States Preventive Services Task Force (USPSTF).

Box 2-1. Objectives of the Preparticipation Physical Evaluation

Primary Objectives
1. Screen for conditions that may be life-threatening or disabling.
2. Screen for conditions that may predispose to injury or illness.

Secondary Objectives
1. Determine general health.
2. Serve as an entry point to the health care system for adolescents.
3. Provide an opportunity to initiate discussion on health-related topics.

■ PRIMARY OBJECTIVES

1. **Detect potentially life-threatening or disabling medical or musculoskeletal conditions.** There is no solid evidence that a screening PPE will reliably identify important but clinically silent conditions (such as hypertrophic cardiomyopathy),[5] yet the consensus panel feels that a comprehensive, uniformly applied approach to the PPE offers the best opportunity to meet this objective. Both absolute and relative contraindications for safe participation are considered. For example, myocarditis is an absolute contraindication for most if not all sports because of the risk of sudden death with exertion. Ventricular septal defect, however, is a relative contraindication, because the athlete may be able to participate, depending on the severity of the defect.

2. **Screen for medical or musculoskeletal conditions that may predispose an athlete to injury or illness during training or competition.** In a survey[3] of 716 athletes, about 66% believed that the PPE was not absolutely necessary to participate safely in sports. However, 90% believed that the PPE could help prevent injury. Though evidence is lacking regarding the ability of the PPE to conclusively meet this objective, there is general agreement that identification of conditions that may predispose an athlete to injury or illness is worthwhile. Such conditions include acute, recurrent, chronic, or untreated injuries or illnesses; inadequately rehabilitated injuries; and congenital or developmental problems.

   Early recognition of any of these problems minimizes time lost from play by initiating evaluation and treatment and completing rehabilitation. For example, an athlete with recurrent ankle sprains who has returned to sports prior to completing ankle rehabilitation will likely benefit from instruction and follow-up regarding appropriate rehabilitation. Similarly, an obese athlete is at an increased risk for heat illness and may benefit from counseling on weight control, acclimatization, and hydration before the season starts. While exercise-induced bronchospasm (EIB) is not reliably picked up by screening questions and examination,[6] identification of those athletes with conditions such as EIB and skin infection allows the physician to initiate treatment or refer the athlete for appropriate care.

■ SECONDARY OBJECTIVES

1. **Determine general health.** Studies have shown that many adolescents do not routinely see a health care provider and, in fact, the only contact many will have with the health care system is via a required PPE.[7] This finding may be especially true of athletes from low-income families who cannot afford routine medical care. One review of the effectiveness of the PPE in identifying abnormalities suggests that yearly examinations of adolescents are not useful or cost-effective.[8] However, the Society for Adolescent Medicine (SAM) estimates that 5% to 10% of adolescents will have a chronic condition that requires ongoing care, and up to half of adolescents will have less severe medical problems.[6] Furthermore, there are other reasons to consider periodic health examinations including general health screening, counseling, and establishing a medical home or primary care relationship. The Guidelines for Adolescent Preventive Services (GAPS) developed by the American Medical Association (AMA) and the Centers for Disease Control and Prevention recommends that all adolescents have an annual routine health examination. A similar recommendation is made by the SAM, American Academy of Pediatrics (AAP), American Academy of Family Physicians (AAFP), and USPSTF.[9,10]

2. **Serve as an entry point into the health care system for adolescents.** The SAM recommends that health care for adolescents be readily available, visible, confidential, affordable, and flexible.[10] A thorough PPE can and ideally should be integrated into a regular examination with the athlete's personal physician. The best practice for performing a preparticipation evaluation is in the context of the patient's medical home. It is in this setting that it is most appropriate to pursue the secondary objectives. The PPE is not intended to replace routine health maintenance visits. However, because the PPE is the only periodic health examination for many athletes, it seems prudent to acknowledge the reality of how and when adolescents receive health care.

   One interesting study[4] notes that up to one-third of parents identify the PPE as their student-athlete's only contact with the health care system; even when up to 90% had an identified primary care provider and their insurance covered yearly health maintenance examinations. While 95% of parents agreed with the primary goals of the PPE (to detect conditions that might affect participation) and 68% believed it should be minimal, one-third thought the PPE should address other health issues and might be a reasonable alternative to routine comprehensive examinations.

Given the above, and viewing the PPE as a point of entry to the health care system, follow-up becomes a critical component of the PPE process. Special attention must be paid to having a careful system to generate necessary referrals; particularly for PPEs not done one-on-one in the private physician's office.

3. **Provide an opportunity for discussion on health and lifestyle issues.** The opportunity to use the PPE as a way to engage adolescents in a discussion on health issues should not be overlooked. There is little solid evidence that supports brief counseling interventions with adolescent lifestyle issues (eg, tobacco and alcohol consumption), but the AAP, SAM, AAFP, AMA, and others recommend such counseling for preventive visits.[11] The PPE provides an opportunity to begin this dialogue.

Seventy percent of adolescents express a desire for more health care information from their personal physician. Despite this statistic, most adolescents also relate that they are not comfortable with questions related to risk behaviors, substance use, sexuality, or weight and diet in the context of a station-based examination.[12] Depending on available time, the PPE, particularly when performed as an office-based or perhaps a modified one-on-one coordinated medical team examination (see Methods and Setting of Evaluation on page 14 of Chapter 3), may provide an opportunity for counseling the athlete and answering health-related questions if patient comfort and reasonable confidentiality are ensured.

Issues that arise may include an explanation of abnormal findings or topics such as proper training techniques, weight-control behaviors, and nutrition. Tobacco use, drinking and driving, drug use, seat belt use, prevention of sexually transmitted infections, and birth control may also be discussed. This objective may be hard to meet, but should be attempted when practical. Using a standardized questionnaire such as the one developed by GAPS allows for a comprehensive overview of many risks faced by the adolescent athlete (http://www.ama-assn.org/ama/pub/physician-resources/public-health/promoting-healthy-lifestyles/adolescent-health/guidelines-adolescent-preventive-services.shtml). The information obtained during the PPE can provide the physician a means to at least initiate discussion with the athlete or to make appropriate referral for health-related and lifestyle issues.

■ REFERENCES

1. Carek P. Evidence-based preparticipation physical examination. In: MacAuley D, ed. *Evidence-Based Sports Medicine.* Malden, MA: Blackwell Pub; 2007:18–35

2. Koester MC, Amundson CL. Preparticipation screening of high school athletes: are recommendations enough? *Phys Sportsmed.* 2003;31(8):35–38

3. Carek PJ, Futrell M. Athletes' view of the preparticipation physical examination. *Arch Fam Med.* 1999;8(4):307–312

4. Krowchuk DP, Krowchuk HV, Hunter DM, et al. Parents' knowledge of the purposes and content of preparticipation physical examinations. *Arch Pediatr Adolesc Med.* 1995;149(6):653–657

5. Wingfield K, Matheson GO, Meeuwisse WH. Preparticipation evaluation: an evidence-based review. *Clin J Sport Med.* 2004;14(3):109–122

6. Hulkower S, Fagan B, Watts J, Ketterman E, Fox BA. Clinical inquiries: do preparticipation clinical exams reduce morbidity and mortality for athletes? *J Fam Pract.* 2005;54(7):628–632; discussion 628

7. Metzl J. The adolescent preparticipation physical examination: is it useful? *Clin Sports Med.* 2000;19(4):577–590

8. Montalto N. Implementing the guidelines for adolescent preventive services. *Am Fam Physician.* 1998;57(9):2181–2190

9. Rosen DS, Elster A, Hedberg V, et al. Clinical preventive services for adolescents: position paper of the Society for Adolescent Medicine. *J Adolesc Health.* 1997;21(3):203–214

10. United States Preventive Services Task Force. *The Guide to Medical Preventive Services.* 2nd ed. Alexandria, VA: International Medical Publishing Inc; 1996

11. Moyer V, Butler M. Gaps in the evidence for well-child care: a challenge to our profession. *Pediatrics.* 2004;114:1511–1521

12. Klein JD. Access to health care for adolescents: position paper of the Society for Adolescent Medicine. *J Adolesc Health.* 1992;13(2):162–170

Timing, Setting, and Structure

The timing, setting, and structure of the preparticipation physical evaluation (PPE) depends on many factors including the age of the participants (college vs high school), the presence of a team physician, the availability of health care providers trained and willing to do the examinations, and the health insurance available to the athlete.

■ QUALIFICATIONS OF THE EXAMINERS

Physicians with an MD or DO degree have the clinical training and unrestricted medical license that allows them to deal with the broad range of problems that may be encountered during the PPE. For this reason, the PPE writing group concurs that the ultimate responsibility for the PPE should be assigned to a physician with an MD or DO degree.[1-3] Physicians performing PPEs must be able to fulfill the goals and objectives outlined in the previous chapter and should seek consultation with an appropriate specialist to address problems beyond their expertise.[1]

State regulations determine which practitioners are licensed to perform PPEs for public, middle, and high schools, and many states allow health care providers other than physicians to perform the evaluation. Regardless of their training, practitioners performing PPEs should competently screen athletes for problems that would affect participation or place the athlete at undue risk (greater than the inherent risk of the sport). Implementing standardized history forms in paper or electronic format or more comprehensive electronic history forms to gather the appropriate health data prior to the examination would mitigate the variance in training that is permitted by law in some states. At the collegiate, professional, national, and international competition levels, the respective athletic governing bodies determine who may perform the PPE, and standardized formats would likewise benefit those athletes.

When PPEs are done in a group setting, the team physician should coordinate the process and supervise a team of health care professionals to ensure that all appropriate components of the assessment take place as outlined in Table 3-1.

TABLE 3-1. ELEMENTS OF A COORDINATED MEDICAL EVALUATION

Stage	Purpose
Waiting area	Sign-in, registration, and review, including careful instruction about completing required forms.
Vitals station	Height, weight, body mass index,[a] blood pressure, heart rate, and visual acuity may be performed by qualified personnel such as medical assistants, student athletic trainers, medical students, etc.
General medical examination station	History review and physical examination performed by a single physician for a given student-athlete. Clearance status and/or referral plan determined.
Specialty examination stations	Orthopedic assessment, cardiology evaluation, pulmonary function testing, or other systems-based examination.
Optional stations	Education and/or immunization areas.

[a]Body mass index can be calculated from height and weight (see www.cdc.gov/growthcharts).

■ TIMING OF THE EVALUATION

To allow time to further evaluate, treat, or rehabilitate any problem identified in the screening examination, the PPE should ideally be performed at least 6 weeks prior to the start of preseason practice. The PPE writing group feels that student-athletes should ideally schedule this with their personal physician, who has access to medical records, can adjust treatment of chronic medical conditions, and can incorporate the examination into routine well-child examinations. Both the American Academy of Family Physicians and the American Academy of Pediatrics (AAP) endorse the concept of the medical home as a patient-centered model to improve timely, well-organized, and regular care; eliminate barriers to care; and create greater access to preventive care services including the PPE. Whether done by the personal physician or in a group examination, ideal scheduling options include PPEs in midsummer or even at the end of the previous school year. This approach allows the student-athlete to complete any needed evaluations or consultations when they will have less impact on school attendance and sports practice. Athletes examined at the end of the school year for a sport occurring the next fall should report any interval injuries or medical problems that occurred during the summer to the team physician or athletic trainer prior to fall practice to allow needed evaluation. Many collegiate sports medicine programs coordinate the PPE screening process to have these examinations completed before the student-athletes begin practice in their respective sports.

Student-athletes need clear information about how to handle PPE forms so that the clearance forms sent to the school are properly handled and free of confidential information. The history and physical examination forms are intended to remain a part of the confidential medical record at the personal physician's office or in a secure area that can be accessed only by designated medical providers and in accordance with the Health Insurance Portability and Accountability Act (see Chapter 4). Ensuring a secure area in a high school sports setting may be difficult.

For personal physicians to play a greater role in the PPE process, both student-athletes and parents or guardians must assume responsibility for scheduling an appointment with the physician well before the start of the sport season and honestly completing the health history section. Athletes who wait until the week before their season starts may have difficulty being cleared in time for the start of preseason practices, and athletes (and parents or guardians) who do not honestly complete the health history put themselves at unnecessary risk for an adverse outcome.

■ FREQUENCY OF THE EVALUATION

College athletic departments generally determine the PPE frequency policies for their athletes. Since college students typically attend school away from their parents or guardians and their personal physicians and colleges assume some financial risk for athletes during practice and play, more comprehensive health examinations at entry into a collegiate athletic program are the norm. Once a comprehensive evaluation has occurred, student-athletes usually undergo shorter yearly examinations that focus on any injuries and medical problems that may have occurred since the initial comprehensive entry examination. The team physician at the collegiate level needs to become familiar with the health history of the student-athletes and typically will perform many of the examinations as well as review all of the information from completed examinations and yearly updates. This PPE writing group feels this frequency is appropriate for the college age-group.[4]

At the secondary school level, a 2006 survey of all states completed through the Minnesota State High School League Sports Medicine Advisory Committee reveals that the following options are currently used for PPE intervals prior to participation in interscholastic sports activities.

- Thirty-five states require a yearly examination with or without a mandated form.
- Eleven states require every other year comprehensive examinations; 6 with either an interval questionnaire or limited examination and 5 with no interval screening.
- Three states require comprehensive examinations every 3 years with required interval questionnaires in each of the non-examination years.
- Several states do not use a standardized examination form.

The implementation of a nationwide format for PPEs and a data-based recommendation regarding frequency of examination have been delayed by lack of research and other factors. Some issues that have influenced these decisions include (1) the requirements set by each state governing body and by specific schools; (2) the degree of risk of a particular sport; (3) the cost, especially out-of-pocket expenses for students, because costs will be barriers to participation; and (4) the availability of qualified personnel.

No outcome-based research indicates that more frequent PPEs lessen the risk of injury or death in student-athletes, so an optimal frequency for the examination has not been established.[5-10] The consensus of the PPE writing group is

- A comprehensive PPE should be performed every 2 years in younger student-athletes and every 2 to 3 years in older athletes.
- Annual updates should include a comprehensive history questionnaire and a problem-focused examination of any concerns detected in the history.

The basis for this recommendation is that student-athletes pass through stages of development that have both physiologic and psychological changes that merit monitoring. Careful cardiac auscultation on an every other to every third year basis may help screen for previously undetected cardiac conditions. The annual history review also allows an opportunity to address new concerns that may have developed since the time of their comprehensive examination.

One frequent argument for performing a complete PPE annually is that many athletes and parents or guardians use the PPE as their only visit for health care.[11] The AAP recommends routine health screening examinations annually from age 6 to 21 years for healthy children and adolescents,[12] and the Institute for Clinical Systems Improvement recommends periodic health screening elements be integrated into every child and adolescent encounter, acknowledging that there is little evidence to support any of the prescribed interval recommendations for routine health care.[13] When student-athletes have no primary physician, the PPE encounter is unlikely to comprehensively address all health and anticipatory guidance issues, especially when done in a group setting. With this in mind, the examining physician should encourage the student-athlete to establish care with a primary care physician to begin periodic health screening. Conversely, when the student-athlete's personal physician performs annual examinations, required elements of the PPE should be incorporated along with continuity of care and health education so a separate visit for a PPE would not be needed. Incorporating the PPE into the routine health care screening schedule after age 6 may promote physical activity and sports safety in children and adolescents before they reach the age of interscholastic competition and potentially screen for risk of activity-related sudden cardiac death and other medical problems in all children, including those who are not involved in organized sport activities.

■ METHODS AND SETTING OF EVALUATION

The most common methods for performing PPEs are individual examinations or group-based assessments by a coordinated medical team performed in the individual physician's office or a similar private setting. The PPE writing group considers gymnasium/locker room–based examinations as inappropriate to accomplish the goals and objectives of the PPE process. When a group of medical personnel work together to complete the PPE, the history review, physical examination, and sports clearance process should still be a one-on-one examination with a single physician rather than splitting the examination into body system stations where the athlete has the heart and lungs examined at one station, the head and neck at another, and so on. Adolescent athletes should be seen apart from their parents or guardians for at least part of the examination so that the physician can inquire about risk-taking behaviors.

Ideally, the PPE is performed in the athlete's **primary care physician's office,** allowing for better continuity of care. The athlete's personal physician, who has an established relationship, is likely to know the patient's history and have a complete set of medical records, including family history, immunizations, and laboratory studies. Access to the complete medical record during the PPE reduces the possibility that a previously detected abnormality or family risk factor will be missed or omitted that would predispose the athlete to unnecessary risk. The personal physician may be less likely to overlook something that was inadvertently or consciously omitted during completion of the PPE history form. In addition, for student-athletes with known medical problems, the personal physician should have a better sense of the athlete's condition and potential changes in treatment that would allow safer participation. If needed, the personal physician can also coordinate care with consultants. The PPE writing group believes that a personal physician is the ideal person to complete a PPE.

The office setting typically offers privacy and a chance to discuss confidential issues. Familiarity also provides an opportunity to counsel the athlete on sensitive issues and a variety of risk-taking behaviors such as tobacco use, alcohol and recreational drug use, performance enhancement drug use, unsafe nutritional practices, birth control, and prevention of sexually transmitted infections. Young athletes are often more willing to discuss these issues with someone they know and trust rather than a stranger in a group examination.

The only disadvantage to a PPE completed by an athlete's personal physician is the possible lack of understanding the implication of each question or finding in the examination in relation to the athlete at risk. This could reduce the effectiveness of the PPE screening visit. The purpose of this monograph is to close that knowledge gap for primary physicians to improve the quality of the PPE.

Coordinated medical team examinations have a useful role, particularly for student-athletes who do not have a personal physician. Often these examinations are done as a community service and can reduce costs for student-athletes who have limited financial resources, but the team examinations are even more dependent on athletes and parents or guardians accurately completing the health history section. Coordinated medical teams typically are organized by the team physician and often involve both primary care and orthopedic sports medicine specialists, and occasionally activity-oriented cardiologists. Other medical specialists and professionals may allow on-site consultation for a wide range of problems.

In the coordinated medical team approach where multiple physicians are involved (Box 3-1), the PPE writing group recommends that a single physician review the history and perform the examination for a student-athlete. However, on review of the history form, individuals with known medical issues could be directed to the primary care physicians or a medical subspecialty consultant depending on the nature of the condition, and those with known orthopedic issues could be primarily screened by the orthopedists. Colleges typically use a coordinated medical team and may institute special evaluations uniquely useful for a given sport.

Effective coordination of PPEs requires assembling the right mix of personnel. There must be adequate numbers of physicians to comprehensively examine and review each athlete. Primary care and orthopedic physicians can compliment each other's skills in this setting, while cardiologists and other physicians can play a useful role within their particular areas of expertise. By working as a medical team, physicians can also rely on colleagues to help with difficult assessments rather than having to refer the athlete for further assessment and delaying participation clearance. The team physician typically cannot screen all

Box 3-1. Tips to Improve the Coordinated Medical Team Approach to Preparticipation Physical Evaluations

Preparation
Provide the athletes information in advance about the detailed nature of the examination.[a]
Privacy
Ensure separate and private areas for examining male and female athletes.
Require appropriate examination attire (tank tops work well for female athletes).
Ensure a private counseling room for discussion of sensitive issues.
Continuity of care
Enhance familiarity and continuity of care by enlisting the assistance of as many of the athletes' primary physicians and orthopedists as possible for the group being examined.
Referrals
Establish a clear protocol for referral to appropriate primary physicians and specialists for more extensive evaluation or rehabilitation for every student-athlete who is not cleared for participation.
Aid athletes who need help arranging follow-up evaluations (ie, low-income, uninsured, and those without physicians).
Disqualification
Keep a record of athletes who are disqualified or who require further evaluation before final clearance (see Determining Clearance in each system section of Chapter 6). The team physician or PPE site physician coordinator should follow up on the athletes to establish the final disposition.
Counsel the athlete who is not cleared for the desired sport regarding possible alternate activities.

[a]Filling out the history, physical examination, and clearance forms (pages 153–156) carefully can improve the entire process. Therefore, at the start of a coordinated medical team evaluation, explaining to the student-athletes how to correctly complete the forms will result in a more useful completed form. Appropriate privacy, storage, and handling of forms can give the athlete greater confidence in the confidentiality of the process.

individuals but, by coordinating the process, can learn the overall health status of many student-athletes and be brought into the evaluation of all of those with serious problems.

Physical therapists, athletic trainers, nutritionists, and exercise physiologists can be incorporated to help with check-in, check-out, "traffic control," vital sign measurements, patient education, and teaching of rehabilitation exercises. Coaches and school administrators can be enlisted to help maintain order and discipline in what can be a chaotic environment.

The team physician must choose a location that will allow adequate space for the large number of participants and ensure private and quiet space for each individual examination. A number of physicians use their medical offices after hours to conduct these examinations so that individual examiners and athletes have privacy. The rooms can be arranged to allow an orderly flow of athletes and specific consultations to take place.

When a student-athlete merits disqualification, good communication between the evaluating physician, the student-athlete, the athlete's parents or guardians, and coaches is essential. In the medical team setting, the team physician will often lead this discussion. This decision is often not made on the same day of the examination. Rather, it occurs after consulting with medical subspecialists, reviewing risks of participation with the consultant, and then meeting with the athlete (and their family) in a private setting to discuss the specific problem.

For a summary of the PPE administration process, see Box 3-2.

Box 3-2. The Preparticipation Physical Evaluation (PPE) Administration Summary

1. The final responsibility for a PPE lies with the primary or coordinating physician. Some states allow non-physicians to complete the examination and assume the responsibility.
2. The PPE can be done in an individual or a group setting. The individual setting in the primary care office with a personal physician familiar with the athlete is preferred. A group setting requires oversight by a team or coordinating physician to ensure that all mandatory elements are performed.
3. A group setting PPE is not equivalent to the recommended periodic preventive health screening examinations for children and adolescents. Physicians should use the PPE to encourage athletes to seek periodic preventive health examinations.
4. Problems discovered during the PPE that are beyond the expertise of the responsible physician should be directed to an appropriate specialist for referral or consultation.
5. The standardized PPE history form is the preferred format for documentation in either paper or electronic format.
6. The PPE should be performed at least 6 weeks prior to the start of the preseason practice.
7. In a group examination setting, review of the history, physical examination, and clearance should be done by a single physician.
8. Adolescent athletes should be seen apart from their parents or guardians for at least part of the examination so that the physician can inquire about risk-taking behaviors.
9. Defined sections of the PPE are protected health information and require confidential, secure handling and permission of the athlete or parent or guardian to be shared beyond the athlete's health care personnel.
10. Athletes and parents or guardians are responsible for timely scheduling of PPEs and completing the history questions in an honest manner.

■ INTERIM ANNUAL EVALUATIONS

An interim annual evaluation takes place between comprehensive examinations, either face to face or by questionnaire. To complete an evaluation, all student-athletes should complete either a comprehensive or a cardiac-medical risk history questionnaire and undergo a focused examination for any area indicated by the history. The purpose of the interim evaluation is to assess problems that have occurred since the athlete's comprehensive PPE. If this is done in the physician's office, it also serves as a time to reinforce previously discussed lifestyle issues and restate critical questions regarding syncope and concussion that athletes have been known to answer in a way to avoid disqualification.

Ideally, the physician reviews the history form and determines what parts of the physical examination should be performed. While this may be a very brief visit, if the physician identifies potentially serious symptoms, a more detailed examination would be performed. For example, in a student-athlete reporting syncope during exercise, a complete cardiovascular assessment would be required before clearance is granted. In some states, the questionnaire is passed through review by an administrator of the school (school nurse, athletic trainer, or activity director) who sends athletes with positive responses to the clearing physician of record for reevaluation and clearance determination.

■ REFERENCES

1. Team physician consensus statement. *Med Sci Sports Exerc.* 2000;32(4):877–878
2. Team physician consensus statement. *Am J Sports Med.* 2000;28(3):440–441
3. Sideline preparedness for the team physician: a consensus statement. *Med Sci Sports Exerc.* 2001;33(5):846–849
4. Maron BJ, Thompson PD, Ackerman MJ, et al. Recommendations and considerations related to preparticipation screening for cardiovascular abnormalities in competitive athletes: 2007 update: a scientific statement from the American Heart Association Council on Nutrition, Physical Activity, and Metabolism: endorsed by the American College of Cardiology Foundation. *Circulation.* 2007;115(12):1643–1645
5. Wingfield K, Matheson GO, Meeuwisse WH. Preparticipation evaluation: an evidence-based review. *Clin J Sport Med.* 2004;14(3):109–122
6. Brukner P, White S, Shawdon A, et al. Screening of athletes: Australian experience. *Clin J Sport Med.* 2004;14(3):169–177
7. Metzl JD. Preparticipation examinations of the adolescent athlete, part 1. *Pediatr Rev.* 2001;22(6):199–204
8. Stickler GB. Are yearly physical examinations in adolescents necessary? *J Am Board Fam Pract.* 2000;13(3):172–177
9. O'Connor FG, Kugler JP, Oriscello RG. Sudden death in young athletes: screening for the needle in a haystack. *Am Fam Physician.* 1998;57(11):2763–2770
10. Montalto NJ. Implementing the guidelines for adolescent preventive services. *Am Fam Physician.* 1998;57(9):2181–2190
11. Krowchuk DP, Krowchuk HV, Hunter DJ, et al. Parents' knowledge of the purpose and content of preparticipation physical examinations. *Arch Pediatr Adolesc Med.* 1995;149(6):653–657
12. American Academy of Pediatrics. Policy statement: recommendations for preventive pediatric health care. *Pediatrics.* 2007;120(6):1376
13. Institute for Clinical Systems Improvement. *Health Care Guideline: Preventive Services for Children and Adolescents.* 14th ed. http://www.icsi.org/preventive_services_for_children__guideline_/preventive_services_for_children_and_adolescents_2531.html (Accessed October 7, 2009)

CHAPTER 4

Administrative, Ethical, and Legal Concerns

Physicians face several administrative, ethical, and legal issues involving the preparticipation physical evaluation (PPE) process. Contending with these issues in a complex and divergent system is difficult. This chapter will touch on administrative issues such as how to inform schools and coaches of participation decisions in ways that protect an athlete's confidentiality yet ensure proper follow-up. It will also discuss federal privacy laws like the Health Insurance Portability and Accountability Act (HIPAA) and the Federal Education Records Protection Act (FERPA) and review which laws may be applicable in any given situation. This chapter will also explore ethical issues including real or perceived breaches of professional conduct during the examination and discuss dealing with conflicts between the physician's participation recommendations when that decision differs from the athlete's wishes. A physician's and institution's liability surrounding controversial clearance decisions and issues such as informed consent and waivers designed to circumvent medical opinion will be explored.

This chapter is intended as a general overview and *should not* be considered a legal opinion. Many of these issues are complex, and situations may differ depending on jurisdiction.

■ ADMINISTRATIVE

HIPAA regulations. HIPAA protects the privacy of health information through applicable federal privacy and confidentiality requirements in health care settings that use electronic billing.[1] When passed by Congress in 1996, HIPAA was designed to create a single uniform electronic system to check eligibility, record data, exchange information, and pay claims to reduce health care costs. At the same time, HIPAA created new and uniform federal standards for protecting the privacy of patient records and defined protected health information. Protected health information is defined as any information that can potentially identify a patient (in the PPE setting, an athlete) relating to past, present, or future physical or mental health conditions such as name, medical diagnosis, address, phone number, or social security number.[1] These standards for patient privacy are most closely associated with HIPAA. Depending on what setting the PPE is completed in and how the examination is billed, HIPAA regulations may or may not apply.

The HIPAA Privacy Rule expressly allows release of medical information without an individual's authorization in certain circumstances. The "cleared" or "not cleared" decision relayed *without other medical information* falls within this category and can be given to coaches and school administrators who need to know the player's medical eligibility.[2] However, if the school or coach wishes to know more detail beyond the "cleared" or "not cleared" decision, a signed authorization for release of patient information must be obtained in most circumstances. Some states may have regulations that are more stringent than federal HIPAA rules, and in these situations state laws supersede federal regulations. These authorizations can be rescinded at any time by the athlete or an athlete's parent or guardian if the athlete is younger than the age of consent.

FERPA regulations. FERPA was developed in 1974 and is the applicable law when information is considered part of an educational record.[3] FERPA regulations have similar intent to HIPAA and apply to entities like public schools that receive certain government educational funds. FERPA documents are specifically excluded from HIPAA. FERPA potentially allows medical information that is classified as an educational administrative record to be released to parents or guardians or to school personnel without special consent; information that would be protected if these records were HIPAA controlled. Often school-based training room records such as PPEs and training room medical encounters maintained by team physicians or certified athletic trainers are judged to fall under the purview of FERPA.

Whether HIPAA or FERPA regulations apply is a complex legal question and may vary by state and by specific situation. It is prudent to review HIPAA, FERPA, and institutional privacy policies with the educational institution's legal counsel or privacy officer to make sure that proper procedure and applicable laws are followed with regard to the PPE. All coaches, administrators, certified athletic trainers, and school personnel should receive education on privacy regulations that affect athlete care and transfer of health-related information. Sports organizations need to develop educational programs for privacy legislation and legal constraints so all personnel working with athletes follow all state and federal laws.

Confidentiality and PPE forms. The PPE clearance form has a "not cleared for certain sports" and a "not cleared for any sports" check box that will allow the physician to transmit the recommendation about a permanent disorder to the school without breaking the confidentiality rules that govern medical interactions.[2] For the purposes of participation clearance in a private practice setting, it is safest to separate the clearance form from the confidential history and physical portions of the examination. The alternative is to have a clear release of medical information form that is signed by the athlete (and parent or guardian if the athlete has not reached the age of majority) allowing the entire or specific portions of the record that contains private information to go to the school or team. A copy of the history and physical examination form should stay with the athlete's medical record. With or without HIPAA and FERPA regulations, athletes have a right to privacy, and all medical interactions should respect their confidentiality.

For examinations done in a group setting, the issue of confidential storage of the forms must be addressed. The information pertaining to restrictions should be shared only with those in the school administration who need to know. With parent or guardian and athlete permission, a copy of the form should be made available to the athlete's primary physician whenever possible. Giving the athlete or parent or guardian (if the athlete is a minor) a copy of the form to take to their physician will often facilitate this process.

The forms in this monograph reflect the restrictions placed on protected health information and are designed to share essential information regarding athlete evaluation, emergency care, and future sports participation with those who need to know.

Restriction from participation. When an athlete is restricted from participation, the question of who needs to know of the restriction always arises. The only information the coach and administration need to know is if the athlete is eligible to participate. In many cases the athlete or the parent or guardian will share the facts of the case with the coach. A signed medical release form must be obtained for a physician to discuss the case details with the coach or administrator.[4] At schools where there are team physicians, athletes may be required to sign a form that authorizes sharing of essential medical information between the physician, certified athletic trainer, coaches, and school administrators as a condition of participation. In most team circumstances, the certified athletic trainer is considered part of the medical treatment team and may be privy to the essential medical details of the athlete's case on a need-to-know basis.

Sharing emergency and public health information. For athlete safety and quick response to emergency situations or sideline use, the clearance form should include information such as known allergies and tetanus status. The team physician or certified athletic trainer should also have access to a listing of chronic medical problems and medications for emergency care when parents or guardians are not available. When a team physician or certified athletic trainer is not available, one of the coaching staff should have this information.

In some cases the question of whether or not personal health information can or should be shared with officials or coaches without the consent of the athlete will arise. For example, if an athlete develops an infectious disease such as herpes gladiatorum or meningococcal meningitis, the issue of whether there is an obligation to inform others of potential transmission or whether the right of the athlete to keep their personal health information confidential is more important may arise. The answer regarding duty to disclose will vary according to jurisdiction. When these situations arise, legal counsel should be sought regarding responsibilities as a health care provider. In cases where legal consult is not available, every effort should be taken to relay the potential public health risk without divulging the identity of the individual involved. This may involve reporting to the local or state Department of Public Health.

Electronic transmission. When coaches and certified athletic trainers use electronic record systems to store and transport information needed to treat athletes, the information systems must be secure from access by unauthorized people. One example is e-mail communications to and from a coach or certified athletic trainer may not be secure when sent through public communication lines such as the Internet if they are not encrypted and password protected. Athletes need to give permission for physicians to communicate personal health information with coaches and certified athletic trainers via e-mail.

Restricting information. Athletes have the right to request a restriction or limitation on the health information the school uses or discloses.[1] The request must be in writing to the facility where the team records are maintained (see Appendix A on page 159 for an example of a consent form). The request must state (1) what information is to be limited; (2) whether the limit pertains to use, disclosure, or both; and (3) to whom the limits apply. The athlete may also request that all confidential communications be conducted away from the practice sessions, games sites, and locker rooms. For those seeking more detail about HIPAA, the US Department of Health and Human Services Office of Civil Rights maintains a Web site at www.hhs.gov/ocr/hipaa that provides a variety of helpful information, including forms and educational materials about the privacy rule.

Travel. Ideally, the information obtained during the PPE should be available to the team physician, team certified athletic trainer, and emergency medical personnel, who may all be called to render emergency care for an athlete on the sideline or in the training room. Many teams travel with a copy of the PPE medical form should an athlete be injured during an away game. When the team physician performs the PPE, the confidentiality of the PPE record is simplified as long as the records are in a secure storage area during travel.

When high school athletes have examinations completed by their primary care physicians, confidentiality of the record becomes more complicated. A history of diabetes, seizure disorder, asthma, or allergies can be critical in certain instances. The clearance form developed for this monograph attempts to address this issue by including allergies and other emergency information that can be included at the discretion of the athlete and parents or guardians. However, it falls to the athlete and/or parents or guardians to complete that section of the form and inform the on-site physician, certified athletic trainer, or coach of medical conditions that might result in an emergency for the athlete.

■ ETHICAL

Breaches of conduct. The issue of improper professional conduct during the PPE has surfaced on several occasions with allegations of sexual improprieties on the part of the physician.[5] Although most of these complaints have involved male-to-female interactions, any doctor-patient interaction has potential for perceived and real transgressions. The station-based group examination format may present the greatest risk of such claims, given the typical lack of previous relationship between the patient-athlete and the examiner.

There is always risk of false accusations in any patient encounter when the door is closed and the physician is alone with a patient; a chaperone in the room is recommended when this is a concern. Furthermore, athletes may not expect to have a thorough examination, and portions of the PPE, although proper, can be perceived as improper, particularly when the genitalia are involved. Common sense should prevail, and the examination should be tailored to the history.

In every case, the physician should inform the athlete of the extent and purpose of the physical examination prior to performing it; provide an appropriate setting, including chaperones; and use discretion with comments or actions that may be misconstrued. Offering examination stations with physicians of both genders and allowing athletes to choose the examiner during a multiple-physician examination can also decrease the risk of perceived impropriety. Consistency in patient attire during the examination (eg, males in shorts and T-shirts and females in shorts and tank tops under a T-shirt with shirts removed in the privacy of the examination room) and in the examination routine (eg, deferring female genital and breast examinations) will decrease the risk of an athlete comparing his or her examination with those of other athletes and questioning why it might have been different.

Ethical decision-making and restriction from participation. Occasionally, the adage "first, do no harm" conflicts with the athlete's desire to compete when PPE findings lead to a recommendation for "no participation" in the athlete's sport. Although conditions that preclude participation are rare and many are well described, athletes will sometimes challenge activity restrictions, and the physician is confronted with an ethical dilemma that pits "the right to participate" against "do no harm." The decision to restrict participation in selected or all physical activity is seldom made by a single physician and usually requires a thorough educational effort by all involved to explain the decision and the potential consequences of both the activity restriction and a decision to continue on with the restricted activity despite the potential risks. Athletes may seek another medical opinion or pursue legal intervention to allow participation, even when accepted preparticipation recommendations like those of the American Heart Association state that the risk is too great for safe play or participation.[6] The decision to restrict participation is not always clear-cut, and it is important to remember that these decisions are life-altering for affected athletes.

Ideally, the physician who advises restricted participation should seek the opinion of consulting physicians to develop a participation recommendation that reflects the relative risk for the athlete's safety during practice and competition. Following the consultations, it is imperative that the physician fully inform the athlete (and parents or guardians) of potential risks associated with participation based on the disqualifying condition. This will allow the athlete and parents or guardians to make an informed decision regarding participation. It is important to remember that for athletes who have achieved the age of majority, it would be a breach of confidentiality to discuss a disqualifying condition with a parent or guardian without the patient's permission. Part of the difficulty in these conversations arises from the fact that the degree of risk is usually not quantifiable, and there is some degree of risk to participation in all athletics. The degree of acceptable risk may also vary depending on the situation. Such discussions should be clearly documented in the athlete's medical record.

Whether it is ethically right for an athlete to participate should not be confused with the issue of whether it is legally prudent to have an athlete participate for an institution. An institution may wish to clear an athlete to play even though there is significant risk because of a player's ability. They may be motivated to clear an athlete to avoid a potential lawsuit, particularly if there is divergent medical opinion regarding the condition. An institution may also wish to restrict an athlete from participation rather than accept any legal risk from adverse outcome, particularly with a player of limited ability or in a non-revenue sport. These are all reasonable factors for an institutional risk manager to consider but should not factor into the physician's decision to represent the patient's best interest.

The primary consideration of the physician should be if there is a reasonable risk that the athlete will suffer permanent, serious harm if allowed to participate. As the potential consequences of participation become more serious, the level of acceptable reasonable risk decreases. When conditions arise after the athlete has been cleared for participation, the physician may rescind the clearance until the problem is resolved and the potential consequences are completely explained to the athlete and parents or guardians.

■ LEGAL

Legal aspects of restriction from play. A team physician and an institution have the legal right to restrict an individual from participating in athletics as long as the decision is individualized, reasonably made, and based on competent medical evidence.[7] All institutions may not evaluate risk in the same way. In other words, one set of physicians and institution may elect to clear someone for participation while another may not; however, as long as the decision is based on sound medical judgment it is legally acceptable.

This legal precedent was set in 1996 in Knapp v Northwestern University.[8] As a high school senior, Nicholas Knapp suffered a cardiac arrest and was successfully resuscitated. He subsequently had an implantable cardiac defibrillator placed and was cleared to play basketball by 3 cardiologists. He participated without incident during the summer prior to matriculation. At Northwestern, he was not cleared for practice and competition by the team physician based on the opinion of their consulting cardiologist and the 26th Bethesda Guidelines (the most current at the time). Northwestern did agree to honor its commitment for his scholarship. Knapp sued Northwestern citing the Rehabilitation Act of 1973, which compels institutions that receive federal funds to provide disabled persons with an opportunity to participate fully in activities in which they have the physical skills and capabilities to perform.

The courts deemed that playing an intercollegiate sport was not a "major life activity" and therefore the Rehabilitation Act did not apply, and that Northwestern's decision, based on established medical guidelines, was reasonable. Similarly, a federal district court upheld the right of the University of Kansas to restrict a player with cervical spinal stenosis who had had an incident of transient quadriparesis from returning to play even though 3 outside medical specialists had counseled him that he was at no greater risk of permanent paralysis than any other football player.[7]

The decision as to whether an athlete may or may not participate at a particular institution has thus far been left in the hands of the team physicians, their consultants, and the institution. The level of risk that seems reasonable and ethical will vary from institution to institution, but the decision remains individualized and under local control.

Exculpatory waivers. If an athlete wishes to participate despite contrary medical recommendations, the athlete and his or her parents or guardians may suggest an "exculpatory waiver" or "risk release" to clearly indicate that they are fully informed of the inherent risk of participation against medical advice and that they assume this risk. An exculpatory waiver or risk release is a written contract between the athlete and his or her parents or guardians, the physician, and the school or activity sponsor. In it, the athlete promises not to sue the physician or activity sponsor and releases the physician and activity sponsor from liability.[9] Generally, courts have invalidated contracts releasing physicians from liability for negligent medical care of their patients.[5] A waiver of legal rights by an athlete who is a minor is usually not enforceable, even if a waiver is also given by the parents or guardians because minors have only limited legal capacity to enter contracts.[7]

Informed consent. A physician may choose to allow an athlete to participate if the athlete and parents or guardians express a clear understanding of the possible risks for a potentially catastrophic condition and choose to participate anyway—despite the risk. To protect themselves, some legal experts recommend that the physician have the parents or guardians and athlete write, in their own words and in their own handwriting, a signed letter indicating their understanding of the risks of continued participation, and that they understand the risks they are taking, instead of signing a waiver.[10,11] The difference is that a standard waiver is usually a form with blanks that are filled in by the physician and written in language that the parents or guardians or athlete would not normally use. With the standard waiver form, it has been successfully argued in court that, despite having signed a waiver, the parents or guardians and athlete did not fully understand the risks involved. However, with a letter written by the parents or guardians and/or athlete, it would be difficult to convince a jury that the parents or guardians or athlete did not understand the risks prior to any adverse event that might occur from continued participation. A videotape of the athlete and parents or guardians stating that they clearly understand their condition and detailing their understanding of both their condition and associated risks is an alternative to a letter that some institutions have used to document informed decision-making.

Limiting legal risk. In order to limit legal risk, clearance recommendations should be individualized after appropriate studies and consultant opinions are obtained. National guidelines, such as the 36th Bethesda Guidelines[6] (http://www.scribd.com/doc/2353746/36th-BETHESDA-CONFERENCE-JOURNAL-OF-THE-AMERICAN-COLLEGE-OF-CARDIOLOGY), offer helpful information in certain situations regarding clearance recommendations but are necessarily conservative. If one chooses to deviate from consensus guidelines there should be clearly articulated and thought out medical reasons why continuing participation is reasonable in a particular case. Consultant agreement and patient and parent or guardian understanding of the issues involved are essential to limit legal exposure for the primary or team physician.

Legal ramifications of the examination setting. The examination setting will have some bearing on all aspects of the PPE. Physicians who evaluate and recommend sports participation after completing a PPE in the office always face liability issues as they would with any patient encounter. An examination and clearance recommendation completed by the athlete's personal physician continues the physician-patient relationship with access to an ongoing medical record. This method therefore leaves less room for error and misunderstanding and less risk for missed or intentionally omitted medical information compared with group examinations.

Good Samaritan statutes and charitable immunity. The legal liability of those who perform PPEs on a volunteer basis is not easily understood. Good Samaritan statutes vary from state to state and generally apply only to emergency situations and only in regard to persons who render care without compensation or the expectation of compensation. Under a Good Samaritan law, providers are typically protected from all liability except those types associated with gross negligence or willful and wanton acts of malpractice. However, because the PPE is not emergency care, in most states providers should not depend on these statutes for malpractice protection.

In many cases where physicians are doing PPEs on a volunteer basis, charitable immunity statutes are more applicable. In general, these laws apply to licensed health care providers who are volunteering and acting within the scope of their practice. These laws typically make it more difficult for a plaintiff to win a lawsuit and may cap damages or limit noneconomic claims. Historically, state laws control malpractice liability and every state has different laws and different legal precedent. The Volunteer Protection Act of 1997 was designed to encourage volunteerism by health care providers at nonprofit clinics and is a federal law that offers protection to volunteering at a nonprofit institution.[12] It covers people in states where there are no or weak charitable immunity laws. The Volunteer Protection Act protects volunteers from simple negligence and limits allowable damages for gross negligence.

It is important for physicians to know their state's statutes regarding PPEs in volunteer settings. Information on charitable immunity can be found in *Understanding Charitable Immunity Legislation: A Volunteers in Health Care Guide* (www.volunteersinhealthcare.org/manuals/charit.imm.man.12.02.pdf). Physicians who volunteer as examiners in mass screening PPE sessions that are not covered under Good Samaritan or charitable immunity statutes must address the issue of malpractice insurance coverage. It is prudent for physicians to check with their insurance carrier before volunteering at PPE sessions.

Due to limitations of protection offered by Good Samaritan acts, Charitable Immunity statutes, and the federal Volunteer Protection Act, all physicians volunteering as a team physician or providing PPEs outside of the traditional office setting should obtain confirmation of coverage from their professional liability insurers prior to participating in the activity.

■ REFERENCES

1. Summary of the HIPAA privacy rule. Washington, DC: US Department of Health and Human Services; 2003. http://www.hhs.gov/ocr/privacy/hipaa/understanding/summary/
2. Magee JT, Almekinders LC, Taft TN. HIPAA and the team physician. *Sports Med Update.* March–April 2003:4–7
3. Family Educational Rights and Privacy Act (FERPA). http://www.ed.gov/policy/gen/guid/fpco/ferpa/index.html. Accessed February 2, 2009
4. Pearsall AW IV, Kovaleski JE, Madanagopal SG. Medicolegal issues affecting sports medicine practitioners. *Clin Orthop Relat Res.* 2005;433:50–57
5. Herbert DL. Prospective releases: will their use protect sports medicine physicians from suit? *Sports Med Stand Malpract Rep.* 1994;6(3):35–36
6. Maron BJ, Zipes DP. Introduction: eligibility recommendations for competitive athletes with cardiovascular abnormalities—general considerations. *J Am Coll Cardiol.* 2005;45(8):1318–1321
7. Mitten MJ. Emerging legal issues in sports medicine: a synthesis, summary, and analysis. *St Johns Law Rev.* 2002;76(1):100–182
8. Maron BJ, Mitten MJ, Quandt EF, Zipes DP. Competitive athletes with cardiovascular disease: the case of Nicholas Knapp. *N Engl J Med.* 1998;339(22):1632–1635
9. Gallup EM. *Law and the Team Physician.* Champaign, IL: Human Kinetics; 1995
10. Jones C. College athletes: illness or injury and the decision to return to play. *Buffalo Law Rev.* 1992;40:113–115
11. Mitten MJ. Team physicians and competitive athletes: allocating legal responsibility for athletic injuries. *Univ Pittsbg Law Rev.* 1993;55(1):129–169
12. Hattis PA, Walton J. *Understanding Charitable Immunity Legislation: A Volunteers in Health Care Guide.* Providence, RI: Volunteers in Health Care; 2003

CHAPTER 5

General Considerations of the History, Physical Examination, and Clearance

In order to achieve the specific goals and objectives of the preparticipation physical evaluation (PPE) described in Chapter 2, a thorough and systematic approach to the administration of the history, physical examination, and clearance determination is necessary. In this monograph, the history, physical examination, and clearance considerations that pertain to specific organ systems and medical aspects of the PPE are detailed in Chapter 6. This chapter presents a discussion of the primary issues regarding these components of the PPE.

■ HISTORY

The medical history is the most important element of the PPE. Studies investigating the value of the medical history in general medicine demonstrate that 76% to 90% of diagnoses are based on this aspect of the patient evaluation[1-5] and, likewise, studies assessing the PPE in high school and collegiate athletes show that the medical history identifies 65% to 77% of conditions.[6-9] More specifically, the medical history alone leads to the diagnosis of 88% of medical conditions and 67% of musculoskeletal conditions detected during the PPE.[9]

Obtaining an accurate medical history is therefore essential to an optimum examination outcome. However, given that there are more than 7 million athlete seasons annually at the high school level[10] and an estimated 30 million athletes younger than 18 years who play on some sort of organized sports team in the United States, devising a screening tool that will be efficient, thorough, understandable, and user-friendly is a significant challenge. Compounding this challenge is the fact that the medical history portion of the PPE should be designed to screen for conditions that could place the athlete at unacceptable medical risk, but it has not been proven. Further, it is not possible to achieve a zero-risk circumstance in competitive sports.[11]

Previous studies of the PPE have highlighted the difficulties in obtaining an accurate medical history. For example, in studies of high school students undergoing a PPE, only 19% to 39% of the athletes' responses agreed with information given by their parents or guardians completing the same form.[7,12] Other issues, such as illiteracy or English as a second language, may play a role and may further diminish the accuracy of responses to the medical history questions. For non–English-speaking athletes or athletes who are not fluent in English, using the assistance of a medical interpreter and/or a PPE form in the athlete's native language should help to accurately complete the history.

It is important that a physician review the history in a private setting with the athlete. Any positive responses on the history form should prompt further questions by the examining physician to clarify the issue of concern. The questions that comprise the history portion of the PPE form should be considered primary questions. These questions attempt to address fundamental issues of greatest concern for sports participation and general health risk during physical activity. Background information and rationale for the inclusion of the primary questions are available in this monograph. Where possible, validated questions from sources such as the Youth Risk Behavior Surveillance System have been used.[13] The secondary questions provided in the monograph are intended to serve as a guide for physicians to gather more in-depth information regarding a positive response to a primary question. Secondary questions appear within the text but not on the form.

In addition, the physical examination form (page 155) includes questions to be pursued by the physician on high-risk behaviors. Because it would be difficult to glean truthful information to written questions on such sensitive topics, these questions have been placed on the physical examination form rather than on the history form so that the patient will not complete them individually in the section that requires their signature or that of a parent or guardian. This information can be obtained verbally by the physician. A teen screen (Appendix B, page 160) is designed to guide the examiner regarding inquiries into high-risk behaviors and is not intended to be included on the PPE form. Other questionnaires (such as Guidelines for Adolescent Preventive Services, www.ama-assn.org) may be considered when evaluating these issues as long as the athlete is allowed to complete these questionnaires confidentially.

■ PHYSICAL EXAMINATION

Although the medical history has been established to be the key element of the PPE, the importance of the physical examination cannot be discounted. Blood pressure measurement and testing of visual acuity are essential. In fact, elevated blood pressure and abnormal vision are 2 of the most common findings reported in studies of the PPE.[6-8,14-20]

With respect to musculoskeletal conditions, the history remains of primary importance, and one study identified 92% of musculoskeletal problems on the basis of the history.[21] Nonetheless, the physical examination may yield unique information, and another study diagnosed 33% of musculoskeletal conditions during the physical examination.[9]

Another important aspect of the physical examination pertains to screening for cardiovascular conditions and is detailed in the cardiovascular section of Chapter 6. This monograph incorporates the American Heart Association recommendations for cardiac screening of competitive athletes.[22]

The components of each segment of the examination are discussed in the systems-based evaluation sections that follow.

■ DETERMINING CLEARANCE

Determining clearance is an important and sometimes difficult decision. Studies of the PPE show that 3.1% to 13.9% of athletes require further evaluation before a final clearance status can be determined.[6–8,14–18,23,24]

The initial clearance status for an athlete can be divided into 4 categories
- Cleared for all activities without restriction
- Cleared with recommendations for further evaluation or treatment (eg, "recheck blood pressure in 1 month")
- Not cleared—clearance status to be reconsidered after completion of further evaluation, treatment, or rehabilitation
- Not cleared for certain types of sports or for any sports
Forms for recording clearance status are available on pages 155 and 156.

■ CLEARANCE CONSIDERATIONS

It must be emphasized that the PPE is not intended to discourage or prevent participation in competitive sports. All athletes deserve a diligent and thorough assessment of any issues that could lead to denial of participation. Should such an evaluation result in restriction from participation in the sport of choice, the physician must consider alternative forms of physical activity based on the static and dynamic demands of participation that the athlete can tolerate. Limiting or withholding an athlete from athletic participation is a complicated and difficult decision and will often require consultation with other specialists in the area of concern. The decision to restrict participation may prevent an individual from reaping the many health benefits of regular physical exercise and may cause significant psychological consequences. For young competitive athletes, being an "athlete" is often a large part of their self-identity, and restricting their participation in sports may have other negative consequences on their self-esteem and overall health that should be anticipated and considered in the final decision. One study emphasized the importance of participation by pointing out that adolescents rank failure to make a team worse than the death of a close friend, failure to pass a grade in school, and separation of parents.[25] Any athlete withheld from athletic participation should receive ongoing follow-up to monitor their psychological and physical condition.

When an abnormality or condition is found that may limit an athlete's participation or predispose him or her to further injury, the physician must consider the following questions:
- Does the problem place the athlete at increased risk for injury or illness?
- Is another participant at risk for injury or illness because of the problem?
- Can the athlete safely participate with treatment (such as medication, rehabilitation, bracing, or padding)?
- Can limited participation be allowed while treatment is being completed?
- If clearance is denied only for certain sports or sport categories, in what activities can the athlete safely participate?
When a potentially disqualifying issue is identified during the PPE, clearance to participate in a particular sport should be based on a review of the pertinent current literature. Examples include guidelines

established by the American Academy of Pediatrics Committee on Sports Medicine and Fitness and the 36th Bethesda Conference guidelines on cardiovascular abnormalities.[26,27]

These recommendations classify sports according to the degree of contact and the level of dynamic and static stress. Contact categories are based on the potential for injury from collision (Box 5-1). High-impact contact-collision sports, such as football and ice hockey, have a higher risk of serious injury, and also have higher static and dynamic demands, than do noncontact sports, such as golf.

Box 5-1. Classification of Sports According to Contact[a]

Contact or Collision	Limited Contact	Noncontact
Basketball	Adventure racing[b]	Badminton
Boxing[c]	Baseball	Body building[d]
Cheerleading	Bicycling	Bowling
Diving	Canoeing or kayaking (white water)	Canoeing or kayaking (flat water)
Extreme sports[e]	Fencing	Crew or rowing
Field hockey	Field events	Curling
Football, tackle	High jump	Dance
Gymnastics	Pole vault	Field events
Ice hockey[f]	Floor hockey	Discus
Lacrosse	Football, flag or touch	Javelin
Martial arts[g]	Handball	Shot-put
Rodeo	Horseback riding	Golf
Rugby	Martial arts[g]	Orienteering[h]
Skiing, downhill	Racquetball	Power lifting[d]
Ski jumping	Skating	Race walking
Snowboarding	Ice	Riflery
Soccer	In-line	Rope jumping
Team handball	Roller	Running
Ultimate Frisbee	Skiing	Sailing
Water polo	Cross-country	Scuba diving
Wrestling	Water	Swimming
	Skateboarding	Table tennis
	Softball	Tennis
	Squash	Track
	Volleyball	
	Weight lifting	
	Windsurfing or surfing	

[a]Adapted with permission from: Rice SG, American Academy of Pediatrics Council on Sports Medicine and Fitness. Medical conditions affecting sports participation. *Pediatrics.* 2008;121(4):841–848.

[b]Adventure racing is defined as a combination of 2 or more disciplines, including orienteering and navigation, cross-country running, mountain biking, paddling, and climbing and rope skills.

[c]The American Academy of Pediatrics opposes participation in boxing for children, adolescents, and young adults.

[d]The American Academy of Pediatrics recommends limiting bodybuilding and power lifting until the adolescent achieves sexual maturity rating 5 (Tanner stage V).

[e]Extreme sports has been added since the previous statement was published.

[f]The American Academy of Pediatrics recommends limiting the amount of body checking allowed for hockey players 15 years and younger to reduce injuries.

[g]Martial arts can be subclassified as judo, jujitsu, karate, kung fu, and tae kwon do; some forms are contact sports and others are limited-contact sports.

[h]Orienteering is a race (contest) in which competitors use a map and a compass to find their way through unfamiliar territory.

Distinctions based on cardiovascular demands (Figure 5-1) are particularly relevant for athletes with cardiovascular or pulmonary disease. Static exercise causes a pressure load, whereas dynamic exercise causes a volume load on the left ventricle.[28] In all cases, the physician's judgment is essential in applying these recommendations to a specific patient.

It is the opinion of the author societies that clearance status is best determined when the PPE is conducted using the single-physician examiner model. If the PPE is performed with multiple examiners, clearance should be determined by a physician who has reviewed the entire history and physical examination. In either PPE format, a physician who is familiar with the demands of the activities, the limitations that result from various problems associated with the activities, and the current medical literature on what affects safe participation during the activity is in the best position to establish clearance to participate for the athlete. The physician determining clearance should refer to the relevant recommendations needed to establish the clearance status of the athlete or seek appropriate consultation when needed (Table 5-1). The clearing physician may also find that a specific problem discovered during the PPE may warrant additional follow-up and evaluation, whether or not the problem affects participation clearance.

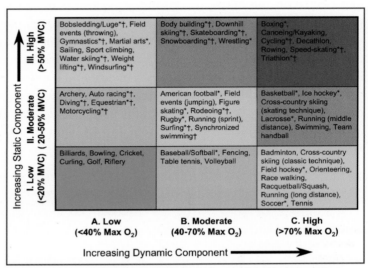

Figure 5-1. Classification of sports. This classification is based on peak static and dynamic components achieved during competition. It should be noted, however, that higher values may be reached during training. The increasing dynamic component is defined in terms of the estimated percent of maximal oxygen uptake (MaxO$_2$) achieved and results in an increasing cardiac output. The increasing static component is related to the estimated percent of maximal voluntary contraction (MVC) reached and results in an increasing blood pressure load. The lowest total cardiovascular demands (cardiac output and blood pressure) are shown in green and the highest in red. Blue, yellow, and orange depict low moderate, moderate, and high moderate total cardiovascular demands. *Danger of bodily collision. †Increased risk if syncope occurs. Reprinted with permission from: Maron BJ, Zipes DP. 36th Bethesda Conference: eligibility recommendations for competitive athletes with cardiovascular abnormalities. *J Am Coll Cardiol.* 2005;45(8):1317–1375.

When participation clearance status is not full and unrestricted, it is extremely important to ensure that any restrictions, workup and treatment, and alternative activities in which the athlete may participate are completely understood by the athlete and parents or guardians. While athletic trainers, coaches, and school administrators can be informed of the general participation status of the athlete, confidentiality regarding the medical reasons for the restrictions must be maintained. The dissemination of any medical information must be done in accordance with federal laws concerning privacy or medical records (see Chapter 4).

Using a clearance form that is separate from the history and physical examination form, such as that on page 156, will protect the confidentiality of athletes' history and physical findings. The physician should provide the school with a copy of clearance decisions and the parents or guardians a copy of the form and follow-up recommendations.

In some cases, the school or organization may have a designated team physician who was not part of the PPE process. In such situations, it may be appropriate for the physician who performed the PPE to seek permission from the student-athlete and parents or guardians to communicate to the team physician any ongoing problems that could affect safe participation.

After the initial clearance, the clearing physician should modify the athlete's level of participation as new or changing medical conditions arise. Following injury that requires medical intervention, a return to play evaluation and subsequent clearance to participate signed by a physician is required by high school governing bodies in some states and also in some sports programs before the athlete can return to practice or competition. Likewise, a new heart murmur or episode of syncope may require a change in the participation status until the athlete has had a complete evaluation and is deemed safe to return to activity. Finally, the primary care or team physician may find it necessary to rescind participation clearance based on changes in the athlete's health status that would affect the initial clearance decisions. This includes contacting school officials and/or the athletic trainer at an institution to inform them of the change in the athlete's clearance status. The specifics of the condition do not need to be shared unless the patient and family grant their permission.

TABLE 5-1. MEDICAL CONDITIONS AND SPORTS PARTICIPATION[a,b]

Condition	May Participate
Atlantoaxial instability (instability of the joint between cervical vertebrae 1 and 2) *Explanation:* Athlete (particularly if he or she has Down syndrome or juvenile rheumatoid arthritis with cervical involvement) needs evaluation to assess risk of spinal cord injury during sports participation, especially when using a trampoline.	Qualified yes
Bleeding disorder *Explanation:* Athlete needs evaluation.	Qualified yes
Cardiovascular disease Carditis (inflammation of the heart) *Explanation:* Carditis may result in sudden death with exertion.	No
Hypertension (high blood pressure) *Explanation:* Those with severe hypertension (>99th percentile for age plus 5 mm Hg) should avoid heavy weight and power lifting, bodybuilding, strength training, and high-static component sports (Figure 5-1). Those with sustained hypertension (>95th percentile for age) need evaluation. The National High Blood Pressure Education Program working group report defined prehypertension and stage 1 and stage 2 hypertension.	Qualified yes
Congenital heart disease (structural heart defects present at birth) *Explanation:* Consultation with a cardiologist is recommended. Those with mild forms may participate fully in most cases; those with moderate or severe forms or who have undergone surgery need evaluation. The 36th Bethesda Conference defined mild, moderate, and severe disease for common cardiac lesions.	Qualified yes

Dysrhythmia (irregular heart rhythm)
   Long QT syndrome
   Malignant ventricular arrhythmias
   Symptomatic Wolff-Parkinson-White syndrome
   Advanced heart block
   Family history of sudden death or previous sudden cardiac event
   Implantation of a cardioverter-defibrillator
     Explanation: Consultation with a cardiologist is advised. Those with symptoms (chest pain, syncope, near syncope, dizziness, shortness of breath, or other symptoms of possible dysrhythmia) or evidence of mitral regurgitation (leaking) on physical examination need evaluation. All others may participate fully.
	Qualified yes

TABLE 5-1. MEDICAL CONDITIONS AND SPORTS PARTICIPATION[a,b], CONTINUED

Condition	May Participate
Cardiovascular disease, continued	
Heart murmur	Qualified yes
Explanation: If the murmur is innocent (does not indicate heart disease), full participation is permitted. Otherwise, the athlete needs evaluation (see congenital heart disease, structural heart disease [especially hypertrophic cardiomyopathy and mitral valve prolapse]).	
Structural/acquired heart disease	Qualified no
Hypertrophic cardiomyopathy	Qualified no
Coronary artery anomalies	Qualified no
Arrhythmogenic right ventricular cardiomyopathy	Qualified no
Acute rheumatic fever with carditis	Qualified no
Ehlers-Danlos syndrome, vascular form	Qualified yes
Marfan syndrome	Qualified yes
Mitral valve prolapse	Qualified yes
Anthracycline use	
Explanation: Consultation with a cardiologist is recommended. The 36th Bethesda Conference provided detailed recommendations. Most of these conditions carry a significant risk of sudden cardiac death associated with intense physical exercise. Hypertrophic cardiomyopathy requires a thorough workup and repeated evaluations, because disease may change manifestations during later adolescence. Marfan syndrome with an aortic aneurysm can also cause sudden death during intense physical exercise. An athlete who has ever received chemotherapy with anthracyclines may be at increased risk of cardiac problems because of the cardiotoxic effects of the medications, and resistance training in this population should be approached with caution; strength training that avoids isometric contractions may be permitted. Athlete needs evaluation.	
Vasculitis/vascular disease	Qualified yes
Kawasaki disease (coronary artery vasculitis)	
Pulmonary hypertension	
Explanation: Consultation with a cardiologist is recommended. Athlete needs individual evaluation to assess risk on the basis of activity of disease, pathologic changes, and medical regimen.	
Cerebral palsy	Qualified yes
Explanation: Athlete needs evaluation to assess functional capacity to perform sports specific activity.	
Diabetes mellitus	Yes
Explanation: All sports can be played with proper attention to diet, blood glucose concentration, hydration, and insulin therapy. Blood glucose concentration should be monitored before exercise, every 30 minutes during continuous exercise, 15 minutes after completion of exercise, and at bedtime.	
Diarrhea, infectious	Qualified no
Explanation: Unless symptoms are mild and the athlete is fully hydrated, no participation is permitted, because diarrhea may increase the risk of dehydration and heat illness. See fever.	
Eating disorders	Qualified yes
Explanation: Athlete with an eating disorder needs medical and psychiatric assessment before participation.	

TABLE 5-1. MEDICAL CONDITIONS AND SPORTS PARTICIPATION[a,b], CONTINUED

Condition	May Participate

Eyes
Functionally one-eyed athlete
Loss of an eye
Detached retina or family history of retinal detachment at a young age
High myopia
Connective tissue disorder, such as Marfan or Stickler syndromes
Previous intraocular eye surgery or serious eye injury
    Explanation: A functionally one-eyed athlete is defined as having a best-corrected visual acuity of less than 20/40 in the eye with worse acuity. Such an athlete would suffer significant disability if the better eye were seriously injured, as would an athlete with loss of an eye. Specifically, boxing and full-contact martial arts are not recommended for functionally one-eyed athletes, because eye protection is impractical and/or not permitted. Some athletes who previously have undergone intraocular eye surgery or had a serious eye injury may have an increased risk of injury because of weakened eye tissue. Availability of eye guards approved by the American Society for Testing and Materials and other protective equipment may allow participation in most sports, but this must be judged on an individual basis.
Conjunctivitis, infectious
    Explanation: An athlete with active infectious conjunctivitis should be excluded from swimming.
	Qualified yes
	
	Qualified no

Fever *Explanation:* Fever can increase cardiopulmonary effort, reduce maximum exercise capacity, make heat illness more likely, and increase orthostatic hypertension during exercise. Fever may rarely accompany myocarditis or other conditions that may make exercise dangerous.	No

Gastrointestinal
Malabsorption syndromes (celiac disease, cystic fibrosis)
    Explanation: Athlete needs individual assessment for general malnutrition or specific deficits resulting in coagulation or other defects; with appropriate treatment, these deficits can be adequately treated to permit normal activities.
Short bowel syndrome or other disorders requiring specialized nutritional support including parenteral or enteral nutrition
    Explanation: Athlete needs individual assessment for collision, contact, or limited-contact sports. Presence of a central or peripheral indwelling venous catheter may require special considerations for activities and emergency preparedness for unexpected trauma to the device(s).
	Qualified yes

Heat illness, history of *Explanation:* Because of the likelihood of recurrence, the athlete needs individual assessment to determine the presence of predisposing conditions and to develop a prevention strategy, which includes sufficient acclimatization, conditioning, hydration, and salt intake as well as other effective measures to improve heat tolerance and reduce heat injury risk.	Qualified yes
Hepatitis, infectious (primarily hepatitis C) *Explanation:* All athletes should have received Hep B vaccination prior to participation. Because of the apparent minimal risk to others, all sports may be played that the athlete's state of health allows. In all athletes, skin lesions should be covered properly, and athletic personnel should use universal precautions when handling blood or body fluids with visible blood.	Yes
Human immunodeficiency virus infection *Explanation:* Because of the apparent minimal risk to others, all sports may be played that the athlete's state of health allows (especially if the viral load is undetectable or very low). In all athletes, skin lesions should be covered properly, and athletic personnel should use universal precautions when handling blood or body fluids with visible blood. However, certain sports (such as wrestling or boxing) may create a situation that may favor viral transmission (likely bleeding plus skin breaks). If a viral load is detectable, these athletes should be advised to avoid such high-contact sports.	Yes

TABLE 5-1. MEDICAL CONDITIONS AND SPORTS PARTICIPATION[a,b], CONTINUED

Condition	May Participate
Kidney, absence of one *Explanation:* Athlete needs individual assessment for contact, collision, and limited-contact sports. Protective equipment may reduce risk of injury to the remaining kidney sufficiently to allow participation in most sports, providing such equipment remains in place during activity.	Qualified yes
Liver, enlarged *Explanation:* If the liver is acutely enlarged, participation should be avoided because of risk of rupture. If the liver is chronically enlarged, individual assessment is needed before collision, contact, or limited-contact sports are played. Patients with chronic liver disease may have changes in liver function that may affect stamina, mental status, coagulation, or nutritional status.	Qualified yes
Malignant neoplasm *Explanation:* Athlete needs individual assessment.	Qualified yes
Musculoskeletal disorders *Explanation:* Athlete needs individual assessment.	Qualified yes
Neurologic disorders History of serious head or spine trauma or abnormality, including craniotomy, epidural bleeding, subdural hematoma, intracerebral hemorrhage, second-impact syndrome, vascular malformation, and neck fracture. *Explanation:* Athlete needs individual assessment for collision, contact, or limited-contact sports.	Qualified yes
History of simple concussion (mild traumatic brain injury), multiple simple concussions, and/or complex concussion. *Explanation:* Athlete needs individual assessment. Research supports a conservative approach to concussion management, including no athletic participation while symptomatic or when deficits in judgment or cognition are detected, followed by a graduated, sequential return to full activity.	Qualified yes
Myopathies *Explanation:* Athlete needs individual assessment.	Qualified yes
Recurrent headaches *Explanation:* Athlete needs individual assessment.	Yes
Recurrent plexopathy (burner or stinger) and cervical cord neuropraxia with persistent defects *Explanation:* Athlete needs individual assessment for collision, contact, or limited-contact sports; regaining normal strength is an important benchmark for return to play.	Qualified yes
Seizure disorder, well-controlled *Explanation:* Risk of seizure during participation is minimal.	Yes
Seizure disorder, poorly controlled *Explanation:* Athlete needs individual assessment for collision, contact, or limited-contact sports. The following noncontact sports should be avoided: archery, riflery, swimming, weight or power lifting, strength training, or sports involving heights. In these sports, occurrence of a seizure during the activity may pose a risk to self or others.	Qualified yes
Obesity *Explanation:* Because of the increased risk of heat illness, the obese athlete particularly needs careful acclimatization, sufficient hydration, and potential activity and recovery modifications during competition and training.	Yes
Organ transplant recipient (and those taking immunosuppressive medications) *Explanation:* Athlete needs individual assessment for contact, collision, and limited-contact sports. In addition to the potential risk of infections, some medications (eg, prednisone) may increase tendency for bruising.	Qualified yes
Ovary, absence of one *Explanation:* Risk of severe injury to the remaining ovary is minimal.	Yes

TABLE 5-1. MEDICAL CONDITIONS AND SPORTS PARTICIPATION[a,b], CONTINUED

Condition	May Participate
Pregnancy/postpartum *Explanation:* Athlete needs individual assessment. As pregnancy progresses, modifications to usual exercise routines will become necessary. Activities with a high risk of falling or abdominal trauma should be avoided. Scuba diving and activities posing a risk of altitude sickness should also be avoided during pregnancy. Postpartum, physiologic, and morphologic changes of pregnancy take 4 to 6 weeks to return to baseline.	Qualified yes

Respiratory conditions
Pulmonary compromise, including cystic fibrosis
    Explanation: Athlete needs individual assessment, but generally, all sports may be played if oxygenation remains satisfactory during a graded exercise test. Athletes with cystic fibrosis need acclimatization and good hydration to reduce the risk of heat illness.
Asthma
    Explanation: With proper medication and education, only athletes with the most severe asthma will need to modify their participation. For those using inhalers, recommend having a written action plan and using a peak flow meter daily. Athletes with asthma may encounter risks when scuba diving.
Acute upper respiratory infection
    Explanation: Upper respiratory obstruction may affect pulmonary function. Athlete needs individual assessment for all but mild disease. See fever.
	Qualified yes
	
	Yes
	
	Qualified yes

Rheumatologic diseases
Juvenile rheumatoid arthritis
    Explanation: Athletes with systemic or polyarticular juvenile rheumatoid arthritis and history of cervical spine involvement need radiographs of vertebrae C1-C2 to assess risk of spinal cord injury. Athletes with systemic or HLA B27-associated arthritis require cardiovascular assessment for possible cardiac complications during exercise. For those with micrognathia (open bite and exposed teeth), mouth guards are helpful. If uveitis is present, the risk of eye damage from trauma is increased; ophthalmologic assessment is recommended, and if visually impaired, guidelines for functionally one-eyed athletes should be followed.
Juvenile dermatomyositis (JDM), idiopathic myositis
Systemic lupus erythematosis (SLE)
Raynaud phenomenon
    Explanation: Athlete with JDM or SLE with cardiac involvement requires cardiology assessment before participation. Athletes on systemic corticosteroids are at higher risk of osteoporotic fractures and avascular necrosis, which should be assessed before clearance; those on immunosuppressive medication are at higher risk of serious infection. Sports activity should be avoided when myositis is active. Rhabdomyolysis during intensive exercise may cause renal injury in athletes with idiopathic myositis and other myopathies. Because of photosensitivity with JDM and SLE, sun protection is necessary during outdoor activity. With Raynaud phenomenon, exposure to the cold presents risk to hands and feet.
	Qualified yes
	
	Qualified yes

Sickle cell disease *Explanation:* Athlete needs individual assessment. In general, if status of the illness permits, all sports may be played; however, any sport or activity that entails overexertion, overheating, dehydration, and chilling should be avoided. Participation at high altitude, especially when not acclimatized, also poses risk of sickle cell crisis.	Qualified yes

TABLE 5-1. MEDICAL CONDITIONS AND SPORTS PARTICIPATION[a,b], CONTINUED

Condition	May Participate
Sickle cell trait *Explanation:* Athletes with sickle cell trait generally do not have an increased risk of sudden death or other medical problems during athletic participation under normal environmental conditions. However, when high exertional activity is performed under extreme conditions of heat and humidity or increased altitude, such catastrophic complications have occurred rarely. Athletes with sickle cell trait, like all athletes, should be progressively acclimatized to the environment and to the intensity and duration of activities and should be sufficiently hydrated to reduce the risk of exertional heat illness and/or rhabdomyolysis. According to NIH management guidelines, sickle cell trait is not a contraindication to participation in competitive athletics and there is no requirement for screening prior to participation. More research is needed to fully assess potential risks and benefits of screening athletes for sickle cell trait.	Yes
Skin infections Herpes simplex, molluscum contagiosum, verrucae (warts), staphylococcal and streptococcal infection (furuncle [boils], carbuncle, impetigo, methicillin-resistant *Staphylococcus aureus* [cellulitis, abscess, necrotizing fasciitis]), scabies, tinea Explanation: During contagious period, participation in gymnastics with mats; martial arts; wrestling; or other collision, contact, or limited-contact sports is not allowed.	Qualified yes
Spleen, enlarged *Explanation:* If the spleen is acutely enlarged, participation should be avoided because of risk of rupture. If the spleen is chronically enlarged, individual assessment is needed before collision, contact, or limited-contact sports are played.	Qualified yes
Testicle, undescended or absence of one *Explanation:* Certain sports may require a protective cup.	Yes

[a]Adapted with permission from: Rice SG, American Academy of Pediatrics Council on Sports Medicine and Fitness. Medical conditions affecting sports participation. *Pediatrics.* 2008;121(4):841–848.

[b]This table is designed for use by medical and nonmedical personnel. "Needs evaluation" means that a physician with appropriate knowledge and experience should assess the safety of a given sport for an athlete with the listed medical condition. Unless otherwise noted, this need for special consideration is because of variability of the severity of the disease, the risk of injury for the specific sports listed in Box 5-1, or both.

■ REFERENCES

1. Platt R. Two essays of the practice of medicine. *Manchester Univ Med Sch Gazette.* 1947;27:139–145
2. Hampton JR, Harrison MJ, Mitchell JR, Prichard JS, Seymour C. Relative contributions of medical history-taking, physical examination, and laboratory investigation to diagnosis and management of medical outpatients. *BMJ.* 1975;2(5969):486–489
3. Gruppen LD, Wooliscroft JO, Wolf FM. The contribution of different components of the clinical encounter in generating and eliminating diagnostic hypotheses. *Res Med Educ.* 1988;27:242–247
4. Peterson MC, Holbrook JH, Von Hales D, Smith NL, Staker LV. Contributions of the history, physical examination, and laboratory investigation in making medical diagnoses. *West J Med.* 1992;156(2):163–165
5. Roshan M, Rao AP. A study on relative contributions of the history, physical examination and investigations in making medical diagnosis. *J Assoc Physicians India.* 2000;48(8):771–775
6. Goldberg B, Saraniti A, Witman P, Gavin M, Nicholas JA. Preparticipation sports assessment: an objective evaluation. *Pediatrics.* 1980;66(5):736–745
7. Risser WL, Hoffman HM, Bellah GG Jr. Frequency of preparticipation sports examinations in secondary school athletes: are the University Interscholastic League guidelines appropriate? *Tex Med.* 1985;81(7):35–39
8. Lively MW. Preparticipation physical examinations: a collegiate experience. *Clin J Sport Med.* 1999;9(1):3–8
9. Chun J, Haney S, DiFiori J. The relative contributions of the history and physical examination in the preparticipation evaluation of collegiate student-athletes. *Clin J Sport Med.* 2006;16(5):437–438

10. National Federation of State High School Associations. 2006–2007 high school athletics participation survey. http://www.nfhs.org/web/2007/09/high_school_sports_participation.aspx. Accessed June 8, 2008

11. Maron BJ, Poliac LC, Roberts WO. Risk for sudden cardiac death associated with marathon running. *J Am Coll Cardiol.* 1996;28(2):428–431

12. Carek PJ, Futrell M, Hueston WJ. The preparticipation physical examination history: who has the correct answers? *Clin J Sport Med.* 1999;9(3):124–128

13. Grunbaum JA, Kann L, Kinchen SA. Youth risk behavior surveillance—United States, 2001. *MMWR Surveil Summ.* 2002;51(4):1–62

14. Linder CW, DuRant RH, Seklecki RM, Strong WB. Preparticipation health screening of young athletes. Results of 1268 examinations. *Am J Sports Med.* 1981;9(3):187–193

15. Tennant FS Jr, Sorenson K, Day CM. Benefits of preparticipation sports examinations. *J Fam Pract.* 1981;13(2):287–288

16. Thompson TR, Andrish JT, Bergfeld JA. A prospective study of preparticipation sports examinations of 2670 young athletes: method and results. *Cleve Clin Q.* 1982;49(4):225–233

17. DuRant RH, Seymore C, Linder CW, Jay S. The preparticipation examination of athletes. Comparison of single and multiple examiners. *Am J Dis Child.* 1985:139(7):657–661

18. Magnes SA, Henderson JM, Hunter SC. What conditions limit sports participation: experience with 10,540 athletes. *Phys Sportsmed.* 1992;20(5):143–158

19. Fuller CM, McNulty CM, Spring DA, et al. Prospective screening of 5,615 high school athletes for risk of sudden cardiac death. *Med Sci Sports Exerc.* 1997;29(9):1131–1138

20. Dixit S, DiFiori J. Prevalence of hypertension and prehypertension in collegiate student athletes. *Clin J Sport Med.* 2006;16(5):440

21. Gomez JE, Landry GL, Bernhardt DT. Critical evaluation of the 2-minute orthopedic screening examination. *Am J Dis Child.* 1993;147(10):1109–1113

22. Maron BJ, Thompson PD, Ackerman MJ, et al. Recommendations and considerations related to preparticipation screening for cardiovascular abnormalities in competitive athletes: 2007 update: a scientific statement from the American Heart Association Council on Nutrition, Physical Activity, and Metabolism. *Circulation.* 2007;115(12):1643–1655

23. Rifat SF, Ruffin MT IV, Gorenflo DW. Disqualifying criteria in a preparticipation sports evaluation. *J Fam Pract.* 1995;41(1):42–50

24. Smith J, Laskowski ER. The preparticipation physical examination: Mayo Clinic experience with 2,739 examinations. *Mayo Clin Proc.* 1998;73(5):419–429

25. Coddington RD. The significance of life events as etiologic factors in the disease of children. II. A study of a normal population. *J Psychosom Res.* 1972;16:205–213

26. Rice SG, American Academy of Pediatrics Council on Sports Medicine and Fitness. Medical conditions affecting sports participation. *Pediatrics.* 2008;121(4):841–848

27. Maron BJ, Zipes DP. 36th Bethesda Conference: eligibility recommendations for competitive athletes with cardiovascular abnormalities. *J Am Coll Cardiol.* 2005;45(8):1317–1375

28. Mitchell JH, Haskell WL, Raven PB. Classification of sports. *Med Sci Sports Exerc.* 1994;26(10 suppl):S242–S245

CHAPTER 6

Systems-Based Examination

A: Cardiovascular Problems

■ HISTORY FORM QUESTIONS

5. *Have you ever passed out or nearly passed out DURING or AFTER exercise?*

6. *Have you ever had discomfort, pain, tightness, or pressure in your chest during exercise?*

7. *Does your heart ever race or skip beats (irregular beats) during exercise?*

8. *Has a doctor ever told you that you have any heart problems (high blood pressure, high cholesterol, a heart murmur, a heart infection, Kawasaki disease, or other)?*

9. *Has a doctor ever ordered a test for your heart (for example, ECG/EKG or echocardiogram)?*

10. *Do you get lightheaded or feel more short of breath than expected during exercise?*

11. *Have you ever had an unexplained seizure?*

12. *Do you get more tired or short of breath more quickly than your friends during exercise?*

13. *Has any family member or relative died of heart problems or had any unexpected or unexplained sudden death before age 50 (including drowning, unexplained car accident, or sudden infant death syndrome)?*

14. *Does anyone in your family have hypertrophic cardiomyopathy, Marfan syndrome, arrhythmogenic right ventricular cardiomyopathy, long QT syndrome, short QT syndrome, Brugada syndrome, or catecholaminergic polymorphic ventricular tachycardia?*

15. *Does anyone in your family have a heart problem, pacemaker, or implanted defibrillator?*

16. *Has anyone in your family had unexplained fainting, unexplained seizures, or near drowning?*

■ KEY POINTS

- Sudden cardiac death (SCD) in young athletes and children is caused by a diverse etiology of structural and electrical diseases of the heart.
- A detailed patient and family history may identify athletes at risk for SCD.
- Warning symptoms that require cardiac workup before returning to exercise include exertional chest pain, exertional syncope or near-syncope, unexplained seizures, excessive dyspnea or fatigue disproportionate to the level of exertion, and palpitations or irregular heart beats.

- A family history of sudden unexpected or unexplained death, sudden death before the age of 50 due to cardiac problems, sudden infant death, unexplained drowning, near drowning, or unexplained seizures may indicate the presence of a genetic cardiovascular disorder placing the athlete at increased risk for SCD.
- Physical examination should focus on detecting the heart murmur of left ventricular outflow tract obstruction and the physical findings suggestive of Marfan syndrome.
- Patients or families suspected or identified to be at risk of SCD should be referred to a cardiovascular specialist for further evaluation.

Cardiovascular disorders are the leading cause of sudden death in young athletes[1-3] and account for approximately 75% of all sudden death in athletes.[3] Healthy-appearing athletes may harbor unsuspected cardiovascular disease, making identification of athletes at risk of sudden death more difficult.[4]

Preparticipation cardiovascular screening is the systematic practice of evaluating athletes before participation in sports for the purpose of identifying or raising suspicion of abnormalities that could provoke disease progression or sudden death.[5] The American Heart Association (AHA) states that the principal objective of screening is to reduce the cardiovascular risks associated with physical activity and enhance the safety of athletic participation.[5] The American College of Cardiology also contends that the ultimate objective of preparticipation screening of athletes is the detection of silent cardiovascular abnormalities that can lead to sudden death.[6] In 2007 the AHA updated its consensus statement on preparticipation cardiovascular screening in athletes with specific recommendations for a detailed personal and family history and physical examination.[5]

This section
- Reviews the incidence and etiologies of SCD in young athletes
- Defines a comprehensive cardiovascular assessment of athletes using personal and family history and appropriate physical examination
- Discusses the proper diagnostic investigation for concerning history or examination findings
- Explores the role of noninvasive cardiovascular screening in athletes, such as electrocardiogram (ECG)
- Provides guidelines and resources for the management and clearance decisions for athletes identified with cardiovascular disorders

■ INCIDENCE OF SUDDEN CARDIAC DEATH IN YOUNG ATHLETES

The exact incidence of SCD in athletes is unknown in the United States. Studies to date have relied on survey or non-mandatory reporting systems that may underestimate the true incidence.[4,5,7] Initial studies estimated the annual incidence of SCD to be 1:100,000 to 1:200,000 in high school–aged athletes and 1:65,000 to 1:69,000 in college-aged athletes.[2,4,5,8-10] The US Sudden Death in Young Athletes Registry has identified more than 100 cases of SCD per year in young competitive athletes participating in organized sports at the middle school, high school, college, and professional level.[3,11] Approximately 80% of these cases occur in a high school or college athlete.[3] With approximately 5 million competitive high school athletes and 500,000 competitive collegiate athletes in the United States, a more current estimate of the annual incidence of SCD in high school and college athletes is about 1:75,000 athletes.

In Italy, with a mandatory reporting system for juvenile sudden death, the baseline incidence of SCD in young competitive athletes (age 12–35) was 1:25,000 prior to the implementation of a national screening program.[12] In US military recruits (median age 19, range 18–35 years), the incidence of exercise-related SCD was found to be 1:9,000.[13,14]

Sudden cardiac death in athletes occurs more commonly in males, with male:female differences ranging from 5:1 to 9:1.[1,15] Although SCD can occur in any sport, these deaths occur most frequently in basketball and football in the United States (sports that have the highest levels of participation). A disproportionate amount (>40%) of SCD in US athletes occurs in African American athletes, greater than the proportion of African Americans participating in athletics.

■ ETIOLOGY OF SUDDEN CARDIAC DEATH IN YOUNG ATHLETES

Sudden cardiac death in young athletes is due to a heterogeneous group of structural cardiovascular abnormalities and primary electrical diseases that typically go undetected in otherwise healthy-appearing athletes (Box 6A-1).[1,4,5,7,9,16–19] Vigorous exercise seems to be a trigger for lethal arrhythmias in athletes with occult heart disease.[1] In the United States, hypertrophic cardiomyopathy and congenital coronary artery anomalies are the most common etiologies of SCD. The combined prevalence of all cardiovascular disorders known to cause SCD in the young athletic population is estimated to be 3:1,000.[5]

HYPERTROPHIC CARDIOMYOPATHY

Hypertrophic cardiomyopathy (HCM) accounts for about one-third of SCD deaths in US athletes younger than 30 years.[1,4,5] The characteristic morphologic features of HCM include asymmetric left ventricular (LV) hypertrophy (usually involving the ventricular septum), LV wall thickness of 16 mm or more (normal <12 mm; borderline 13–15 mm), a ratio between the septum and free wall thickness of more than 1.3, and a non-dilated LV with impaired diastolic function.[20] Histologic analysis shows a disorganized cellular architecture with cardiac myocyte disarray and intramural tunneling (myocardial bridging) in which a segment of coronary artery is completely surrounded by myocardium in about one-third of cases.

Box 6A-1. Causes of Sudden Cardiac Death in Young Athletes

Structural/Functional	• Hypertrophic cardiomyopathy[a] • Idiopathic left ventricular hypertrophy • Coronary artery anomalies • Myocarditis • Arrhythmogenic right ventricular cardiomyopathy[a] • Dilated cardiomyopathy[a] • Aortic rupture/Marfan syndrome[a] • Aortic stenosis • Coronary artery atherosclerotic disease[a] • Postoperative congenital heart disease
Electrical	• Long QT syndrome[a] • Catecholaminergic polymorphic ventricular tachycardia[a] • Wolff-Parkinson-White syndrome • Brugada syndrome[a] • Short QT syndrome[a]
Other	• Drugs and stimulants • Primary pulmonary hypertension[a] • Commotio cordis

[a]Familial/genetic.

The prevalence of HCM is 1:500 in the general population and approximately 1:1,000 to 1:1,500 in competitive athletes.[21-23] It is inherited as an autosomal dominant disorder with variable expression in more than half of cases.[24] Morphologic expression of HCM may appear in childhood, but typically develops in early adolescence to young adulthood and is characteristically present by the end of physical maturity in most individuals who are genetically predisposed for the disorder. The phenotypic expression of HCM in adolescence is the primary rationale supporting the recommendation that preparticipation cardiovascular screening be performed every other year while in high school and on matriculation to college.[5,9]

Most athletes with HCM are asymptomatic, and sudden death is often the sentinel event of their disease. In one study, only 21% of athletes who died from HCM had any signs or symptoms of cardiovascular disease in the 36 months prior to their death.[4] Symptoms may include exertional chest pain, dyspnea, light-headedness, or syncope. On physical examination, the characteristic murmur of HCM is a harsh systolic ejection murmur (best heard at the right upper sternal border) that increases with maneuvers that decrease venous return (ie, Valsalva or moving from squatting to standing) and diminishes with maneuvers that increase venous return (ie, lying supine or moving from standing to a squatting position). Because only 25% of patients with HCM have a murmur,[24] most athletes will have a normal cardiac examination.

An ECG will be abnormal in up to 95% of patients with HCM,[25,26] with prominent Q waves, deep negative T waves, or dramatic increases in QRS voltage associated with ST depression or T-wave inversion. Echocardiography remains the standard to confirm the diagnosis of HCM by identifying pathologic LV wall thickness (>16 mm) and a non-dilated LV with impaired diastolic function. In cases where the diagnosis of HCM is uncertain (ie, borderline LV wall thickness of 13–15 mm), repeat echocardiography or magnetic resonance imaging (MRI) after 4 to 6 weeks of deconditioning should resolve the hypertrophy and may help in distinguishing HCM from athletic heart syndrome.

CORONARY ARTERY ANOMALIES

Coronary artery anomalies are the second-leading cause of SCD in athletes and account for approximately 17% of cases.[1,5] The most common coronary anomaly is an abnormal origin of the left coronary artery arising from the right sinus of Valsalva. Impingement of the anomalous artery as it traverses between the expanding great vessels during exercise may lead to ischemia and a subsequent arrhythmia. Other features that may contribute to ischemia during exercise include an acute angled take-off, a hypoplastic ostium, or an intramyocardial course of the anomalous artery.

Less than half of SCD cases from coronary anomalies have prodromal symptoms that may be identified by a preparticipation history.[13,27] In one study, only 12 out of 27 athletes (44%) who died of an anomalous coronary artery had prodromal symptoms such as exertional syncope, chest pain, or palpitations in the 24 months prior to their death.[27] If suspected, transthoracic echocardiography can identify the coronary artery origins in about 95% of patients. Advanced cardiac imaging such as computed tomography (CT) angiography, cardiac MRI, or coronary angiography may be needed in some cases to detect anomalous origins and can also identify other coronary anomalies such as an acute angled take-off, intramyocardial course, and hypoplastic coronary arteries.

MYOCARDITIS

Myocarditis accounts for 6% of SCD in US athletes.[5] Acute inflammation of the myocardium may lead to an arrhythmogenic focus and sudden death. Coxsackievirus B is implicated in more than 50% of cases, but echovirus, adenovirus, influenza, and *Chlamydia pneumoniae* have also been associated with myocarditis. The acute phase of myocarditis presents with a flu-like illness that may lead to dilated cardio-myopathy and signs and symptoms of congestive heart failure. Histologic analysis shows a lymphocytic infiltrate of the myocardium with necrosis or degeneration of adjacent myocytes.

Characteristic symptoms of myocarditis include a prodromal viral illness followed by progressive exercise intolerance and congestive symptoms of dyspnea, cough, and orthopnea.

If suspected, ECG may show diffuse low voltage, ST-T wave changes, heart block, or ventricular arrhythmias. Serologic testing may show leukocytosis, eosinophilia, an elevated sedimentation rate or C-reactive protein, and increased myocardial enzymes. Echocardiography will confirm the diagnosis within the right clinical context showing a dilated LV, global hypokinesis or segmental wall abnormalities, and decreased LV ejection fraction.

ARRHYTHMOGENIC RIGHT VENTRICULAR CARDIOMYOPATHY

Arrhythmogenic right ventricular cardiomyopathy (ARVC) represents 4% of SCD in the United States,[5] but was reported as the leading cause of SCD (22%) in the Veneto region of northeastern Italy.[21] Arrhythmogenic right ventricular cardiomyopathy is characterized by a progressive fibro-fatty replacement of the right ventricular myocardium causing wall thinning and right ventricular dilatation. The estimated prevalence is 1 in 5,000 in the general population and results from mutations in genes encoding for des-mosomal (cell adhesion) proteins.[28]

Arrhythmogenic right ventricular cardiomyopathy can present with myocardial electrical instability leading to ventricular arrhythmias that precipitate cardiac arrest, especially during physical activity.[28] In a review of SCD from ARVC, 68% of athletes who died from ARVC had prodromal symptoms such as syncope, chest pain, or palpitations.[29] Physical examination is typically normal. The ECG may show right precordial T-wave inversion (beyond V1), an epsilon wave (small terminal notch seen just beyond the QRS in V1 or V2), prolongation of QRS duration greater than 110 ms, or right bundle branch block pattern. Echocardiogram, cardiac MRI, or CT may demonstrate right ventricular dilatation and wall thinning, reduced right ventricular ejection fraction, focal right ventricular wall motion abnormalities, or right ventricular aneurysms. Fibro-fatty infiltration of the right ventricle is best seen on cardiac MRI or by histologic analysis in selected cases.

AORTIC RUPTURE/MARFAN SYNDROME

Marfan syndrome is the most common inherited disorder of connective tissue that affects multiple organ systems, with a reported incidence of 2 to 3 in 10,000 individuals.[30] Marfan syndrome causes a progressive dilatation and weakness (cystic medial necrosis) of the proximal aorta that can lead to rupture and sudden death. Myxomatous degeneration of the mitral and aortic valves may also lead to valvular dysfunction. Marfan syndrome is caused by mutations in the fibrillin-1 gene, with 75% of cases inherited through autosomal dominant transmission with variable expression and 25% of cases from de novo mutations.[30]

Cardiovascular complications are the major cause of morbidity and mortality in patients with Marfan syndrome. The risk of aortic rupture or dissection increases during adolescence, and 50% of undiagnosed patients with Marfan syndrome die by 40 years of age.[30] Symptoms of aortic dissection typically include sudden, excruciating chest or thoracic pain, often described as tearing or ripping. Heart failure also occurs secondary to aortic valve incompetence.

Physical examination findings include highly variable clinical features usually manifested in adolescence and young adulthood. Diagnosis of Marfan syndrome is primarily based on the Ghent criteria.[31] These criteria rely on the recognition of both "major" and "minor" clinical manifestations involving the skeletal, cardiovascular, and ocular systems (Box 6A-2).

Box 6A-2. Physical Findings Suggestive of Marfan Syndrome[a]

Skeletal	
Major	**Minor**
Need 4 • Arm span to height ratio >1.05 • Arachnodactyly (long slender fingers and toes) • Scoliosis >20 degrees or spondylolisthesis • Pectus carinatum (pigeon chest) • Pectus excavatum (requiring surgery) • Reduced extension of elbows <170 degrees • Pes planus • Protrusio acetabuli of any degree (ascertained on radiographs)	• Pectus excavatum (moderate severity) • Joint hypermobility • High arched palate • Facial appearance (dolichocephaly, malar hypoplasia, enophthalmos, retrognathia, down-slating palpebral fissures)

Cardiovascular	
Major	**Minor**
Need 1 • Dilatation of the ascending aorta involving the sinuses of Valsalva, with or without aortic regurgitation • Dissection of the ascending aorta	• Mitral valve prolapse with or without mitral regurgitation • Dilatation of the pulmonary artery • Calcification of the mitral annulus • Dilatation or dissection of the descending thoracic or abdominal aorta

Ocular	
Major	**Minor**
Need 1 • Ectopia lentis (dislocated lens)	• Flat cornea • Increased axial globe length • Hypoplastic iris • Myopia • Retinal detachment

Other Findings	
Major	**Minor**
Need 1 • Lumbosacral dural ectasia by computed tomography or magnetic resonance imaging	• Spontaneous pneumothorax • Apical blebs • Stretch marks • Recurrent incisional hernias

[a]Ghent criteria[31] for the diagnosis of Marfan syndrome: Major criteria are clinical features that are highly specific for Marfan syndrome and rarely occur in the general population. Minor criteria are features that are present in individuals with Marfan syndrome, but are also often present in the general population. The diagnosis requires that at least 2 of the major manifestations of the condition be present in patients without other affected family members. In families in which Marfan syndrome is known to occur, only one major criterion is required.

AORTIC STENOSIS

Aortic stenosis (AS) accounts for 3% of SCD in US athletes. The most common etiology of AS in youth is a bicuspid aortic valve, which occurs in 1% to 2% of the general population and was found in 2.5% of competitive athletes investigated by echocardiography.[22] Congenital narrowing of the aortic valve causes elevation of LV systolic pressure and cardiac work, leading to LV hypertrophy without a compensatory increase in coronary blood supply. Ischemia can develop secondary to increased LV cardiac mass, coupled with poor coronary artery supply and decreased diastolic filling time (because of a prolonged systolic phase) that is worsened with physical exertion.

Athletes with aortic stenosis are usually asymptomatic, and only about 5% will develop chest pain, angina, or syncope. Physical examination reveals a systolic ejection murmur at the upper right sternal border and an apical ejection click. The murmur of AS typically diminishes with maneuvers that decrease venous return (ie, Valsalva or moving from squatting to standing), and thus has the opposite characteristics of the murmur associated with HCM. Aortic stenosis is confirmed by echocardiography, which shows narrowing of the aortic valve with an elevated pressure gradient and LV hypertrophy.

CORONARY ARTERY DISEASE

Atherosclerotic coronary artery disease accounts for only 3% of SCD in athletes younger than 35 years but is the most frequent cause of SCD in athletes older than 35 years.[5] Atherosclerotic plaque development is progressive and related to coronary risk factors such as hypertension, diabetes, dyslipidemia, tobacco use, illicit drug or anabolic steroid use, and a family history of premature atherosclerotic disease. Homozygous familial hypercholesterolemia is a very rare autosomal dominant disease characterized by accelerated severe atherosclerosis and coronary artery obstruction presenting at an early age (adolescence).[32] Exercise may cause myocardial ischemia or may be a stimulus for plaque disruption with symptoms of exertional chest pain (typical angina), lightheadedness, palpitations, dyspnea, or even sudden death.

ION CHANNEL DISORDERS

Ion channel disorders are primary electrical diseases of the heart predisposing to potentially lethal ventricular arrhythmias and are characterized by mutations in ion channel proteins leading to dysfunctional sodium, potassium, calcium, and other ion transport across cell membranes. Confirmed channelopathies account for approximately 3% of SCD in US athletes.[5] In an additional 3% of SCD in athletes, routine postmortem examination fails to identify a structural cardiac cause of death[1,5] that may be due to inherited arrhythmia syndromes and ion channel disorders such as long QT syndrome (LQTS), short QT syndrome, Brugada syndrome, or familial catecholaminergic polymorphic ventricular tachycardia (CPVT).[1]

The prevalence of ion channel disorders as a cause of SCD in US athletes may be underestimated because autopsy-negative sudden unexplained death (SUD) represents a substantially larger proportion of SCD in the young in other study populations, and the accurate diagnosis of ion channelopathies postmortem is still limited. In Australia, autopsy-negative SUD represents approximately 30% of SCD in individuals younger than 35 years,[18,19] and in US military recruits autopsy-negative SUD accounts for 35% of non-traumatic sudden deaths.[13,14] In studies performing postmortem genetic testing (so-called molecular autopsy) in cases of autopsy-negative SUD, more than one-third of cases were found to have a pathogenic cardiac ion channel mutation.[33,34]

Sudden death is often the sentinel cardiovascular event in autopsy-negative SUD. Sudden death was found to represent the initial event in more than 80% of mutation-positive cases[34] and in more than 90% of US military recruits with autopsy-negative SUD.[13] In 2007 Tester et al[34] reported a family history of

SCD or syncope documented by a medical examiner in 26 of 49 cases (53%) of SUD (average age of 14.2 ± 10.9 years). A personal history of syncope, seizure-like activity, and/or cardiac arrest before these SUDs was reported in 7 of the 49 cases.[34] The high frequency of familial SCD or syncope in presumed primary arrhythmia syndromes emphasizes the need for a careful family history of SUD to identify athletes at risk.

Long QT syndrome is the most common ion channelopathy and characterized by prolongation of ventricular repolarization as measured by the QT interval corrected for heart rate (QTc). There are 10 recognized gene abnormalities for LQTS involving potassium and sodium ion channels important in cardiac repolarization.[35] Most arrhythmias from LQTS are triggered by emotional or physical stress and present with syncope or near-syncope, seizures, or sudden death (Table 6A-1). Syncope is usually due to Torsades des pointes, a specific form of polymorphic ventricular tachycardia. Up to 20% of patients who have LQTS and present with syncope (but are not diagnosed and treated) will experience SCD in the first year after their syncope, and 50% will have SCD by 5 years.[36]

A history of syncope, seizures, or arrhythmias in the patient, or a family history of unexpected or unexplained sudden death, drowning or near drowning, unexplained motor vehicle accident, unexplained seizures (collapse with myoclonic activity), or sudden infant death requires exclusion of an ion channel disorder. The diagnosis of LQTS involves measurement of the QT interval in lead II (alternate leads V_5 or V_6) on ECG and calculating the QTc interval (using the Bazett formula) to compensate for heart rate–related changes. The upper limit of normal for the QTc is 0.46 seconds in individuals younger than 15 years. After age 15 (post puberty), the upper limit is 0.47 seconds in women (due to hormonal changes) and 0.45 seconds in men.[37] Patients with LQTS may also have bizarre, flat, or peaked T wave morphology, alternating T wave polarity (T wave alternans), or prominent U waves or T-U wave complexes.[38] The resting ECG may be normal in up to 30% of patients who are genetically positive for LQTS, and a significant proportion of the normal population will have QTc intervals up to 0.47 seconds.[39] QTc intervals greater than 0.5 seconds are associated with an increased risk of SCD.[36] A QTc greater than 0.5 seconds, with or without symptoms and regardless of family history, distinguishes individuals most at risk for a cardiac event, thus limiting athletic participation. These individuals should be denied clearance from sports until final evaluation by an electrophysiologist or cardiologist experienced with LQTS. Relying on the computer-generated QTc interval is not appropriate because it is frequently inaccurate and the interval should be confirmed by a cardiologist. Within the "gray zone" range of 0.44 to 0.50 sec, there will be both unaffected and potentially affected individuals, making the determination of eligibility for sports participation very difficult.

Catecholaminergic polymorphic ventricular tachycardia is a familial disorder characterized by stress-induced ventricular arrhythmias that result in SCD in children and young adults and most commonly involves a cardiac ryanodine receptor/calcium release channel mutation. Catecholaminergic polymorphic ventricular

TABLE 6A-1. SIGNS AND SYMPTOMS OF CARDIAC ION CHANNEL DISORDERS

Disorder	Trigger	Event
LQTS-1	Emotional stress, physical exercise, swimming, and diving into water	Syncope, sudden death, seizure, drowning or near drowning, motor vehicle accident
LQTS-2	Emotional stress, physical exercise, auditory stimuli (loud noises)	Syncope, sudden death, seizure, motor vehicle accident
LQTS-3	Rest or sleep	Sudden death or sudden infant death
CPVT	Emotional stress, vigorous physical exercise	Syncope, sudden death, seizure, drowning or near drowning

Abbreviations: LQTS, long QT syndrome; CPVT, catecholaminergic polymorphic ventricular tachycardia.

tachycardia can present with syncope, drowning or near drowning, seizure, or sudden death triggered by vigorous physical exertion or acute emotion. Leenhardt et al[40] reported that syncope was a presenting symptom for 20 of 21 CPVT patients, with the first syncopal event occurring at 7.8 ± 4 years of age and a family history of syncope or sudden death was present in 30%. Physical effort or emotion usually triggered symptoms, and the diagnosis of CPVT was generally delayed due to the misdiagnosis of epilepsy or vasovagal events.

HYPERTENSION

Hypertension is the most common cardiovascular disease encountered in the athletic population, and an elevated blood pressure (BP) was found in 6.4% of athletes presenting for routine preparticipation physical evaluation (PPE).[41] Athletes with persistently elevated BP should be questioned about a family history of hypertension and the use of stimulants (such as caffeine, nicotine, or ephedrine) or anabolic steroids. Young athletes (< age 25) with upper extremity hypertension should also have a lower extremity BP checked to exclude coarctation of the aorta.

The *Seventh Report of the Joint National Committee on Prevention, Detection, Evaluation, and Treatment of High Blood Pressure (JNC 7)*[42] has established a BP classification for adults including: normal less than 120/80; pre-hypertension 120–139/80–89; stage 1 hypertension 140–159/90–99; and stage 2 hypertension 160/100 or greater. The Fourth Report on the Diagnosis, Evaluation, and Treatment of High Blood Pressure in Children and Adolescents[43] has established BP standards for pediatric and adolescent patients based on gender, age, and height. The Fourth Report also classifies hypertension in athletes younger than 18 years as pre-hypertension, stage 1 hypertension, and stage 2 hypertension and mirrors the taxonomy used for adults.[43] The diagnosis of hypertension in athletes younger than 18 years requires at least 3 BP measurements with values from 90% to 95% of age-, gender-, and height-based norms defined as pre-hypertension; values from 95% to 99% plus 5 mm Hg of norms defined as stage 1 hypertension; and values greater than 99% plus 5 mm Hg defined as stage 2 hypertension. A convenient pocket guide to BP measurement in children is available at http://www.nhlbi.nih.gov/health/public/heart/hbp/bp_child_pocket/bp_child_pocket.pdf, with tables based on gender, age, and height with systolic BP and diastolic BP values listed for prehypertension, stage 1 hypertension, and stage 2 hypertension.

All children and adolescents diagnosed with hypertension require a careful evaluation for secondary causes of hypertension and target organ disease. This includes blood chemistries (glucose, creatinine, electrolytes, lipid profile, and thyroid function), hematocrit, urinalysis, and ECG. A renal ultrasound is also recommended for all children with stage 1 or stage 2 hypertension. Evaluation of target organ disease including an echocardiogram and retinal examination is recommended in all athletes with comorbid risk factors of diabetes mellitus or renal disease associated with a BP between the 90th to 94th percentile and in all patients with blood pressure in the 95th percentile or higher with stage 2 hypertension.[43] Athletes found to have stage 2 hypertension or findings of end-organ damage should not be allowed to participate in any competitive sport until their BP is further evaluated, treated, and under control, at which time eligibility for participation can be reevaluated.[6]

■ PERSONAL AND FAMILY HISTORY

A comprehensive personal and family history is critical to identifying a proportion of asymptomatic athletes at risk because a normal examination is common with many of the conditions that may result in SCD. The cardiovascular questions of the PPE were developed to elicit responses that may indicate the presence of a serious cardiac condition and lead to further investigation. Parent/guardian verification of personal and family history is recommended for high school and middle school athletes. Use of a standardized and detailed questionnaire (such as the History Form on page 153) is strongly recommended to assist health care providers in performing a comprehensive cardiovascular risk assessment.

PERSONAL HISTORY

The medical history should focus on exertional-related symptoms that suggest underlying cardiovascular disease. The AHA recommends the personal medical history include specific questions on (1) exertional chest pain/discomfort, (2) unexplained syncope/near-syncope, (3) excessive exertional and/or unexplained dyspnea/fatigue associated with exercise, (4) prior recognition of a heart murmur, and (5) a history of elevated systemic blood pressure.[5] A history of palpitations or an irregular heart beat related to exercise (which is not included in the AHA recommendations) is also relevant. Other questions with the potential to affect cardiovascular risks include current or past illicit drug use, ergogenic supplement use (ie, anabolic steroids, human growth hormone, and stimulants), and a recent acute viral syndrome (risk of myocarditis).

Exertional chest discomfort, pain, pressure, or tightness may indicate the presence of myocardial ischemia with exercise, but in athletes is more likely due to exercise-induced asthma or gastroesophageal reflux. Congenital coronary artery anomalies, such as anomalous origin of the left coronary artery or myocardial bridging (intramyocardial course) and left ventricular hypertrophy from aortic stenosis or HCM (LV wall thickness outgrows its blood supply) may produce ischemic chest pain during exercise. Advanced atherosclerotic disease is unusual before age 40 except when associated with abnormal lipid metabolism, but must be considered in any athlete presenting with typical angina, especially if risk factors for atherosclerosis are present. Chest pain associated with other symptoms, such as syncope, near-syncope, or palpitations, is very concerning and warrants a careful cardiac investigation.

Exertional syncope can occur during or immediately following exercise and involves a transient loss of consciousness and postural tone. Exertional syncope that occurs during exercise is a red flag symptom and an ominous sign of potential underlying cardiovascular disease warranting a thorough investigation before allowing an athlete to return to sport.[44] Careful questioning of the athlete should be made to distinguish between syncope occurring *during* exercise (ie, the athlete collapses while running toward the finish line or during play) and syncope occurring *after* exercise (ie, the athlete collapses shortly after crossing the finish line). The absence of prodromal symptoms before a syncopal event also warrants a higher level of suspicion for a pathologic etiology, because a sudden, abrupt loss of consciousness is more likely associated with the sudden onset of a ventricular arrhythmia as seen in patients with LQTS and CPVT. In a review of 474 athletes with a history of syncope or near-syncope found during the PPE, 33% with syncope occurring during exercise had structural cardiac disease known to cause SCD.[45] The diagnostic workup is usually performed in consultation with a cardiologist and includes ECG, echocardiogram, stress ECG, and possibly advanced cardiac imaging (such as MRI or CT) to rule out rare structural abnormalities such as ARVC or congenital coronary artery anomalies.

Syncope or near-syncope (dizziness or lightheadedness) occurring after exercise is much more common and unlikely to represent underlying cardiovascular disease. Syncope preceded by lightheadedness, diaphoresis, nausea, and tunnel vision suggests a neurally mediated event (so-called vasovagal syncope) and is less likely to represent a cardiovascular disorder. An example is exercise-associated collapse (EAC) commonly observed at endurance events. Exercise-associated collapse involves athletes who are unable to stand or walk unaided as a result of lightheadedness, faintness, dizziness, or syncope.[46] During exercise, increases in heart rate and stroke volume result in a substantial rise in cardiac output and offset diminished systemic vascular resistance from vasodilatation to exercising muscles. After exercise, without the muscular activity (muscle pump) to maintain venous return, cardiac filling may reduce dramatically. Forceful ventricular contractions against a diminished ventricular volume are postulated to excessively stimulate ventricular mechanoreceptors causing reflex vasodilatation and bradycardia, and subsequent hypotension and possibly syncope.[44] This neurally mediated syncope, also known as neurocardiogenic syncope, is generally regarded as the most common mechanism of syncope in young adults and can be triggered by situational as well as exercise stressors. Nonetheless, EAC or any suspected neurocardiogenic syncope **associated with a complete loss of consciousness** deserves a diagnostic workup to exclude an underlying cardiac disorder. In addition, recurrent cases of apparently benign vasovagal syncope should be investigated with an ECG at minimum.

Excessive unexplained dyspnea or fatigue associated with exercise may also indicate a cardiovascular condition such as myocarditis, and hypertrophic or dilated cardiomyopathy. **Palpitations or irregular beats** may signify arrhythmias or conduction abnormalities, such as supraventricular tachyarrhythmias, ion channel disorders, or Wolff-Parkinson-White syndrome. Such symptoms may mandate further investigation before medical clearance for sports participation. A clear history of an abrupt increase in heart rate disproportional to activity, and palpitations associated with syncope or near-syncope, requires further investigation usually involving ECG, echocardiogram, cardiac event monitoring, stress ECG, and consultation with an electrophysiologist.

Heart tests such as ECG, echocardiogram, and exercise treadmill testing performed previously on an athlete may indicate a history of a cardiac disorder or suspected disorder. A history of prior cardiac testing should be investigated fully, and review of past medical records is recommended.

FAMILY HISTORY

A detailed family history may help identify asymptomatic athletes with underlying cardiac disease. The AHA recommends that the family history include specific questions on (1) premature death (sudden and unexpected, or otherwise) before age 50 years due to heart disease in 1 or more relatives, (2) disability from heart disease in a close relative younger than 50 years, and (3) specific knowledge of certain cardiac conditions in family members known to cause SCD in athletes.[5] A family history of sudden death before age 50 is significant because it indicates that the cause, absent trauma, was most likely cardiac related and may be familial, including HCM, Marfan syndrome, ARVC, LQTS, Brugada syndrome, CPVT, and lipid abnormalities causing premature coronary artery disease. In addition, a family history of unexplained syncope, unexplained near-drowning or drowning, unexplained motor vehicle accident, unexplained seizure activity, or sudden infant death syndrome may indicate the presence of an ion channel disorder such as LQTS or CPVT.

■ PHYSICAL EXAMINATION

The AHA recommends the PPE include (1) auscultation for heart murmurs, (2) palpation of femoral pulses to exclude aortic coarctation, (3) examination for the physical stigmata of Marfan syndrome, and (4) a brachial artery blood pressure taken in the sitting position.[5]

Auscultation of the heart should be performed in both the supine and standing positions (or with Valsalva maneuver), specifically to identify murmurs of dynamic LV outflow tract obstruction. Particular attention should be paid to the presence and character of any murmurs, the timing of murmurs in relation to S_1 and S_2, extra heart sounds (S_3, S_4), and clicks (Table 6A-2). Standing is preferred to sitting because the diagnostic murmur of HCM (if present) becomes louder when the patient is standing due to decreased venous return.

TABLE 6A-2. SIGNIFICANCE OF ABNORMAL HEART MURMURS

Auscultatory Finding	Significance
• Harsh, loud (usually grade ≥3), systolic ejection murmur • Loudest right upper sternal border • Increases with maneuvers that decrease venous return (ie, Valsalva, or moving from squatting to standing)	HCM-associated LV outflow tract obstruction
• Systolic ejection murmur heard best at right upper sternal border • Radiation to neck • Diminishes with maneuvers that decrease venous return (ie, Valsalva) and increases with maneuvers that increase venous return (ie, squatting)	Aortic stenosis
• Holosystolic murmur heard best at the apex • Radiation to axilla	Mitral valve regurgitation, possible dilated cardiomyopathy or HCM
• Diastolic murmur heard at right upper sternal border • Murmur accentuated with hand grip (increased systemic vascular resistance)	Aortic valve insufficiency, possible Marfan syndrome or bicuspid aortic valve
• High-frequency diastolic murmur heard best at left upper sternal border	Pulmonary valve insufficiency from primary pulmonary hypertension (Graham-Steele murmur)
• Soft early systolic murmur heard best at the upper sternal border while supine (increased venous return) • Murmur often absent or diminished when standing or sitting and with Valsalva	Physiologic (hyperdynamic) "flow" murmur in a well-trained athlete

Abbreviations: HCM, hypertonic cardiomyopathy; LV, left ventricular.

Significant murmurs that may indicate LV outflow tract obstruction are typically early systolic, harsh, and usually grade 3/6 or higher in thin-chested individuals, heard best at the right upper sternal border, that increases with Valsalva or moving from squatting to standing. However, in heavier individuals, the murmur may be only grade 1/6 or 2/6. In contrast, the murmur of aortic stenosis typically diminishes with maneuvers that decrease venous return and increases with maneuvers that increase venous return (ie, squatting). Both pathologic entities are important to recognize. A holosystolic murmur heard best at the apex with radiation to the axilla may indicate mitral valve regurgitation and could be related to a dilated cardiomyopathy. Systolic ejection or midsystolic clicks typically are abnormal at any age. A diastolic murmur heard at the right upper sternal border may represent aortic regurgitation and indicate an incompetent aortic valve, such as that present in Marfan syndrome and sometimes with a bicuspid aortic valve. If suspected, aortic regurgitation can be accentuated by hand grip, which increases systemic vascular resistance. A high-frequency diastolic murmur may also represent pulmonary hypertension with pulmonic insufficiency (Graham-Steele murmur). Any diastolic murmur should be considered pathologic.

Soft early systolic murmurs (grade 1 or 2) and mid-systolic vibratory or musical-type (Still) murmurs likely represent innocent murmurs. A common murmur heard in well-trained athletes is a physiologic (hyperdynamic) "flow" murmur. These are characterized by a grade 1/6 or 2/6 soft early systolic murmur heard best at the upper sternal border. The murmur results from an overall increase in plasma volume and thus stroke volume that occurs as a physiologic adaptation to regular physical training. Often the murmur is only heard when the athlete is supine (increased venous return) and absent when standing or sitting, and should diminish with the strain phase of a Valsalva maneuver. In the absence of concerning symptoms or family history, innocent murmurs require no further investigation. If doubt persists, referral for an echocardiogram or referral to a cardiovascular specialist is recommended.

Palpation of femoral artery pulses is also an important component of the physical examination. Delayed femoral artery pulses compared to radial artery pulses (palpated simultaneously) may indicate the presence of coarctation of the aorta and should be investigated if present.

Recognition of the physical stigmata of Marfan syndrome is critical in the screening of young athletes. Physical examination findings that suggest Marfan syndrome include kyphoscoliosis, high-arched palate, pectus carniatum or excavatum, arachnodactyly (long slender fingers), arm span greater than height (ratio >1.05), mitral valve prolapse, aortic insufficiency murmur, myopia, and generalized hyperlaxity. As noted earlier in the chapter, the diagnosis of Marfan syndrome is based on the Ghent criteria[31] (Box 6A-2) and is confirmed by the presence of typical skeletal manifestations, ectopia lentis (lens dislocation detected by slit-lamp examination), aortic root dilatation or dissection (detected on echocardiography), or lumbosacral dural ectasia (detected by CT or MRI).

Brachial artery blood pressure should be measured on a bare upper arm supported at heart level in the sitting position with the back supported. Use of an appropriate cuff size is of paramount importance, because obese or large athletes may require a large adult cuff or thigh cuff used on the arm to obtain an accurate BP measurement. The most frequent error in measuring BP in the outpatient setting is undersizing the cuff on large arms, and the error in BP measurement is greater when the cuff is too small relative to the patient's arm circumference rather than when the cuff is too large.[47] The "ideal" cuff should have a bladder length that encircles at least 80% of the arm circumference.[47] If the BP is initially elevated, the athlete should sit or lie quietly for 5 to 10 minutes before repeating the measurement.

■ INVESTIGATION OF ATHLETES WITH CARDIOVASCULAR SYMPTOMS

Athletes identified with cardiovascular symptoms such as exertional syncope or near-syncope, chest pain, palpitations, or excessive exertional dyspnea require a careful and thorough cardiovascular evaluation to exclude underlying heart disease before allowing an athlete to return to sport. Syncope occurring during exercise is an ominous sign and warrants a high index of suspicion for underlying cardiac disease. The diagnostic workup of exertional syncope is usually performed in consultation with a cardiologist and may include ECG, echocardiogram, stress ECG, and possibly advanced cardiac imaging (such as MRI or CT) to rule out rare structural abnormalities such as ARVC or congenital coronary artery anomalies. The investigation of rapid or irregular heart beats associated with supraventricular tachyarrhythmias, ion channel disorders, or Wolff-Parkinson-White syndrome may include an ECG, echocardiogram, Holter monitoring, stress ECG, and consultation with a cardiologist and/or electrophysiologist.

■ LIMITATIONS OF THE PREPARTICIPATION CARDIOVASCULAR EVALUATION

No outcomes-based study exists that demonstrates the PPE is effective in preventing or detecting athletes at risk for sudden death. The disease-specific presentations described earlier strongly support that warning symptoms and/or a concerning family history will be present in a significant proportion of athletes at risk for SCD. However, successful detection of athletes at risk of SCD requires that physicians ask the appropriate questions. Unfortunately, standardized questionnaire forms developed to assist health care providers in performing a comprehensive PPE have been grossly underused in the primary care and scholastic communities.[48–50]

NONINVASIVE CARDIOVASCULAR SCREENING IN ATHLETES

The added value of noninvasive screening tests such as ECG or echocardiography to the screening process in athletes is a highly debated topic in sports medicine and sports cardiology.[51,52] Recent articles by Myerburg and Vetter[51] (pro) and Chaitman[52] (con) highlight the controversy regarding routine use of ECG in the preparticipation screening of athletes. The AHA recommended against cardiovascular screening of asymptomatic athletes with ECG or echocardiography because of a poor sensitivity, high false-positive rate, poor positive predictive value, poor cost-effectiveness, and the total cost of implementation.[9] The AHA also contends that ECG is not practical for mass, universal screening due to the size of the athlete cohort, low prevalence of disease, limited resources, absence of a physician cadre to interpret the ECG, and the potential to create anxiety in athletes with false-positive test results.[5] These recommendations were based in part on a small study of 501 collegiate athletes undergoing ECG screening that yielded a 15% false-positive rate and no definitive cases of potentially lethal cardiovascular disease.[53]

In contrast, the European Society of Cardiology,[54] International Olympic Committee,[55] and the governing associations of several US and international professional sports leagues[56] support the routine use of ECG, in addition to personal and family history and physical examination, in the preparticipation screening of athletes. These recommendations are supported by studies showing the higher sensitivity of a standardized history, physical examination, and 12-lead ECG in identifying athletes with underlying cardiovascular disease compared to history and physical alone.[12,21,57,58] In 1998 Corrado et al[21] found that the ECG had a 77% greater power to detect HCM than history and physical examination. In 2006 Corrado et al[12] reported a 25-year experience in 42,386 athletes using a national preparticipation screening program in Italy. In their study, the use of a standardized history, physical examination, and 12-lead ECG provided a 10-fold reduction in the incidence of SCD in young competitive athletes, and an 89% reduction of SCD due to cardiomyopathies.[12] Although only 0.2% of athletes were disqualified with potentially lethal cardiovascular conditions, the study reported a 7% false-positive rate and a 2% overall disqualification rate,[12] raising concerns that adoption of such a program in the United States would lead to an unacceptable number of disqualifications in athletes that may be at low risk of SCD.

Recent studies are helping to refine the ECG criteria used to distinguish normal from abnormal findings in athletes and suggest that a prolonged PR interval, incomplete right bundle branch block, early repolarization, isolated voltage criteria for LV hypertrophy (Sokolow-Lyon criteria), and isolated increases in QRS amplitude (without associated ST-T changes, pathologic Q waves, left atrial enlargement, or left axis deviation) are not indicative of underlying cardiovascular disease in a young athlete.[26,59] Contemporary studies using modified ECG criteria based on the Italian[12,59] studies are demonstrating improved accuracy of ECG screening with lower total positive and false-positive rates. A study of 2,720 competitive athletes and physically active school children in the United Kingdom reported a total positive rate of only 1.5% through ECG screening using updated ECG criteria.[58] Preliminary findings of ECG screening in 9,125 young adults (aged 14–18) from the Midwest region of the United States[60] found only 2% (138) of ECGs to be abnormal using modified Corrado[12] ECG criteria.

The cost-effectiveness of mass ECG screening in athletes is also highly disputed. Fuller[61] estimated a cost per life year saved of $44,000 if ECG screening was used in high school athletes. In contrast, the AHA estimated a cost of $330,000 for each athlete detected with cardiac disease and $3.4 million for each death prevented.[5] The differences in cost-effectiveness estimates lie in the baseline statistics used for SCD incidence and the false-positive rate requiring further cardiovascular workup at additional cost. The AHA calculations are based on an SCD incidence of 1 in 200,000 and a false-positive rate of 15%.[8,53] More recent studies suggest the actual incidence of SCD in young competitive athletes is substantially higher and may approximate 1 in 75,000.[3,11] Using stricter, more accurate ECG criteria (yielding a total positive rate of about 2%–5%) and assuming a higher incidence of detectable and preventable SCD may make the cost-effectiveness estimates more favorable for ECG screening.[62]

However, feasibility and practical concerns still exist regarding large-scale implementation of ECG screening in the United States. Who will pay for and interpret the ECGs? What is the long-term result of disqualifying athletes with cardiovascular disease at an increased but unquantifiable risk for sudden cardiac arrest (SCA)? Clearly, large-scale outcomes-based research is needed in a US population of athletes to better define the true prevalence of disease, cost of investigating false-positives, and reduction of SCD through withdrawal from athletic participation. Education of US primary care providers, sports medicine physicians, and cardiologists in ECG interpretation in athletes is also needed. Until then, the debate on ECG screening and discordance between recommendations from US and European authorities will surely continue.

Recommendations for or against ECG screening in athletes are beyond the scope of this monograph. The writing group acknowledges that there are conflicting consensus recommendations and studies, further highlighting the complexity of this topic. For individual practitioners interested in including the ECG in the preparticipation evaluation or in offering ECG screening within the model of informed decision-making with patients and families, suggested ECG criteria are listed in Table 6A-3.

■ CLEARANCE RECOMMENDATIONS FOR ATHLETES WITH IDENTIFIED CARDIOVASCULAR DISEASE

Careful activity recommendations involving temporary or permanent sports disqualification for athletes with identified cardiovascular disease should be made in consultation with a cardiologist. The 36th Bethesda Conference sponsored by the American College of Cardiology provides eligibility recommendations for competitive athletes with cardiovascular abnormalities.[6] These expert consensus recommendations provide a framework in which to base clearance decisions once a cardiovascular abnormality is identified. The 36th Bethesda recommendations take into account the severity of disease, potential for sudden death or disease progression, and the type and intensity of exercise involved in a particular sport.[6]

Withdrawal from athletic training and competition can reduce a portion of sudden deaths in athletes who have disorders predisposing them to SCA.[12] Early detection of clinically significant cardiovascular disease through preparticipation screening will, in some cases, permit timely therapeutic interventions that may alter clinical course and significantly prolong life. For example, high-risk individuals with genetic heart disease may be eligible for implantable cardioverter-defibrillators or other therapeutic interventions. These recommendations are predicated on the likelihood that intense athletic training and competition act as a trigger to increase the risk for SCD or disease progression in susceptible athletes with underlying heart disease.[6]

Box 6A-3. ECG Interpretation in Athletes 12 Years or Older

ABNORMAL **Findings strongly suggest underlying cardiovascular disease.**
ST segment depression (≥0.1 mV) in ≥2 leads
Deep negative T waves (≥0.2 mV) in ≥2 leads
Romhilt-Estes voltage criterion for LVH (R or S wave ≥2.0 mV in any limb lead, or S wave in V1 or V2 ≥3.0 mV or R wave in V5 or V6 ≥3.0 mV) with ST segment depression or T wave inversion
Pathologic Q wave patterns (≥0.04 s in duration or depth >25% of the height of the ensuing R wave or QS pattern in ≥2 leads)
Complete right or left bundle branch block (QRS duration ≥0.12 s)
R or R′ wave in V1 ≥0.5 mV in amplitude and R:S ratio ≥1
ST segment elevation in V1 to V3 with the right bundle branch block pattern (Brugada-like pattern)
Prolonged QTc interval measured in leads II, V5, or V6 (≥0.50 s)
Short QTc interval (≤0.33 s)
Ventricular preexcitation (short PR <0.12 s) with or without delta wave
Epsilon wave (small negative deflection or terminal notch just beyond the QRS in V1 or V2, found in ARVC)
Left atrial enlargement (negative portion of P wave in V1 ≥0.1 mV in depth and ≥0.04 s in duration)
Right atrial enlargement (P wave ≥0.25 mV in leads II and III or V1)
Left axis deviation (-30 degrees to -90 degrees)
Right axis deviation (≥120 degrees)
Third degree atrioventricular block
Second degree Mobitz II atrioventricular block
Complex ventricular arrhythmias
Atrial tachydysrhythmias (supraventricular tachycardia, atrial flutter, atrial fibrillation)
POSSIBLY ABNORMAL **Findings may suggest underlying cardiovascular disease.**
Romhilt-Estes voltage criterion for LVH (R or S wave ≥2.0 mV in any limb lead, or S wave in V1 or V2 ≥3.0 mV or R wave in V5 or V6 ≥3.0 mV) without ST segment depression or T wave inversion
QTc interval in males 0.44–0.50 s and females 0.46–0.50 s
Second degree Mobitz I (Wenckebach) atrioventricular block
QRS duration ≥0.11 s and <0.12 s
Left anterior fascicular block
Premature ventricular contractions (≥3 PVCs per tracing)

Box 6A-3. ECG Interpretation in Athletes 12 Years or Older, continued

PROBABLY NORMAL **Findings common in well-conditioned athletes.**
Sinus bradycardia (<60 beats/min)a
Sinus arrhythmiaa
Prolonged PR interval or first degree atrioventricular blocka
Junctional rhythma
Early repolarization pattern (J-point ST segment elevation)a
Tall T waves
Incomplete right bundle branch block (RSR′ pattern in precordial leads with QRS duration <0.11 s)
Isolated Sokolow voltage criterion for LVH (S wave in V1 + R wave in V5 or V6 ≥3.5 mV) without ST depression or T wave inversion

Abbreviations: ECG, electrocardiogram; LVH, left ventricular hypertrophy; ARVC, arrhythmogenic right ventricular cardiomyopathy

aChanges normalize with exercise.

■ REFERENCES

1. Maron BJ. Sudden death in young athletes. *N Engl J Med.* 2003;349(11):1064–1075

2. Van Camp SP, Bloor CM, Mueller FO, Cantu RC, Olson HG. Nontraumatic sports death in high school and college athletes. *Med Sci Sports Exerc.* 1995;27(5):641–647

3. Maron BJ, Doerer JJ, Haas TS, Tierney DM, Mueller FO. Profile and frequency of sudden death in 1463 young competitive athletes: from a 25 year US national registry: 1980–2005. *Circulation.* 2006;114:II(18):830

4. Maron BJ, Shirani J, Poliac LC, Mathenge R, Roberts WC, Mueller FO. Sudden death in young competitive athletes. Clinical, demographic, and pathological profiles. *JAMA.* 1996;276(3):199–204

5. Maron BJ, Thompson PD, Ackerman MJ, et al. Recommendations and considerations related to preparticipation screening for cardiovascular abnormalities in competitive athletes: 2007 update: a scientific statement from the American Heart Association Council on Nutrition, Physical Activity, and Metabolism: endorsed by the American College of Cardiology Foundation. *Circulation.* 2007;115(12):1643–1455

6. Maron BJ, Zipes DP. 36th Bethesda Conference: eligibility recommendations for competitive athletes with cardiovascular abnormalities. *J Am Coll Cardiol.* 2005;45(8):1318–1321

7. Drezner JA, Courson RW, Roberts WO, et al. Inter-association task force recommendations on emergency preparedness and management of sudden cardiac arrest in high school and college athletic programs: a consensus statement. *Heart Rhythm.* 2007;4(4):549–565

8. Maron BJ, Gohman TE, Aeppli D. Prevalence of sudden cardiac death during competitive sports activities in Minnesota high school athletes. *J Am Coll Cardiol.* 1998;32(7):1881–1884

9. Maron BJ, Thompson PD, Puffer JC, et al. Cardiovascular preparticipation screening of competitive athletes. A statement for health professionals from the Sudden Death Committee (clinical cardiology) and Congenital Cardiac Defects Committee (cardiovascular disease in the young), American Heart Association. *Circulation.* 1996;94(4):850–856

10. Drezner JA, Rogers KJ, Zimmer RR, Sennett BJ. Use of automated external defibrillators at NCAA Division I Universities. *Med Sci Sports Exerc.* 2005;37(9):1487–1492

11. Maron BJ. Hypertrophic cardiomyopathy and other causes of sudden cardiac death in young competitive athletes, with considerations for preparticipation screening and criteria for disqualification. *Cardiol Clin.* 2007;25(3):399–414, vi

12. Corrado D, Basso C, Pavei A, Michieli P, Schiavon M, Thiene G. Trends in sudden cardiovascular death in young competitive athletes after implementation of a preparticipation screening program. *JAMA.* 2006;296(13):1593–1601

13. Eckart RE, Scoville SL, Campbell CL, et al. Sudden death in young adults: a 25-year review of autopsies in military recruits. *Ann Intern Med.* 2004;141(11):829–834

14. Eckart RE, Scoville SL, Shry EA, Potter RN, Tedrow U. Causes of sudden death in young female military recruits. *Am J Cardiol.* 2006;97(12):1756–1758

15. Drezner JA, Chun JS, Harmon KG, Derminer L. Survival trends in the United States following exercise-related sudden cardiac arrest in the youth: 2000–2006. *Heart Rhythm.* 2008;5(6):794–799

16. Maron BJ, Carney KP, Lever HM, et al. Relationship of race to sudden cardiac death in competitive athletes with hypertrophic cardiomyopathy. *J Am Coll Cardiol.* 2003;41(6):974–980

17. Corrado D, Basso C, Thiene G, et al. Spectrum of clinicopathologic manifestations of arrhythmogenic right ventricular cardiomyopathy/dysplasia: a multicenter study. *J Am Coll Cardiol.* 1997;30(6):1512–1520

18. Doolan A, Langlois N, Semsarian C. Causes of sudden cardiac death in young Australians. *Med J Aust.* 2004;180(3):110–112

19. Puranik R, Chow CK, Duflou JA, Kilborn MJ, McGuire MA. Sudden death in the young. *Heart Rhythm.* 2005;2(12):1277–1282

20. Maron BJ, Pelliccia A, Spirito P. Cardiac disease in young trained athletes. Insights into methods for distinguishing athlete's heart from structural heart disease, with particular emphasis on hypertrophic cardiomyopathy. *Circulation.* 1995;91(5):1596–1601

21. Corrado D, Basso C, Schiavon M, Thiene G. Screening for hypertrophic cardiomyopathy in young athletes. *N Engl J Med.* 1998;339(6):364–369

22. Stefani L, Galanti G, Toncelli L, et al. Bicuspid aortic valve in competitive athletes. *Br J Sports Med.* 2008;42(1):31–35; discussion 35

23. Basavarajaiah S, Wilson M, Whyte G, Shah A, McKenna W, Sharma S. Prevalence of hypertrophic cardiomyopathy in highly trained athletes: relevance to pre-participation screening. *J Am Coll Cardiol.* 2008;51(10):1033–1039

24. Maron BJ. Hypertrophic cardiomyopathy. *Lancet.* 1997;350(9071):127–133

25. Maron BJ, Roberts WC, Epstein SE. Sudden death in hypertrophic cardiomyopathy: a profile of 78 patients. *Circulation.* 1982;65(7):1388–1394

26. Melacini P, Cianfrocca C, Calore C, et al. Abstract 3390: marginal overlap between electrocardiographic abnormalities in patients with hypertrophic cardiomyopathy and trained athletes: implications for preparticipation screening. *Circulation.* 2007;116(II):765

27. Basso C, Maron BJ, Corrado D, Thiene G. Clinical profile of congenital coronary artery anomalies with origin from the wrong aortic sinus leading to sudden death in young competitive athletes. *J Am Coll Cardiol.* 2000;35(6):1493–1501

28. Basso C, Corrado D, Thiene G. Arrhythmogenic right ventricular cardiomyopathy in athletes: diagnosis, management, and recommendations for sport activity. *Cardiol Clin.* 2007;25(3):415–422, vi

29. Corrado D, Basso C, Fontaine G, et al. Abstract session 15: clinical electrophysiology II: clinical profile of young competitive athletes who died suddenly of arrhythmogenic right ventricular cardiomyopathy/dysplasia: a multicenter study. *Pacing Clin Electrophysiol.* 2002;25:544

30. Ammash NM, Sundt TM, Connolly HM. Marfan syndrome-diagnosis and management. *Curr Probl Cardiol.* 2008;33(1):7–39

31. De Paepe A, Devereux RB, Dietz HC, Hennekam RC, Pyeritz RE. Revised diagnostic criteria for the Marfan syndrome. *Am J Med Genet.* 1996;62(4):417–426

32. Brook GJ, Keidar S, Boulos M, et al. Familial homozygous hypercholesterolemia: clinical and cardiovascular features in 18 patients. *Clin Cardiol.* 1989;12(6):333–338

33. Tester DJ, Ackerman MJ. The role of molecular autopsy in unexplained sudden cardiac death. *Curr Opin Cardiol.* 2006;21(3):166–172

34. Tester DJ, Spoon DB, Valdivia HH, Makielski JC, Ackerman MJ. Targeted mutational analysis of the RyR2-encoded cardiac ryanodine receptor in sudden unexplained death: a molecular autopsy of 49 medical examiner/coroner's cases. *Mayo Clin Proc.* 2004;79(11):1380–1384

35. Lehnart SE, Ackerman MJ, Benson DW Jr, et al. Inherited arrhythmias: a National Heart, Lung, and Blood Institute and Office of Rare Diseases workshop consensus report about the diagnosis, phenotyping, molecular mechanisms, and therapeutic approaches for primary cardiomyopathies of gene mutations affecting ion channel function. *Circulation.* 2007;116(20):2325–2345

36. Hobbs JB, Peterson DR, Moss AJ, et al. Risk of aborted cardiac arrest or sudden cardiac death during adolescence in the long-QT syndrome. *JAMA.* 2006;296(10):1249–1254

37. Goldenberg I, Moss AJ, Zareba W. QT interval: how to measure it and what is "normal." *J Cardiovasc Electrophysiol.* 2006;17(3):333–336

38. Vetter VL. Clues or miscues? How to make the right interpretation and correctly diagnose long-QT syndrome. *Circulation.* 2007;115(20):2595–2598

39. Priori SG, Napolitano C, Schwartz PJ. Low penetrance in the long-QT syndrome: clinical impact. *Circulation.* 1999;99(4):529–533

40. Leenhardt A, Lucet V, Denjoy I, Grau F, Ngoc DD, Coumel P. Catecholaminergic polymorphic ventricular tachycardia in children. A 7-year follow-up of 21 patients. *Circulation*. 1995;91(5):1512–1519

41. DiFiori J, Haney S. Preparticipation evaluation of collegiate athletes. *Med Sci Sports Exerc*. 2004;36(5):S102

42. Chobanian AV, Bakris GL, Black HR, et al. The seventh report of the Joint National Committee on Prevention, Detection, Evaluation, and Treatment of High Blood Pressure: the JNC 7 report. *JAMA*. 2003;289(19):2560–2572

43. National High Blood Pressure Education Program Working Group on High Blood Pressure in Children and Adolescents. The fourth report on the diagnosis, evaluation, and treatment of high blood pressure in children and adolescents. *Pediatrics*. 2004;114(2 suppl 4th report):555–576

44. O'Connor FG, Oriscello RG, Levine BD. Exercise-related syncope in the young athlete: reassurance, restriction or referral? *Am Fam Physician*. 1999;60(7):2001–2008

45. Colivicchi F, Ammirati F, Santini M. Epidemiology and prognostic implications of syncope in young competing athletes. *Eur Heart J*. 2004;25(19):1749–1753

46. Roberts WO. Exercise-associated collapse in endurance events: a classification system. *Physician Sportsmed*. 1989;15(5):49–50, 52–54, 59

47. Pickering TG, Hall JE, Appel LJ, et al. Recommendations for blood pressure measurement in humans and experimental animals: part 1: blood pressure measurement in humans: a statement for professionals from the Subcommittee of Professional and Public Education of the American Heart Association Council on High Blood Pressure Research. *Circulation*. 2005;111(5):697–716

48. Gómez JE, Lantry BR, Saathoff KN. Current use of adequate preparticipation history forms for heart disease screening of high school athletes. *Arch Pediatr Adolesc Med*. 1999;153(7):723–726

49. Pfister GC, Puffer JC, Maron BJ. Preparticipation cardiovascular screening for US collegiate student-athletes. *JAMA*. 2000;283(12):1597–1599

50. Glover DW, Glover DW, Maron BJ. Evolution in the process of screening United States high school student-athletes for cardiovascular disease. *Am J Cardiol*. 2007;100(11):1709–1712

51. Myerburg RJ, Vetter VL. Electrocardiograms should be included in preparticipation screening of athletes. *Circulation*. 2007;116(22):2616–2626; discussion 2626

52. Chaitman BR. An electrocardiogram should not be included in routine preparticipation screening of young athletes. *Circulation*. 2007;116(22):2610–2614; discussion 2615

53. Maron BJ, Bodison SA, Wesley YE, Tucker E, Green KJ. Results of screening a large group of intercollegiate competitive athletes for cardiovascular disease. *J Am Coll Cardiol*. 1987;10(6):1214–1221

54. Corrado D, Pelliccia A, Bjornstad HH, et al. Cardiovascular pre-participation screening of young competitive athletes for prevention of sudden death: proposal for a common European protocol. Consensus Statement of the Study Group of Sport Cardiology of the Working Group of Cardiac Rehabilitation and Exercise Physiology and the Working Group of Myocardial and Pericardial Diseases of the European Society of Cardiology. *Eur Heart J*. 2005;26(5):516–524

55. International Olympic Committee Medical Commission. Sudden cardiovascular death in sport: Lausanne recommendations on preparticipation cardiovascular screening. December 10, 2004. http://multimedia.olympic.org/pdf/en_report_886.pdf. Accessed October 1, 2008

56. Harris KM, Sponsel A, Hutter AM Jr, Maron BJ. Brief communication: cardiovascular screening practices of major North American professional sports teams. *Ann Intern Med*. 2006;145(7):507–511

57. Fuller CM, McNulty CM, Spring DA, et al. Prospective screening of 5,615 high school athletes for risk of sudden cardiac death. *Med Sci Sports Exerc*. 1997;29(9):1131–1138

58. Wilson MG, Basavarajaiah S, Whyte GP, Cox S, Loosemore M, Sharma S. Efficacy of personal symptom and family history questionnaires when screening for inherited cardiac pathologies: the role of electrocardiography. *Br J Sports Med*. 2008;42(3):207–211

59. Pelliccia A, Culasso F, Di Paolo FM, et al. Prevalence of abnormal electrocardiograms in a large, unselected population undergoing pre-participation cardiovascular screening. *Eur Heart J*. 2007;28(16):2006–2010

60. Nora M, Zimmerman F, Ow P, Fenner P, Marek J. Abstract 3718: preliminary findings of ECG screening in 9,125 young adults. *Circulation*. 2007;116(II):845

61. Fuller CM. Cost effectiveness analysis of screening of high school athletes for risk of sudden cardiac death. *Med Sci Sports Exerc*. 2000;32(5):887–890

62. Drezner JA. Contemporary approaches to the identification of athletes at risk for sudden cardiac death. *Curr Opin Cardiol*. 2008;23(5):494–501

B: Central Nervous System

The neurologic conditions that may affect an athlete's ability to participate in sports or require additional workup, rehabilitation, or informed decision-making prior to sports participation include a history of previous concussions or head injuries, seizure disorders, frequent or exertional headaches, problems with recurrent stingers or burners, or a previous episode of transient quadriparesis or cervical cord neuropraxia. This section will review the questions on the preparticipation physical evaluation (PPE) form designed to elicit previous neurologic issues, provide a brief framework of pertinent issues, and discuss appropriate workup as well as treatment and clearance concerns for each topic.

■ CONCUSSIONS

HISTORY FORM QUESTIONS

34. *Have you ever had a head injury or concussion?*

35. *Have you ever had a hit or blow to the head that caused confusion, prolonged headache, or memory problems?*

KEY POINTS

- Concussions are common, underrecognized, and underreported.
- Concussions usually do not involve a loss of consciousness.
- No one should return to a contact or collision sport after sustaining a concussion until completely asymptomatic.
- Once asymptomatic, athletes should undergo a graded return to exercise (Box 6B-1).
- Athletes younger than 18 years take longer to recover after concussion than older athletes.
- Sequelae of concussion may include
  — Second impact syndrome if a second head injury occurs while the athlete is still symptomatic
  — Postconcussion syndrome that can last for weeks to months
  — Permanent neurologic deficits such as decreased cognitive functioning or not reaching cognitive potential
- Computerized neuropsychological testing is an evaluation tool that is most helpful when a baseline, pre-injury test is available.
- Return to play after concussion decisions must be individualized.

It is estimated that somewhere between 300,000[1] and 2 million sport-related concussions occur each year,[2,3] but it is difficult to estimate the true incidence of concussion because of inconsistent data reporting. Concussions are most common in football, with about 40,000 per year in US high schools.[4]

Box 6B-1. Graded Return to Exercise

No activity
Light aerobic activity
Sport-specific exercise
Noncontact training drills
Full-contact practice
Return to play

Concussions are also common in soccer, basketball, unorganized free play, extreme sports, ice hockey, and wrestling. It is estimated that by the time an adolescent reaches high school, 53% will have reported a history of concussion and by the time they reach college, 36% will report a history of multiple concussions.[5]

There are many complex definitions of concussion. A straightforward and easily understandable definition is "a traumatically induced transient disturbance of central neurologic function."[6] A loss of consciousness is not required to make the diagnosis of concussion, and in about 90% of concussions there *will be no* loss of consciousness. Typical signs and symptoms associated with a concussion are listed in Box 6B-2. Posttraumatic (either retrograde or antegrade) amnesia has been associated with more severe concussions and longer recoveries.[7–9] Many times athletes who are unaware that they have suffered a concussion or never receive a diagnosis of concussion will report symptoms when specifically questioned.[10] Careful follow-up of questions 34 and 35 should help ascertain whether or not an athlete has had concussive symptoms.

A history of concussions, previously diagnosed or not, is important.[11] If an athlete has had a concussion, he or she is more likely to suffer a second concussion.[10,12,13] Subsequent concussions may result in a longer time for recovery or occur with less trauma.[12,14–16] There is reasonable evidence that athletes younger than 18 years take longer to recover and may be at higher risk for permanent neurologic deficits, particularly with repeat injury.[3,5,17–19] All of these issues need to be factored into clearance or return-to-play recommendations.

There are essentially 3 main issues to consider when deciding whether it is reasonable to clear someone or return them to play after a concussion: second impact syndrome (SIS), postconcussion syndrome, and persistent neurologic deficit.

Box 6B-2. Signs and Symptoms of Concussion

Cognitive
Confusion
Posttraumatic amnesia
Retrograde amnesia
Loss of consciousness
Disorientation
Feeling "foggy" or "out of it"
Vacant stare
Difficulty focusing
Delayed verbal and motor responses
Slurred/incoherent speech
Excessive drowsiness
Somatic
Headache
Fatigue
Disequilibrium
Nausea/vomiting
Visual disturbance
Phonophobia
Affective
Emotional lability
Irritability

Second impact syndrome is hypothesized to occur when a player sustains a second, sometimes low–velocity, blow to the head before full recovery from a previous concussion. The second impact induces a cascade of events that causes a loss of brain blood flow autoregulation leading to pancerebral edema, brain stem herniation, and death. The existence of SIS has been questioned,[20] and the definition continues to evolve. The cerebral edema may represent a variant of malignant brain edema seen in young children after relatively minor head trauma.[21,22] Second impact syndrome may be more likely to occur in athletes younger than 20 years. There is also new review evidence showing that some previous SIS cases may have been misdiagnosed.[23] Despite this, recent basic science research in animal models clearly shows that the brain is more susceptible to secondary injury after concussive injury.[17,24,25] It seems clear that an injured human brain is more vulnerable to repetitive injury and symptoms correlate to functional changes in the brain.[26] Given this, an athlete should never return to play while symptomatic.

Postconcussion syndrome is the persistence of headaches, dizziness, fatigue, depression, or cognitive impairment after a mild traumatic brain injury or concussion.[27] Where postconcussion syndrome begins and the normal course of a concussion ends is not clear. Postconcussion syndrome can occur after a single blow to the head and may last weeks to years. Athletes should not be allowed to participate in contact sports while experiencing symptoms consistent with postconcussion syndrome; however, a return to exercise may be reasonable.

Permanent neurologic deficit is defined as a decrease in cognitive functioning or not reaching full cognitive potential in pediatric patients. This may be more likely to occur with repetitive concussions or in concussions sustained by younger athletes. There may be a genetic predisposition for long-term neurologic sequelae, but there are no clinically available markers to suggest who may be at risk.[28] Recent research indicates that some professional football players who have a history of concussions are more likely than their non-concussed peers to be depressed and suffer from early mild cognitive impairment.[29,30]

Additionally, autopsies of brains of former NFL football players suffering from neuropsychiatric symptoms showed changes consistent with chronic traumatic encephalopathy thought to possibly be secondary to years of repetitive head trauma.[31,32] The specter of long-term neurologic sequelae support the use of caution in clearance and return-to-play recommendations.

HISTORY

The key history in determining further follow-up and clearance recommendations are listed in Box 6B-3.

Box 6B-3. Concussion History

- How many previous head injuries has the athlete experienced or suffered?
- How did it occur?
- What type of symptoms
- How long did each last?
- Was there retrograde or posttraumatic amnesia?
- How long were they held from practice?
- Did they miss any competitions?
- Did they have any difficulty in their classes?
- Were their grades typical for them that semester?
- How long did it take them to feel 100% normal?
- Are there other "dings," hits to the head, or dazed episodes not considered concussions?

PHYSICAL EXAMINATION

The physical examination at the time of PPE should be normal. The typical postconcussion physical examination is done to assess cognitive function. Although rare, findings of a cranial nerve injury, findings of other neurologic deficits, or findings related to a mass lesion, such as a subdural bleed, must also be assessed (Box 6B-4).

DIAGNOSTIC TESTING

Concussions are diffuse axonal injuries that are not associated with abnormalities on conventional imaging tests such as magnetic resonance imaging (MRI) or computed tomography. These should be performed if other diagnoses, such as a bleed or mass, are being considered. Positron emission tomography scans and functional MRIs will show changes after concussion as they measure the metabolic activity of the brain. Their use as a routine clinical test has yet to be defined.

NEUROPSYCHOLOGICAL TESTING

Neuropsychological tests can be used to quantitatively assess the cognitive function, either with pencil and paper or as computerized test batteries. These tests are most useful when a concussed athlete has a pre-injury baseline test for comparison. Some high school and college programs perform relatively brief baseline computerized neuropsychological testing on all high-risk athletes (football, soccer, ice hockey, wrestling, basketball, gymnastics, pole vaulters, and those with prior concussions). Commercially available computer neuropsychological tests are listed in Box 6B-5. Other baseline assessment tools such as the Standardized Assessment of Concussion[33,34] or Standardized Concussion Assessment Test 2[19] (see Appendix C on page 161) are also available for sideline and office assessment.

CLEARANCE FOR PARTICIPATION

A number of concussion management and return-to-play guidelines, consensus statements, and consensus conferences have been published.[6,19,35–40] All guidelines recommend that athletes should never be cleared to participate while still symptomatic. Assessment by a physician familiar with the evaluation and

Box 6B-4. Concussion-Specific Physical Examination

```
Cranial nerve examination
Speech
Gait
Romberg's test
Pronator drift
Mental status examination
   Memory function
         "What venue are we at?"
         "Which half is it?"
         "Who scored last?"
         "What team did we play last?"
         "Did we win?"
   3-word recall
   Name months forward then backward
   Digit sequencing forward and backward up to 5
         1-3-6          6-3-1
         7-4-1-5        5-1-4-7
         5-1-0-6-7      7-6-0-1-5
```

Box 6B-5. Commercially Available Computerized Neuropsychological Tests

Impact (www.impact.com)
Cogsport (www.cogstate.com)
Automated Neuropsychological Assessment Metrics
   (www.armymedicine.army.mil/prr/anam.html)
Headminders (www.headminder.com)

management of concussion should be considered for a concussion that is not straightforward and rapidly resolving. Concussions that raise greater concern include prolonged, severe, or multiple symptoms; prolonged loss of consciousness; a concussive convulsion; repeated or recent concussions; concussions occurring with progressively less trauma; or concussion in athletes younger than 18 years, with depression or other mental health issues, migraine headaches, attention-deficit disorder, or sleep disorders.

Disqualification from contact or high-risk sports may be considered in athletes with persistent post-concussion syndrome or serious head injury. While there are no data to show that restriction is warranted in athletes with multiple concussions who return to baseline function between episodes, most expert guidelines also consider the number, frequency, and severity of symptoms as well as the circumstances in which the concussions occur. For younger athletes, a more conservative approach should be followed. Disqualification from contact sports or sports at high risk for concussion does not mean disqualification from all physical activity, and athletes should be directed toward lower-risk activities.

■ SEIZURES

HISTORY FORM QUESTIONS

36. Do you have a history of seizure disorder?

KEY POINTS

- Seizures should not preclude athletes from physical activity.

Seizures are not very common among athletes, in part because patients with seizure disorder may have been discouraged from participating in strenuous exercise and team sports out of fear that physical activity will exacerbate the disorder.[41,42] However, if athletes have good seizure control, they can participate in both collision and contact sports without adversely affecting seizure frequency.[41]

A history of new-onset seizure or those occurring after head injury requires thorough review of the medical evaluation and treatment prior to clearance for sport. Syncope with myoclonic activity can easily be confused with seizure, and potential cardiac causes of syncope should be ruled out prior to making the diagnosis of seizure disorder (see Chapter 6A: Cardiovascular Problems). Some antiepileptic drugs have side effects that may affect performance, including rash, hirsutism, weight gain, nausea, and both behavioral and cognitive impairment.[43] The World Anti-Doping Agency (WADA) and the NCAA do not ban most antiepileptic drugs but, as with all medications, athletes should keep up to date with current banned medication lists.

Water sports can present unique challenges for athletes with seizures, and limitations may be indicated for some athletes. Precautions must be taken and risks of drowning discussed with the athlete and parents or guardians. Coaches should be informed so they are aware of the risks. The athlete must never swim or train in the water alone. Athletes should be counseled to inform their physician about any seizure activity so that further evaluation and treatment alterations can be implemented.

■ HEADACHES

HISTORY FORM QUESTION

37. Do you have headaches with exercise?

KEY POINTS

- Headaches can be triggered or worsened by exercise and may prohibit physical activity.
- Migraine headache triggers should be identified and avoided.
- Cough headache (benign exertional headache) occurs in sports with frequent and prolonged valsalva.
- Primary exertional headache (effort headache) occurs with aerobic exercise.
- The initial presentation of a subarachnoid hemorrhage or arterial dissection may present with severe headaches related to exertion.

In a survey regarding sports-related headaches, 35% of both male and female athletes reported having headache during activity.[44,45] Frequent headaches can interfere with sports participation and be either caused or worsened by physical activity. Physicians should consider the common causes and sport-specific causes when evaluating an athlete headache. In 2004 the International Headache Society revised their diagnostic criteria for the classification of headaches as primary or secondary as outlined in Box 6B-6.[46] Physical examination should focus on ruling out secondary causes of headache by assessing blood pressure, examining the retina for papilledema, and evaluating cranial nerve and cerebellar function.

Migraine headaches frequently develop during adolescence, occurring more often in females,[47] with a community prevalence of 12% to 18%.[48] Migraines are not a disqualifier for sports participation but certainly may hamper performance and participation. Migraines may be triggered by the heightened stress of competition, by head impact such as heading a soccer ball or head trauma, or simply by physical exertion. Athletes should be questioned about triggers so preventive strategies can be implemented.

Box 6B-6. International Headache Society Classification of Headaches

Primary Headaches

1. Migraine[a]
2. Tension-type headache
3. Cluster headaches and other trigeminal autonomic cephalagias
4. Other headaches
    a. Primary cough headache (benign exertional headache)
    b. Primary exertional headache (effort headache)

Secondary Headaches
5. Headaches attributed to head/neck trauma (post-concussive headache) 6. Headaches attributed to cranial or cervical vascular disorder 7. Headache attributed to nonvascular intracranial disorder 8. Headache attributed to substance or its withdrawal 9. Headache attributed to infection 10. Headache attributed to disorders of homeostasis 11. Headache or facial pain attributed to disorders of cranium, neck, eyes, ears, sinuses, teeth, mouth, or other facial or cranial structure 12. Headache attributed to psychiatric disorder

[a]May be triggered by exercise.

Ergot derivatives and the triptans are not banned by either WADA or the NCAA; however, other commonly used medications like beta-blockers and narcotics are banned. Some medications used in migraine treatment may impair performance or slow reaction time, increasing the risk of some sports. Most athletes can compete effectively and safely after taking a triptan. If an athlete has a headache requiring treatment pre-competition, an injectable form of a triptan may facilitate quicker return to play because of its quicker onset of action. If migraines are a frequent occurrence, prophylactic medications may be indicated.

There are 2 categories of headaches that relate strictly to exercise. They are the cough headache, which has also been termed the *benign exertional headache* in other classification schemes, and the primary exertional headache, which has also been referred to as an *effort headache*.[48]

Primary cough headache is brought on suddenly by coughing, straining, or the valsalva maneuver in the absence of other intracranial pathology such as cerebral aneurysm or Arnold-Chiari malformation.[46] Imaging, particularly of the posterior fossa, is required to rule out secondary forms of cough headache. Treatment strategies include nonsteroidal anti-inflammatory drugs such as indomethacin and altering breathing patterns during weight lifting.

Primary exertional headache is classically triggered by aerobic physical exercise, is pulsating in quality, and lasts anywhere from 5 minutes to 48 hours. Subarachnoid hemorrhage and arterial dissection must be ruled out after any new or different acute onset exertional headache.[45] Prophylactic treatment strategies for recurrent exertional headaches include indomethacin and graduated exercise programs that stay slightly below the onset threshold.

An athlete with effort-related headaches must also be questioned regarding prior concussion and head injury. Following the concussion, an athlete may continue to have headaches with exertion related to the head injury; the presence of these headaches indicates that the concussion is not completely healed and the athlete should be restricted from activity until the symptoms have resolved.[35]

■ STINGERS OR BURNERS

HISTORY FORM QUESTION

38. Have you ever had numbness, tingling, or weakness in your arms or legs after being hit or falling?

KEY POINTS

- Stingers or burners are always unilateral.
- Athletes may return to play when asymptomatic.

Stingers or burners are terms used to describe transient unilateral upper extremity pain and parasthesias following a blow to the neck or shoulders. This phenomenon is also sometimes referred to as *transient brachial plexopathy*. Stingers are most common in football, occurring in 50% to 65% of college football players and 30% of high school football athletes.[49,50] Stingers also occur in wrestling and other contact sports. Athletes will typically complain of burning dysethesias beginning in the shoulder region and radiating down the hand and arm.

The mechanism of injury in stingers is typically described as either tensile or compressive. In tensile injuries the neck is forcibly stretched away from the ipsilateral shoulder. These injuries are more common in high school or younger athletes. In college athletes, where degenerative disks and foraminal narrowing occur more frequently, a compressive mechanism is more often the cause. The neck is forcibly flexed in a posterolateral direction toward the symptomatic upper extremity in a pinching mechanism.[51]

The etiology of stingers is likely an injury to the proximal nerve root-spinal nerve complex. Anatomically, the cervical nerve roots do not have protective epineurium or perineurium to aid in absorbing either compressive or tensile forces. In addition, degenerative changes in the spine may place the nerve root at even more risk.[52] The brachial plexus itself can be injured; however, because of its plexiform nature it is more resistant to stretch.

HISTORY

At the time of the PPE, the examiner should clarify the frequency of previous episodes, the preventive strategies currently employed, and that symptoms are unilateral. The athlete may, at separate times, have stingers in different arms; however, concurrent bilateral symptoms suggest spinal cord pathology. Recurrent stingers are more common in the presence of degenerative disc disease.[51] Anyone with potential spinal cord pathology, such as recurrent or prolonged symptoms, should be fully evaluated before participation clearance is granted.

PHYSICAL EXAMINATION

Pertinent physical examination includes upper extremity assessment of muscle strength, sensation in all dermatomes, reflexes, and muscle mass symmetry (no atrophy); neck range of motion; and Spurling's test. Spurling's test, performed by extending the head in a lateral direction and then rotating it while applying axial pressure (Figure 6B-1), is positive when there is radicular or pain radiation down the arm with the maneuver. When the head is extended, the potential space in the posterior foramina is decreased by 30%, and narrowing or impingement of a cervical nerve root will be exacerbated, usually by a herniated cervical disc.

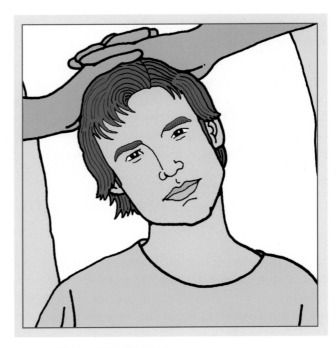

Figure 6B-1. Spurling's test

DIAGNOSTIC IMAGING

If an athlete has frequent stingers, x-rays should be considered to look for degenerative changes. An MRI will better define the anatomical changes contributing to the recurrent stingers and should also be considered. When numbness, weakness, or both persist for longer than 3 to 4 weeks an electromyography should be contemplated to help define the nature of injury. Electromyography done prior to this generally is not helpful and can be falsely negative.

CLEARANCE FOR PARTICIPATION

An athlete who has had only a few stingers that have cleared quickly should be cleared without restrictions. In athletes who have had several episodes, additional imaging for secondary causes should be completed. Those who have degenerative disc disease, osteophytes, or spinal stenosis will likely suffer repetitive stingers and should be counseled in the informed decision-making process. Long-term, significant nerve injury is a rare outcome, but does occur.

A neck strengthening program should be instituted in an athlete with a history of a stinger. In addition, protective equipment that limits lateral neck flexion and hyperextension may be helpful. Tackling technique should be reviewed by knowledgeable coaching staff to prevent dangerous practices, in particular, spearing or "leading with the head."

■ CERVICAL CORD NEURAPRAXIA

HISTORY FORM QUESTION

39. *Have you ever been unable to move your arms or legs after being hit or falling?*

KEY POINTS

- Cervical spinal cord neurapraxia (CCN) presents with motor and/or sensory changes in more than one extremity (bilateral arms or legs or one arm and one leg) and is a spinal cord injury.
- An athlete with CCN should be evaluated for cervical spinal stenosis.
- Return to play with cervical spinal stenosis is controversial.

Cervical spinal cord neurapraxia, also called *transient quadriplegia,* is characterized by an acute, transient impairment of sensory and/or motor function in more than one extremity. Symptoms include burning pain, numbness, tingling, or loss of sensation with or without motor weakness or paralysis. Symptoms usually resolve within 10 to 15 minutes but may last up to 48 hours.[53] The most common cause of CCN is cervical spinal stenosis due to narrowing of the spinal canal that can be congenital or developmental (degenerative changes, cervical instability, or intervertebral disc protrusion).

PHYSICAL EXAMINATION

Unless examined at the time of injury, the physical examination should be normal.

EVALUATION

An MRI of the cervical spine should be obtained to evaluate for an underlying spinal abnormality such as cervical spinal stenosis.[54] Cervical spinal stenosis can be defined by a cervical canal measurement of less than 14 mm at C4. However, the concept of functional spinal stenosis or a canal so small as to obliterate the protective cerebral spinal fluid cushion is more frequently used.[54,55]

CLEARANCE FOR PARTICIPATION

There is considerable controversy regarding return to play after CCN. Torg et al[56] reviewed MRI images of 110 athletes with CCN and followed them for 3 years, concluding that cervical spinal stenosis was a risk factor for CCN and the risk of a recurrent episode strongly correlated with the degree of stenosis. There was a 56% chance of a recurrent episode of CCN in this group, but a single, uncomplicated episode of CCN did not increase the risk of incurring permanent neurologic sequele.[56] Other experts strongly disagree and contend that functional spinal stenosis is an absolute contraindication to play after an episode of CCN[54,55] (Table 6B-1). Given the medicolegal risk and controversy, it would be well-advised to seek neurosurgical consultation prior to allowing return to play following an episode of CCN with documented cervical spinal stenosis.

TABLE 6B-1. GUIDELINES FOR RETURN TO PLAY AFTER TRANSIENT CERVICAL CORD NEURAPRAXIA

	Torg et al[53]	Cantu and Cantu[54]
No restriction	1. No history of CCN and spinal canal-vertebral body ratio ≤0.8	1. One episode of TQ with full recovery and normal workup without functional spinal stenosis
Relative restriction	1. One episode of CCN and spinal canal-vertebral body ratio ≤0.8 2. One episode of CCN with intervertebral disc disease or degenerative changes 3. One episode of CCN with MRI evidence of cord deformation	1. One episode of TQ as a result of minimal contact 2. One episode of TQ and evidence of disc bulging or herniation without functional spinal stenosis
Absolute contraindication	1. CCN with ligamentous instability, neurologic symptoms >36 hours, and/or more than one episode 2. CCN and MRI evidence of cord defect or edema	1. TQ with functional spinal stenosis documented by myelography, CT, or MRI 2. Any permanent neurologic injury, ligamentous instability, or spinal cord contusion following cervical spine trauma

Abbreviations: CCN, cervical cord neurapraxia; CT, computed tomography; MRI, magnetic resonance imaging; TQ, transient quadriplegia.

■ REFERENCES

1. Gessel LM, Fields SK, Collins CL, Dick RW, Comstock RD. Concussions among United States high school and collegiate athletes. *J Athl Train.* 2007;42(4):495–503

2. Reddy CC, Collins MW, Gioia GA. Adolescent sports concussion. *Phys Med Rehabil Clin N Am.* 2008;19(2):247–269

3. Lovell MR, Fazio V. Concussion management in the child and adolescent athlete. *Curr Sports Med Rep.* 2008;7(1):12–15

4. Powell JW, Barber-Foss KD. Traumatic brain injury in high school athletes. *JAMA.* 1999;282(10):958–963

5. Field M, Collins MW, Lovell MR, Maroon J. Does age play a role in recovery from sports-related concussion? A comparison of high school and collegiate athletes. *J Pediatr.* 2003;142(5):546–553

6. Practice parameter: the management of concussion in sports (summary statement). Report of the Quality Standards Subcommittee. *Neurology.* 1997;48(3):581–585

7. Bleiberg J, Cernich AN, Cameron K, et al. Duration of cognitive impairment after sports concussion. *Neurosurgery.* 2004;54(5):1073–1078; discussion 1078–1080

8. Cantu RC. Posttraumatic retrograde and anterograde amnesia: pathophysiology and implications in grading and safe return to play. *J Athl Train.* 2001;36(3):244–248

9. Collins MW, Iverson GL, Lovell MR, McKeag DB, Norwig J, Maroon J. On-field predictors of neuropsychological and symptom deficit following sports-related concussion. *Clin J Sport Med.* 2003;13(4):222–229

10. Delaney JS, Lacroix VJ, Leclerc S, Johnston KM. Concussions among university football and soccer players. *Clin J Sport Med.* 2002;12(6):331–338

11. McCrory P. Preparticipation assessment for head injury. *Clin J Sport Med.* 2004;14(3):139–144

12. Guskiewicz KM, McCrea M, Marshall SW, et al. Cumulative effects associated with recurrent concussion in collegiate football players: the NCAA Concussion Study. *JAMA.* 2003;290(19):2549–2555

13. Guskiewicz KM, Weaver NL, Padua DA, Garrett WE Jr. Epidemiology of concussion in collegiate and high school football players. *Am J Sports Med.* 2000;28(5):643–650

14. Collins MW, Lovell MR, Iverson GL, Cantu RC, Maroon JC, Field M. Cumulative effects of concussion in high school athletes. *Neurosurgery.* 2002;51(5):1175–1179; discussion 1180–1181

15. Iverson GL, Gaetz M, Lovell MR, Collins MW. Cumulative effects of concussion in amateur athletes. *Brain Inj.* 2004;18(5):433–443

16. Slobounov S, Slobounov E, Sebastianelli W, Cao C, Newell K. Differential rate of recovery in athletes after first and second concussion episodes. *Neurosurgery.* 2007;61(2):338–344; discussion 344

17. Giza CC, Hovda DA. The neurometabolic cascade of concussion. *J Athl Train.* 2001;36(3):228–235

18. Giza CC, Mink RB, Madikians A. Pediatric traumatic brain injury: not just little adults. *Curr Opin Crit Care.* 2007;13(2):143–152

19. McCrory P, Meeuwisse W, Johnston K, et al. Consensus statement on concussion in sport: 3rd International conference on concussion in sport held in Zurich, November 2008. *Clin J Sport Med.* 2008;19(3):185–200

20. McCrory P. Does second impact syndrome exist? *Clin J Sport Med.* 2001;11(3):144–149

21. Bruce DA, Alavi A, Bilaniuk L, Dolinskas C, Obrist W, Uzzell B. Diffuse cerebral swelling following head injuries in children: the syndrome of "malignant brain edema." *J Neurosurg.* 1981;54(2):170–178

22. Aldrich EF, Eisenberg HM, Saydjari C, et al. Diffuse brain swelling in severely head-injured children. A report from the NIH Traumatic Coma Data Bank. *J Neurosurg.* 1992;76(3):450–454

23. Mori T, Katayama Y, Kawamata T. Acute hemispheric swelling associated with thin subdural hematomas: pathophysiology of repetitive head injury in sports. *Acta Neurochir Suppl.* 2006;96:40–43

24. Hovda DA, Yoshino A, Kawamata T, Katayama Y, Becker DP. Diffuse prolonged depression of cerebral oxidative metabolism following concussive brain injury in the rat: a cytochrome oxidase histochemistry study. *Brain Res.* 1991;567(1):1–10

25. Vagnozzi R, Signoretti S, Tavazzi B, et al. Hypothesis of the postconcussive vulnerable brain: experimental evidence of its metabolic occurrence. *Neurosurgery.* 2005;57(1):164–171; discussion 164–171

26. Chen JK, Johnston KM, Collie A, McCrory P, Ptito A. A validation of the post concussion symptom scale in the assessment of complex concussion using cognitive testing and functional MRI. *J Neurol Neurosurg Psychiatry.* 2007;78(11):1231–1238

27. Ryan LM, Warden DL. Post concussion syndrome. *Int Rev Psychiatry.* 2003;15(4):310–316

28. Cantu RC. Athletic concussion: current understanding as of 2007. *Neurosurgery.* 2007;60(6):963–964

29. Guskiewicz KM, Marshall SW, Bailes J, et al. Association between recurrent concussion and late-life cognitive impairment in retired professional football players. *Neurosurgery.* 2005;57(4):719–726; discussion 719–726

30. Guskiewicz KM, Marshall SW, Bailes J, et al. Recurrent concussion and risk of depression in retired professional football players. *Med Sci Sports Exerc.* 2007;39(6):903–909

31. Omalu BI, DeKosky ST, Hamilton RL, et al. Chronic traumatic encephalopathy in a national football league player: part II. *Neurosurgery.* 2006;59(5):1086–1092; discussion 1092–1093

32. Omalu BI, DeKosky ST, Minster RL, Kamboh MI, Hamilton RL, Wecht CH. Chronic traumatic encephalopathy in a National Football League player. *Neurosurgery.* 2005;57(1):128–134; discussion 128–134

33. McCrea M, Kelly JP, Kluge J, Ackley B, Randolph C. Standardized assessment of concussion in football players. *Neurology.* 1997;48(3):586–588

34. McCrea M, Kelly JP, Randolph C, et al. Standardized assessment of concussion (SAC): on-site mental status evaluation of the athlete. *J Head Trauma Rehabil.* 1998;13(2):27–35

35. McCrory P, Johnston K, Meeuwisse W, et al. Summary and agreement statement of the 2nd International Conference on Concussion in Sport, Prague 2004. *Br J Sports Med.* 2005;39(4):196–204

36. Guidelines for assessment and management of sport-related concussion. Canadian Academy of Sport Medicine Concussion Committee. *Clin J Sport Med.* 2000;10(3):209–211

37. Concussion (mild traumatic brain injury) and the team physician: a consensus statement. *Med Sci Sports Exerc.* 2006;38(2):395–399

38. Aubry M, Cantu R, Dvorak J, et al. Summary and agreement statement of the First International Conference on Concussion in Sport, Vienna 2001. Recommendations for the improvement of safety and health of athletes who may suffer concussive injuries. *Br J Sports Med.* 2002;36(1):6–10

39. Cantu RC, Aubry M, Dvorak J, et al. Overview of concussion consensus statements since 2000. *Neurosurg Focus.* 2006;21(4):e3

40. Guskiewicz KM, Bruce SL, Cantu RC, et al. Research based recommendations on management of sport related concussion: summary of the National Athletic Trainers' Association position statement. *Br J Sports Med.* 2006;40(1):6–10

41. Dubow JS, Kelly JP. Epilepsy in sports and recreation. *Sports Med.* 2003;33(7):499–516

42. Howard GM, Radloff M, Sevier TL. Epilepsy and sports participation. *Curr Sports Med Rep.* 2004;3(1):15–19

43. Hirtz D, Berg A, Bettis D, et al. Practice parameter: treatment of the child with a first unprovoked seizure: report of the Quality Standards Subcommittee of the American Academy of Neurology and the Practice Committee of the Child Neurology Society. *Neurology.* 2003;60(2):166–175

44. Williams S, Nukada H. Sport and exercise headache. Part 2: diagnosis and classification. *Br J Sports Med.* 1994;28:96–100

45. Williams S, Nukada H. Sport and exercise headache. Part 1: prevalence amongst university students. *Br J Sports Med.* 1994;28:90–95

46. Lipton RB, Bigal ME, Steiner TJ, Silberstein SD, Olesen J. Classification of primary headaches. *Neurology.* 2004;63(3):427–435

47. Lewis DW. Headaches in children and adolescents. *Am Fam Physician.* 2002;65(4):625–632

48. McCrory P. Headaches and exercise. *Sports Med.* 2000;30(3):221–229

49. Clancy WG Jr, Brand RL, Bergfield JA. Upper trunk brachial plexus injuries in contact sports. *Am J Sports Med.* 1977;5(5):209–216

50. Sallis RE, Jones K, Knopp W. Burners: offensive strategy in an underreported injury. *Physician Sportsmed.* 1992;20(11):47–55

51. Levitz CL, Reilly PJ, Torg JS. The pathomechanics of chronic, recurrent cervical nerve root neurapraxia. The chronic burner syndrome. *Am J Sports Med.* 1997;25(1):73–76

52. Weinberg J, Rokito S, Silber JS. Etiology, treatment, and prevention of athletic "stingers." *Clin Sports Med.* 2003;22(3):493–500, viii

53. Torg JS, Pavlov H, Genuario SE, et al. Neurapraxia of the cervical spinal cord with transient quadriplegia. *J Bone Joint Surg Am.* 1986;68(9):1354–1370

54. Cantu RV, Cantu RC. Current thinking: return to play and transient quadriplegia. *Curr Sports Med Rep.* 2005;4(1):27–32

55. Cantu RC. The cervical spinal stenosis controversy. *Clin Sports Med.* 1998;17(1):121–126

56. Torg JS, Corcoran TA, Thibault LE, et al. Cervical cord neurapraxia: classification, pathomechanics, morbidity, and management guidelines. *J Neurosurg.* 1997;87(6):843–850

C: General Medical

■ MEDICAL HISTORY

HISTORY FORM QUESTIONS

1. *Has a doctor ever denied or restricted your participation in sports for any reason?*
2. *Do you have any ongoing medical conditions? If so, please identify (asthma, anemia, diabetes, infections, other)?*
3. *Have you ever spent the night in the hospital?*

SECONDARY QUESTIONS

- When and why were you disqualified from participation?
- Have you seen a doctor for this?
- What has changed since you were disqualified?
- Why were you in the hospital?
- Do you still have that problem?

KEY POINTS

- Only 1% to 2% of screened athletes are completely disqualified from sports participation.
- Chronic medical conditions represent a "big picture" of general health status.
- Obesity is an increasing problem among youth and young athletes.
- The risk of transmitting blood-borne pathogens in sports is not zero, but it has not been quantifiable.

Prior denial or restriction to participation is a significant finding and one that requires investigation. Only 1% to 2% of screened athletes are completely disqualified from sports participation,[1,2] so to have been denied clearance to participate in sports is significant. A history of hospitalization may also be a significant clearance decision if the problem is not fully resolved. In-depth assessment is warranted to determine if the disqualifying condition is still present or has been treated. If the condition is still present, the physician and athlete should discuss issues that will affect safe play, including risks of participation, the use of assistive devices, and alternative sports that may better fit the physical or mental challenges of the athlete.

This will require more in-depth investigation than time permits during a standard screening preparticipation physical evaluation (PPE). When the question of limiting participation arises, scheduling a follow-up appointment or a referral with an appropriate specialist is recommended. If the condition has been treated, determination should be made about the extent of recovery and clearance for participation. Often this clearance will be granted by the treating physician for a specific problem or injury.

Chronic medical conditions must be noted and offer an opportunity for the physician to get a "big picture" of the general health status of the athlete. Such questions can be a springboard for further inquiries and discussions. Chronic medical conditions may affect performance and clearance. Inadequate control of conditions such as asthma, seizures, or even skin disease may affect the ability to play. An athlete who requires frequent hospital admissions for diabetes, seizures, or acute asthma would likely need further medical evaluation before competing. Common medications used to treat many familiar conditions may affect performance or safety and may even be banned, depending on the sport. Some medications may affect judgment, reflexes, or stamina. Athletes should be counseled about the impact of their medical condition on performance even if they are fully cleared for participation.

■ OBESITY

Childhood obesity has reached epidemic proportions.[3] Physicians performing the PPE will undoubtedly encounter athletes who are obese (Table 6C-1), and concerns may arise as to whether to clear them. Although individuals with obesity may have associated conditions (eg, hypertension, exercise-induced asthma, susceptibility to heat injury, diabetes, slipped capital femoral epiphysis), there is no reason to exclude them from sports participation because of their weight alone.

Obesity is particularly dangerous for younger adults. Severely obese white men aged 20 to 30 years live approximately 13 fewer years than others in the general population.[4] Severely obese white women can expect to live 8 fewer years than their non-obese counterparts. Obesity also has a profound effect on the lifespan of younger blacks. Obese black men aged 20 to 30 years lose about 20 years and obese black women lose about 5 years of life, even after adjusting the data for smoking.[4]

Schwarz and Freemark[5] state, "Using BMI criteria, the most recent national surveys demonstrate that 21% to 24% of American children and adolescents are overweight and that 10% to 11% have obesity. These findings indicate that the prevalence of overweight (BMI ≥85th and ≤94th percentile) children and adolescents in the United States has increased by 50% to 60% in a single generation, while the prevalence of obesity (≥95th percentile) has doubled. The prevalence of obesity in American Indians, Hawaiians, Hispanics, and blacks is 10% to 40% higher than that in whites." Finally, preliminary research shows that children with a BMI 95th percentile or greater at 18 years of age will have a 66% to 78% greater risk of being overweight or obese at age 35.[5]

Once underlying causes of obesity have been ruled out (eg, hypothyroidism), every effort should be made to encourage some type of regular physical activity or sports participation. Such athletes, however, should receive counseling on specific strategies to modify their

WHAT IS THE BODY MASS INDEX?

Measuring body mass index (BMI) is an easy screening tool used to determine whether a person is obese. It is important to remember that an athlete with a high lean mass may have an elevated BMI. Thus every elevated BMI in an athletic population will not necessarily equate with overweight or obese status.[6] The BMI is a number representing the ratio of height and weight and is used to assess underweight, healthy weight, overweight, and obese (Table 6C-1). For children, body fat changes with age, growth, and physical maturation. Thus in children, BMI-for-age is both sex and age specific. The BMI-for-age is plotted on sex-specific growth charts for children and teens 2 to 20 years old provided by the Centers for Disease Control and Prevention.

TABLE 6C-1. TERMINOLOGY FOR BODY MASS INDEX (BMI) CATEGORIES[a]

BMI Category-for-Age	Former Terminology	Recommended Terminology
<5th percentile	Underweight	Underweight
5th–84th percentile	Healthy weight	Healthy weight
85th–94th percentile	At risk of overweight	Overweight
≥95th percentile	Overweight or obesity	Obesity

[a]From Barlow SE, Expert Committee. Expert Committee recommendations regarding the prevention, assessment, and treatment of child and adolescent overweight and obesity: summary report. *Pediatrics.* 2007;120(suppl 4):S164–S192.

diet, change their lifestyle, gradually increase their physical activity, prevent heat-related illnesses, and gradually reduce total body fat for future health. Any associated medical conditions must be appropriately treated and monitored.

■ DIABETES MELLITUS

It is important that those with a history of type 1 or type 2 diabetes mellitus be carefully screened for signs of complications that could affect participation status, including cardiovascular disease (hypertension and coronary artery disease), peripheral vascular disease, retinopathy, nephropathy, neuropathy (peripheral and autonomic), and gastrointestinal problems (gastroparesis).[7-9]

For patients with coronary artery disease or peripheral vascular disease, an appropriate level of activity should be determined by the treating primary physician or specialist. In patients with retinopathy, strenuous exercise can cause retinal detachment or vitreal hemorrhage. The American Diabetes Association recommends avoiding activities that significantly elevate blood pressure, such as weight lifting, in those with moderate or severe nonproliferative retinopathy.[9] Athletes with proliferative retinopathy should also avoid these activities, and in addition, high-impact activities (eg, jogging).

There are little data on how strenuous exercise affects diabetic nephropathy, though the presence of this complication may limit exercise capacity. Highly strenuous activities should most likely be restricted, though each case should be managed on an individual basis.[9]

Those with peripheral neuropathy can injure their feet during exercise. Because of this, it is recommended that their activities be limited to those that do not cause repetitive impact to the feet (eg, bicycling and swimming).[9]

Patients with autonomic neuropathy must be screened for coronary artery disease. They can have difficulty exercising in hot or cold environments due to thermoregulatory dysfunction. Postural hypotension may also occur. The activity level of these individuals may therefore be significantly limited. The examining physician may indicate which activities are acceptable on a case-by-case basis.

Diabetic gastroparesis can affect fluid and electrolyte absorption and thus may limit safe participation in strenuous activities, prolonged activities, or activities performed in warm environments.

Because of the risk of hypoglycemia during exercise, sports such as rock climbing, skydiving, and scuba diving are considered high risk for diabetic individuals.[10] Solo endurance activities (eg, ultramarathons, cycling, open water swimming) require proper support available for diabetic athletes to ensure safe participation. Motor sports present a potential risk to other competitors. Although the use of insulin pumps may reduce the frequency of hypoglycemia in type 1 diabetics and are now being used by athletes, such activities remain high risk.[11]

Those with diabetes who are free of complications and who are in good blood glucose control should not be restricted from participation in sports that do not present a high risk. Furthermore, the increasing use of intensive insulin therapy and insulin pumps has given diabetic athletes greater ability in adjusting insulin dosing to suit their activities. Although a complete discussion of the management of diabetes in athletes is beyond the scope of this monograph, the American Diabetes Association provides the following general guidelines for regulating blood glucose in athletes with type 1 diabetes[9]:

1. *Metabolic control before exercise*
   - Avoid exercise if fasting glucose levels are greater than 250 mg/dL and ketosis is present or if glucose levels are greater than 300 mg/dL, regardless of whether ketosis is present.
   - Ingest added carbohydrate if glucose levels are less than 100 mg/dL.

2. *Blood glucose monitoring before and after exercise*
   - Identify when changes in insulin or food intake are necessary.
   - Learn the glycemic response to different exercise conditions.
3. *Food intake*
   - Consume added carbohydrate as needed to avoid hypoglycemia.
   - Carbohydrate-based foods should be readily available during and after exercise.

In addition, the diabetic athlete should be well instructed on maintaining adequate hydration, using proper footwear, and monitoring the feet for skin trauma. All diabetic patients should wear a diabetes identification bracelet or shoe tag.

■ BLOOD-BORNE PATHOGENS: HIV AND HEPATITIS

The blood-borne pathogens of greatest concern in sports are human immunodeficiency virus (HIV) and the hepatitis B and C viruses (HBV and HCV). All can be transmitted through parenteral exposure to blood and blood products, contamination of open wounds or mucous membranes with infected blood, sexual contact, and perinatal spread from an infected mother to her baby. Body piercing and tattoos may also present some risk of contracting HIV and HBV. Further, the sharing of needles during the use of injectable anabolic steroids has been reported to result in HIV transmission and may increase the risk of acquiring HBV and HCV.[12,13]

While HIV is also present in tears, sweat, urine, sputum, vomitus, saliva, and respiratory droplets, only blood is recognized as a threat in the athletic setting. Human immunodeficiency virus transmission during sports has not been documented. One published report described a suspected case in an Italian soccer player.[14] However, this report was poorly documented and has not been accepted as a transmission related to sport. Transmission of HIV has never been shown to occur in the NFL. The *risk* of transmission has been estimated to be less than 1 occurrence per 85 million games.[15]

Although HBV is more concentrated in blood and more easily transmitted than HIV among health care workers, HBV transmission in sports is rare.[16] There have been 2 reports of HBV transmission during sports.[17,18] In the United States, the practice of routine HBV immunization further reduces the risk of transmission.

Hepatitis C virus was recognized as a cause of non-A, non-B hepatitis in 1988.[19] The risk of transmission of HCV to health care workers exposed to infected blood is intermediate to HIV and HBV.[16,19] Transmission of HCV via exposure during sports participation has not been documented.

Thus the risk of transmitting HIV, HBV, and HCV in sports is not zero but, because it is so uncommon, it has not been quantifiable.[20] Sports in which there is close body contact for sustained periods (such as wrestling) are considered to present a relatively higher risk of transmission. Nonetheless, the risk is considered minimal.[16,20,21]

Since HIV, HBV, and HCV seem to present minimal risk to others, the NCAA, American Academy of Pediatrics (AAP), American Medical Society for Sports Medicine, and others do not view the presence of such infections alone as a reason for exclusion from participation.[16,20,21] Asymptomatic individuals may participate in sports under the guidance and ongoing monitoring of a knowledgeable physician. Clinical signs and symptoms should be evaluated in relation to the demands of the sport. The type of athletic activity, health risks of participation, intensity of training, and risk of transmission to others all need to be considered. Changes in the affected athlete's health status mandate reevaluation of the participation level. Finally, confidentiality of the health status of the individual must be maintained.

■ MEDICATIONS AND SUPPLEMENTS

HISTORY FORM QUESTION

Please list all of the prescription and over-the-counter medicines and supplements (herbal and nutritional) that you are currently taking.

SECONDARY QUESTIONS

- Do you take herbs or minerals?
- Do you take any medications for your skin?
- Do you take birth control pills?

KEY POINTS

- Medications may reveal medical problems omitted in the medical history.
- Over-the-counter medications can affect performance.
- Medications may be banned by the sport's national governing body (NGB).

Medications, prescription or nonprescription, taken by athletes may reveal medical problems that the athlete may have omitted in the queries about medical history. Many over-the-counter medications and supplements, herbs, or minerals are not considered important or of consequence by athletes or their parents or guardians. The PPE can be used as an opportunity to discuss and counsel athletes and parents or guardians about the risks of medications, supplements, and ergogenic aids.

In every medical encounter, truthfulness is required for optimal care, and we acknowledge that some athletes may not be forthcoming with information about medications or supplements. However, it is important to inquire and to invite conversation and counseling about substances the athlete may be taking.

Some over-the-counter medications can affect performance and may even be banned by the sport's NGB. For example, antihistamines may cause fatigue and light-headedness. Arrhythmias have been linked to decongestants, methylxanthines, beta-agonists, tricyclic antidepressants, and macrolide antibiotics. Fluoroquinolone antibiotics have been shown to increase the risk of tendinopathy and tendon rupture.[22,23] Supplements are discussed in more detail later in the monograph.

■ ALLERGIES AND ANAPHYLAXIS

HISTORY FORM QUESTION

Do you have any allergies? If yes, please identify specific allergy (medicines, pollens, food, stinging insects)?

SECONDARY QUESTIONS

- Have you ever had a severe allergic reaction (anaphylaxis)?
- Were you hospitalized?
- Have you ever had a breathing tube passed into your lungs or been on a ventilator?
- Do you carry an EpiPen or epinephrine device?

KEY POINTS

- Allergic reactions range from minor rhinitis to anaphylaxis.
- Athletes with a history of anaphylaxis should have injectable epinephrine on-site for immediate use.

Allergic reactions range from minor rhinitis to anaphylaxis. Outdoor environments potentially expose the athlete to stinging insects and allergens. Allergy to hymenoptera (eg, bee, wasp, yellow jacket, or fire ant) envenomation and/or a history of exercise-induced anaphylaxis or exercise-induced urticaria should be noted and aggressive inquiry into details of past events documented so that severity of reaction can be determined and, in the case of anaphylactic reaction, appropriate treatments can be available for practice and competition.

Cholinergic urticaria is an exaggerated cholinergic response to body warming. Urticarial papules may first appear on the upper thorax and neck and then spread to the entire body after exposure to heat and humidity. Individual lesions usually persist for 15 to 20 minutes, but continued reaction and the development of new lesions may affect the athlete for several hours. This is a histamine-mediated reaction that rarely results in vascular collapse.

Anaphylaxis refers to symptoms involving more than one body system and can start as localized erythema and edema followed by generalized urticaria, pruritus, laryngeal edema, and spasm leading to airway obstruction and finally progress to hemodynamic instability and shock. The time course can be very rapid. Insect envenomation or food allergies, especially to shellfish or peanuts, can lead to anaphylaxis. Food sensitivities can also limit calorie sources and affect energy balance in athletes.

Exercise-induced anaphylaxis is a rare form of physical allergy that is induced by exercise and is characterized by a spectrum of symptoms, from a sensation of warmth, pruritus, cutaneous erythema, angioedema, and giant urticaria (>1 cm diameter), to hypotension, shock, and death. The role of exercise in eliciting symptoms remains obscure. Dependent factors include a variety of specific foods (eg, wheat, mushrooms, grapes, wine, onions, snails, corn, garlic, milk, or eggs). There are 2 types of exercise-induced anaphylaxis: classic and variant. Both are immunoglobulin E (IgE)-mediated responses that can result in bronchospasm, pulmonary distress, hemodynamic instability, shock, and even death.

Athletes who are most at risk for serious reaction should be required to have injectable epinephrine (eg, EpiPen) on-site for immediate use. Coaches and medical staff should be aware of the athlete's predisposition to anaphylaxis and be trained and prepared to intervene.

■ SURGICAL HISTORY

HISTORY FORM QUESTIONS

4. *Have you ever had surgery?*

SECONDARY QUESTIONS

- What surgery did you have?
- When did you have it?
- Where did you have it?
- Do you still have problems from your surgery that limit you from participating in certain activities?
- Did you complete a rehabilitation program or see a physical therapist or a certified athletic trainer?

KEY POINTS

- Surgical history may be significant with respect to sports clearance.
- Full recovery with no long-term impact on athletic participation or performance is required for full clearance.

Surgical history is significant and may potentially affect clearance determinations or guide conditioning or rehabilitation programs. The surgeon must clear an athlete who has had recent surgery. For surgeries, such as appendectomy or tonsillectomy, there would be reasonable expectation for full recovery with no long-term impact on athletic participation or performance. Other surgeries, such as colon resection with colostomy or those that remove one of a paired set of organs, such as eye enucleation, may affect clearance or performance and require counseling about risks of further injury and also about protective equipment.

Athletes with illnesses for which surgery and chronic use of medication are aspects of treatment should be advised about the potential impact of medications on athletic performance. For example, where there is no formal drug testing program, such as with most club sports and high schools, the use of narcotics, although not banned, may impair thought processes, reflexes, and stamina.

■ PAIRED ORGANS/ORGANS

HISTORY FORM QUESTION

29. *Were you born without or are you missing a kidney, an eye, a testicle (males), your spleen, or any other organ?*

KEY POINTS

- Absence of a paired organ does not limit the athlete from competing.
- Protective equipment may be advised for missing one of a pair of organs.

■ INFECTIOUS MONONUCLEOSIS

HISTORY FORM QUESTIONS

31. *Have you had infectious mononucleosis (mono) within the last month?*

KEY POINTS

- Fatigue associated with mono may prohibit full activity for several weeks or months.
- Splenomegaly is almost universally present.
- Splenic rupture very rarely occurs beyond 28 days.
- Most athletes are held out of competition for 1 month following onset to reduce risk of splenic rupture.

Mononucleosis is a very common illness among 15- to 35-year-olds and is caused by the Epstein-Barr virus (EBV).[24] It is transmitted through saliva and mucus. Symptoms generally appear 4 to 7 weeks after exposure. Symptoms may be mild or severe and can include severe fatigue, fever, posterior cervical lymphadenopathy, exudative pharyngitis, and left abdominal pain. Atypical activated T lymphocytes (mononuclear cells) appear in the blood. Diagnosis is confirmed with serology testing or an in-clinic Monospot test and an associated increase in atypical lymphocyte cells.[25] If the Monospot test is positive in the setting of atypical symptoms, consider obtaining IgG and IgM testing for EBV to determine the acuity of the illness. The fatigue associated with mononucleosis may prohibit the athlete from engaging fully in sports for several weeks or months after the onset of symptoms. There is no cure for mononucleosis. Care is supportive, with rest, antipyretics, and analgesics forming the basis of treatment.

Splenomegaly is almost universally present in patients who have a confirmed diagnosis of mononucleosis and may persist for several weeks after the onset of initial symptoms. The clinical examination is not sensitive when attempting to assess splenomegaly.[26-29] A recent history of mononucleosis should prompt the physician to advise the athlete, parents or guardians, and coaches about this risk of splenomegaly and adjust activity accordingly. Furthermore, because splenic rupture in infectious mononucleosis (IM) can occur in the absence of trauma, athletes should be restricted from all forms of sports-related activity when an enlarged spleen is suspected.[30,31] The American Medical Society for Sports Medicine Consensus Statement, along with the American Academy of Family Physicians and others, recommend that to minimize the risk of splenic rupture, sports and other physical activities should be avoided during the highest risk period 3 to 4 weeks after the infection starts.[32,33] Determining when it is safe to return the athlete recovering from IM to sports is based on the resolution of clinical symptoms and the risk for splenic rupture.

Once symptoms have resolved, the decision to resume activity is difficult, because there are no prospective studies available that have assessed the spleen. The greatest risk for splenic rupture in those with IM is within the first 21 days of illness in those with splenic enlargement.[30] Splenic rupture very rarely occurs beyond 28 days, but it has been reported.[24]

Complicating the return-to-play decision is that, although acute splenomegaly commonly develops in IM, the physical examination cannot be relied on to determine its presence.[25] Serial ultrasound examination of the spleen in IM patients, however, indicates that spleen size seems to normalize within 28 days.[25] Based on these data, athletes with IM should be restricted from all sports-related activities for the first 21 days of illness. (If the date of symptom onset is not known, the date of the diagnosis should be used as the starting point.) If the patient is asymptomatic by day 21, light activities can be undertaken for the fourth week, with full participation resumed at week 5. Some clinicians employ serial ultrasound measurements as an additional tool in determining return to play. However, it may be difficult to determine when the spleen size has normalized, because parameters for spleen size based on sex, height, weight, and ethnicity have not yet been established, and may vary considerably among individuals.[32]

For individuals with chronic hepatomegaly or splenomegaly, participation in sports should be assessed individually and decisions based on the degree of enlargement and the associated disease state.

■ HEAT ILLNESS

HISTORY FORM QUESTIONS

40. *Have you ever become ill while exercising in the heat?*

41. *Do you get frequent muscle cramps when exercising?*

SECONDARY QUESTIONS

- Did you vomit?
- Did you faint?
- Did you have cramping?
- Did you go to the emergency department?
- Did you have an IV?
- What medications or supplements do you take?
- What do you drink before, during, and after practices/games?

KEY POINTS

- Exertional heat stroke (EHS) can be fatal and is most often seen in preseason football.
- Major EHS risk factors include hot, humid conditions; poor aerobic fitness; football equipment; and inadequate heat acclimatization.
- Maintaining hydration may slow the onset of EHS.

Heat illness (Box 6C-1)[34] adversely affects athletic performance and can be associated with potentially severe morbidity and, occasionally, death from exertional heatstroke. Prior heat illness increases the risk for future heat intolerance or heat illness.[35,36] The PPE should include specific questions regarding possible risk factors including the associated environment, acclimatization status, equipment worn, fluid intake, weight changes during activity, medication and supplement use, and a history of cramping or heat illness.[37,38] The PPE is an opportunity for anticipatory guidance, other prevention measures, and treatment strategies.

Risk factors, including hot, humid conditions; poor aerobic fitness; and inadequate heat acclimatization may contribute to heat illness (Box 6C-2). Other common factors that increase the risk for heat illness include a history of heat illness, dehydration, equipment that inhibits heat loss, excess body fat and large body size, febrile condition, and overexertion.[39] High humidity, even when ambient air temperature is not excessive, may result in high heat stress.[39]

The use of diuretics, caffeine, antihistamines, or stimulants increases the risk of heat illness.[34,37,38] Banned supplements such as ephedra or methamphetamines can increase the risk of heat injury. Athletes should be informed of the increased risk with regard to their medications and supplements.[34]

Box 6C-1. Types of Heat-Related Illness

Heat edema
Heat cramps
Heat syncope/exercise-associated collapse
Heat exhaustion
Heatstroke

Box 6C-2. Possible Factors in Heat-Related Illness

Extrinsic
Environment
Clothing and equipment
Sport
Geography
Certain medications and supplements
Intrinsic
Inadequate acclimatization
Febrile condition or recent viral illness
History of heat illness
Overexertion
Dehydration
Poor aerobic fitness
Excess body fat
Large body size

Young age has been considered a risk factor, but recent studies show that children and adolescents are at similar, if not less, risk for heat stroke than adults. Children can adapt to extremes of temperature as effectively as adults when exposed to high climatic heat stress when hydration and other factors are similarly controlled.[39] Children produce less sweat, have fewer sweat glands, and have a greater body surface area-to-body mass ratio, causing greater heat gain from the environment on a hot day and greater heat loss to the environment on a cold day.[39] They also tend to underestimate body water loss and need encouragement to replace their sweat losses.

Exertional heatstroke and exercise-related collapse in the heat are best prevented by modifying activities in hot, humid conditions to reduce the disparity between body heat production and heat dissipation and allowing time for heat acclimatization, especially in sports with protective equipment. Normal regulatory mechanisms of heat dissipation can be compromised when vapor barrier uniforms and protective equipment such as shoulder pads and helmets are worn.[40] Educating athletes, parents or guardians, and coaches about risk factors and preventive strategies is key to decreasing the incidence of heat illness.

The athlete with a history of heat illness may be at risk for **recurrent heat illness**.[35,36] Because these athletes may have unique characteristics that affect their ability to acclimate to hot environments, they need further assessment to determine the presence of predisposing conditions and to arrange a prevention strategy. On-site monitoring of the practice environment by coaches and athletic trainers that triggers decreasing the intensity and duration of activity when deemed too hot combined with gradual acclimatization and introduction of vapor barrier equipment will decrease the risk. Tracking of fluid losses and monitoring diet and hydration strategies will reduce both acute and cumulative dehydration and the associated risk of hyperthermia. Recurrent heat illness may also be due to a medical condition, such as obesity, febrile illness, or medications, such as antihistamines, antidepressants, or psychomotor stimulants. Poor physical conditioning and wearing dark, heavy clothing or equipment that inhibits heat dissipation are also risk factors.[41] Although a history of heat illness should not disqualify an athlete from participation, a specific prevention strategy should be implemented.

■ SICKLE CELL TRAIT OR DISEASE

HISTORY FORM QUESTION

42. Do you or someone in your family have sickle cell trait or disease?

KEY POINTS
- Sickle cell trait has been associated with sudden deaths in athletes during strenuous activity in high environmental heat or at altitude.
- Universal screening has not been recommended.

Sickle cell disease involves 2 abnormal genes for hemoglobin, which cause a sickling of the red blood cells associated with rhabdomyolysis, splenic rupture, and stroke. Individual assessment must be made to determine clearance as some affected with sickle cell variants are not too anemic, but can have splenomegaly and require close monitoring. Overheating, dehydration, and chilling must be avoided.[42]

Sickle cell disease can become acute with catastrophic consequences if an athlete becomes dehydrated or sustains an internal injury. Such athletes should avoid highly strenuous activities and all contact and collision sports.[42]

Sickle cell trait occurs in approximately 8% of black Americans and 0.01% to 0.05% of caucasians.[43] In ordinary conditions, it is generally thought to be a non–life-threatening condition requiring no special preparticipation assessment.[44] However, recent case reports of sudden deaths in athletes with sickle cell trait during strenuous activity most often accompanied by environmental heat or altitude stress have increased.[42] The US Armed Forces reported more than a 20-fold increase in risk of death among recruits with sickle cell trait engaged in strenuous activity compared with controls without sickle cell trait.[45,46] The threat seems greatest when exercise occurs in high heat and humidity conditions for which the athlete is not acclimated, or altitude greater than 1,500 m, but can occur in less stressful environments also.[47] The risk of heat illness, including heatstroke, for athletes with sickle cell trait is similar to peer group athletes.[44,48,49] Death occurs as a consequence of the complications of sickling, including rhabdomyolysis, profound acidosis, acute renal failure, and multiple-organ system failure.[44]

Athletes of tropical and subtropical descent should be questioned about whether they have sickle cell trait and counseled on recommendations for sports participation. Athletes with sickle cell trait are advised to avoid strenuous activity that leads to muscle pain during early season conditioning sprints beyond 500 yards (cumulative sum).[42] Although there is no clear reason for the response to strenuous activity, one study[50] did observe changes in sickling and an increase in sickle forms after aerobic exercise. It is recommended that athletes with sickle cell trait acclimatize gradually and engage in year-round training to maintain physical conditioning. Athletes and coaches should be instructed regarding the importance of avoiding all-out sprints early in training and preventing dehydration by maintaining adequate fluid intake and not using diuretics.[48]

Athletes with sickle cell trait, even if they have no history of heat illness, should receive specific counseling regarding the prevention of sickling during exertional heat illness. Athletes with a documented history of heatstroke or heat-related rhabdomyolysis merit further investigation. Clearance for these athletes should be individualized.

At this time, there is no clear evidence that screening for sickle cell trait prevents death.[51] Notwithstanding, many collegiate athletic and professional athletic programs have chosen to screen athletes in order to confirm sickle cell trait status. In addition, recent publications from organizations including the NCAA recommend screening for sickle cell trait if sickle cell trait status is not already known.[51,52] The most important aspect of screening is for institutions to educate staff, coaches, and athletes concerning recognition of this condition and prevention of possible complications.[51] Institutions should carefully consider screening when sickle cell trait status is not known.[51,52]

■ EYE DISORDERS AND VISION

HISTORY FORM QUESTIONS

43. *Have you had any problems with your eyes or vision?*

44. *Have you had any eye injuries?*

45. *Do you wear glasses or contact lenses?*

46. *Do you wear protective eyewear, such as goggles or a face shield?*

SECONDARY QUESTIONS

- When was your last eye examination?
- Why don't you wear eye protection? (if applicable)
- Have you had eye surgery (eg, PRK, Lasik)?

KEY POINTS

- Eye injury and loss of vision are always a concern in sports.
- Eye protection should be used in moderate- to high-risk sports.
- Eye injuries increase risk of glaucoma later and need further monitoring.

The potential for loss of vision because of injury is always a concern in sports. Although it is difficult to quantify the relative risk of eye injury for a specific sport, some sports such as basketball, baseball, softball, ice hockey, field hockey, and lacrosse are classified as high risk because of the number of eye injuries reported and the potential for eye impact sufficient to cause injury.[53] The sports with the highest risk of eye injury are baseball and basketball. Risk for injury in a particular sport is categorized into high, moderate, low, and eye safe.[53] Sports with balls or likely risk of being hit are considered to be high risk (eg, softball, martial arts). Track and gymnastics are 2 sports considered "eye safe." Box 6C-3 provides the eye injury risk classification for a variety of sports.

Eye protection is key to preventing eye injuries. In 2000 there were 42,000 eye injuries related to sport and recreation, more than 50% in those younger than 15 years.[54] The AAP and the American Academy of Ophthalmology (AAO) strongly recommend protective eyewear for all participants in sports in which there is risk of eye injury.[55] Both the National Federation of State High School Associations (NFHS) and US Lacrosse mandate the use of protective eyewear for girls' lacrosse, and the full face shield is required in boys' lacrosse.[56] USA Hockey requires face shields for eye protection.[55] The AAO reports that significant eye injury can be reduced at least 90% when properly fitted, appropriate eye protectors are used.[57-59]

Lenses made of polycarbonate or CR-39 are recommended for protection. The AAP recommends that even in low eye–risk sports, athletes use at least approved street-wear frames that meet American National Standards Institute (ANSI) standard Z87.1 with polycarbonate or CR-39 lenses. A strap must secure the frame to the head and must be fitted by an experienced ophthalmologist, optometrist, or optician. For high eye–risk sports, the AAP recommends full sports goggles made of polycarbonate.[60] A list of specific sports and recommendations for eyewear has been developed by the AAP Council on Sports Medicine and Fitness (Table 6C-2). Athletes must be cautioned that contact lenses do not confer any protection from injury and must not be considered eye protectors.

Protective devices exist that can significantly reduce the risk of eye injury, so it is important that all athletes and their parents or guardians are made aware of the types of eye protection available and the risks of the sport. It is essential to consider eye protection for athletes whose vision is already impaired in one eye. A visual acuity of 20/40 or better in at least one eye is considered to provide good vision. An individual is deemed functionally one-eyed if the loss of the better eye would result in a significant change in lifestyle. Consequently, athletes with best corrected vision in one eye of less than 20/40 should be considered functionally one-eyed.[61] The AAO and the AAP recommend mandatory protective eyewear for all functionally one-eyed athletes regardless of sport. Athletes who have had an eye injury or surgery may have a globe that is weakened and therefore more susceptible to injury. Sports in which eye protection cannot be effectively worn are contraindicated for functionally one-eyed athletes. Athletes who are functionally one-eyed and who participate in sports that carry a high risk of eye injury may be individually evaluated and allowed to participate if they wear appropriate protective eyewear (Table 6C-2). The AAO states that such athletes and those who are functionally one-eyed must not participate in boxing, wrestling, or full-contact martial arts.

The athlete, his or her parent(s) or guardian(s), the coach, and school administrators, if necessary, must understand (1) the serious long-term consequences if injury to the better eye were to occur, (2) the level of protection available for the better eye, and (3) the degree of risk of injury—with and without protection—to the better eye. Treatments for injuries that can typically occur in the desired activity should also

Box 6C-3. Categories of Sports-Related Eye Injury Risk to the Unprotected Player[a]

High Risk	*Small, fast projectiles*
	Air rifle
	BB gun
	Paintball
	Hard projectiles, "sticks," close contact
	Baseball/softball
	Basketball
	Cricket
	Fencing
	Hockey (field and ice)
	Lacrosse (men's and women's)
	Racquetball
	Squash
	Intentional injury
	Boxing
	Full-contact martial arts
Moderate Risk	Badminton
	Fishing
	Football
	Golf
	Soccer
	Tennis
	Volleyball
	Water polo
Low Risk	Bicycling
	Diving
	Noncontact martial arts
	Skiing (snow and water)
	Swimming
	Wrestling
Eye Safe	Gymnastics
	Track and field[b]

[a]Adapted with permission from Vinger PF. A practical guide for sports eye protection. *Phys Sportsmed.* 2000;28(6):49–69.

[b]Javelin and discus have a small but definite potential for injury. However, good field supervision can reduce the extremely low risk of injury to nearly negligible.

be discussed. If, after this discussion, the functionally one-eyed athlete still wishes to participate in a given sport, he or she must wear appropriate protective eyewear during participation (see Table 6C-2).

Athletes with eye conditions, including a high degree of myopia; surgical aphakia; retinal detachment; and a history of eye surgery, injury, or infection may be at increased risk for eye injury.[62] Such individuals should be referred to an ophthalmologist for complete evaluation and clearance.

Finally, abnormal visual acuity is among the most frequently reported findings during the PPE.[15,63] Athletes who are identified with abnormal visual acuity at the time of the PPE should be evaluated and treated by an eye-care professional. Visual acuity must be assessed and documented at the time of the PPE. The AAP recommends vision screening at all well-child visits.[60] Vision can slowly deteriorate over time without the athlete being aware of the changes. Poor vision can lead to poor performance and injuries.

TABLE 6C-2. RECOMMENDED EYE PROTECTORS FOR SELECTED SPORTS[a]

Sport	Minimal Eye Protector	Comment
Baseball/softball (youth batter and base runner)	ASTM standard F910	Face guard attached to helmet
Baseball/softball (fielder)	ASTM standard F803 for baseball	ASTM specifies age ranges
Basketball	ASTM standard F803 for basketball	ASTM specifies age ranges
Bicycling	Helmet plus street-wear/fashion eyewear	
Boxing	None available; not permitted in the sport	Contraindicated for functionally one-eyed athletes
Fencing	Protector with neck bib	
Field hockey (men and women)	ASTM standard F803 for women's lacrosse (goalie: full face mask)	Protectors that pass for women's lacrosse also pass for field hockey
Football	Polycarbonate eye shield attached to helmet-mounted wire face mask	
Full-contact martial arts	None available; not permitted in the sport	Contraindicated for functionally one-eyed athletes
Ice hockey	ASTM standard F513 face mask on helmet (goaltenders: ASTM standard F1587)	HECC OR CSA certified full face shield
Lacrosse (men)	Face mask attached to lacrosse helmet	
Lacrosse (women)	ASTM standard F803 for women's lacrosse	Should have option to wear helmet
Paintball	ASTM standard F1776 for paintball	
Racquet sports (badminton, tennis, paddle tennis, handball, squash, and racquetball)	ASTM standard F803 for selected sport	
Soccer	ASTM standard F803 for selected sport	
Street hockey	ASTM standard 513 face mask on helmet	Must be HECC or CSA certified
Track and field	Street-wear with polycarbonate lenses/fashion eyewear[b]	
Water polo/swimming	Swim goggles with polycarbonate lenses	
Wrestling	No standard available	Custom protective eyewear can be made

Abbreviations: ASTM, American Society for Testing and Materials; CSA, Canadian Standards Association; HECC, Hockey Equipment Certification Council.

[a]Adapted with permission from Vinger PF. A practical guide for sports eye protection. *Phys Sportsmed.* 2000;28(6):49–69.

[b]Eyewear that passes ASTM standard F803 is safer than street-wear eyewear for all sports activities with impact potential.

■ IMMUNIZATIONS

Most school districts require standard immunizations for entrance that are independent of sports participation (eg, tetanus, measles, mumps, rubella, diphtheria, varicella, hepatitis B, and *Haemophilus influenzae* type B).[64] For a list of immunizations required for school entry by state, visit www.immunizationinfo.org/vaccineInfo/index.cfm#state.

Whether or not an athlete is up to date regarding immunizations does not affect athletic eligibility. However, the PPE is an opportunity to inquire about the status of elective, but recommended, immunizations such hepatitis A, human papillomavirus, meningococcal, and seasonal influenza (for a complete discussion of immunizations, go to www.cdc.gov/vaccines/recs/schedules/child-schedule.htm or www.cdc.gov/vaccines/recs/schedules).[64] Athletes should be informed of the risk of missed practices and games as a result of contracting influenza, especially for the winter sports where the close proximity of players, coaches, and other team personnel during flu season from November to March or April makes contracting influenza much easier, with potentially devastating effects for the team and on individual performance. Athletes with humoral immune deficiency, sickle cell disease, or functional asplenia may benefit from the 23-valent pneumococcus vaccine (PPSV23) in addition to the influenza immunization. Athletes traveling internationally may have specific vaccination needs and should refer to http://wwwn.cdc.gov/travel/default.aspx for the most current recommendations.

■ QUESTIONS THAT MAY BE PROMPTS DURING THE FOLLOW-UP INTERVIEW

PHYSICAL EXAMINATION FORM QUESTIONS

- *Do you feel stressed out or under a lot of pressure?*
- *Do you ever feel sad, hopeless, depressed, or anxious?*
- *Do you feel safe at your home or residence?*
- *Have you ever tried cigarettes, chewing tobacco, snuff, or dip?*
- *During the past 30 days, did you use chewing tobacco, snuff, or dip?*
- *Do you drink alcohol or use any other drugs?*
- *Have you ever taken anabolic steroids or used any other performance supplement?*
- *Have you ever taken any supplements to help you gain or lose weight or improve your performance?*
- *Do you wear a seat belt, use a helmet, and use condoms?*

These follow-up questions are based on those of the Youth Risk Behavior Surveillance System (www.cdc.gov/HealthyYouth/yrbs), which was developed by the Centers for Disease Control and Prevention (CDC) in 1990 to monitor priority health risk behaviors that contribute markedly to the leading causes of death, disability, and social problems among youth and adults in the United States. Data are compiled from surveys of representative samples of 9th- through 12th-grade students every 2 years.[65,66] They are also based on Healthy People 2010 findings and goals.[67] Athletes should be reassured that conversations are confidential and that the physician is their advocate.

Athletes may have medical or social concerns that they do not feel comfortable being documented on the official form, but about which they would like advice. The questions are designed to invite confidential, non-threatening conversation between the physician and athlete about social concerns that may affect the athlete's overall heath and well-being. They are not listed on the history form and may be best brought up during the physical examination, which is why they are listed on the Physical Examination Form (page 155).

Many schools require student-athletes to sign a contract or agreement attesting that they will not drink alcohol or use tobacco, illicit drugs, or other banned substances. "Zero tolerance" places the offending athlete at risk of immediate dismissal from the athletic team. This risk of dismissal can certainly have the effect of stifling athletes who have a problem or at-risk behavior from being truthful and seeking counseling.

Therefore, we have also included, as an appendix, a Teen Screen, which is designed as a tool to invite dialogue between the physician and the adolescent athlete (see sample in Appendix B). The Teen Screen is not intended to be included in the record of the PPE but rather serve as a template on which conversation can be based. The athlete should be assured that any conversation is entirely confidential and coaches will not have access to this information. Athletes should be assured that the physician is an advocate for them and only wishes to listen and provide information so they can make healthy choices.

STRESS, DEPRESSION, AND FEELING SAFE

Physical Examination Form Question
- *Do you feel stressed out or under a lot of pressure?*
- *Do you ever feel sad, hopeless, depressed, or anxious?*
- *Do you feel safe at your home or residence?*

Stress and school, social, and family pressures can indicate a life out of balance. Depression is common in adolescents, and suicide is a leading cause of death in this age group. Feeling safe is a requisite for mental and physical health. Concerning answers to these questions should trigger a more in-depth psychosocial investigation of the athletes well-being.

CIGARETTES

Physical Examination Form Question
- *Have you ever tried cigarettes, chewing tobacco, snuff, or dip?*

Tobacco use is considered the chief preventable cause of death in the United States, with approximately one-fifth of all death attributable to its use. Cigarette smoking is responsible for heart disease; cancers of the lung, larynx, mouth, esophagus, and bladder; stroke; and chronic obstructive pulmonary disease. In addition, cigarette smokers are more likely to drink alcohol and use marijuana and cocaine as compared with nonsmokers. In 2003 cigarette use among high school students was 21.9%.[68]

SMOKELESS TOBACCO

Physical Examination Form Question
- *During the past 30 days, did you use chewing tobacco, snuff, or dip?*

This question measures smokeless tobacco use. Smokeless tobacco use primarily begins in early adolescence. Approximately 75% of oral cavity and pharyngeal cancers are attributed to the use of smoked and smokeless tobacco. In 2001, 14.8% of male high school students were current smokeless tobacco users.[67]

Many athletes use smokeless tobacco under the mistaken belief that it will improve athletic performance. There is no evidence to support this. Smokeless tobacco does increase heart rate but does not affect reaction time, movement time, or total response time.[69] Tobacco use may be associated with a decrease in maximum voluntary force and maximum rate of force generation.[69] In fact, there is no evidence to support the claim by athletes that neuromuscular performance is enhanced by the use of smokeless tobacco.

The NCAA bans the use of tobacco products by student-athletes and game personnel during practice and competition because of their harmful health effects. The NFHS Coaches Code of Ethics states that coaches shall avoid the use of alcohol and tobacco products when in contact with players.[70]

ALCOHOL

Physical Examination Form Question

- *Do you drink alcohol or use any other drugs?*

The 2003 CDC report shows that 44.9% of 15- to 19-year-olds had one or more drinks of alcohol in the past 30 days, and 28.3% had 5 or more drinks of alcohol on one or more occasions during the past 30 days.[67] Alcohol affects coordination, impairs judgment, and usually does not enhance athletic performance. Motor vehicle crashes are the leading cause of death among youth 15 to 19 years old in the United States, and approximately 30% of all motor vehicle crashes that result in injury involve alcohol.[66] Athletes should be advised against driving while intoxicated or riding in a car with an intoxicated driver. In 2003, 12.1% of high school students nationwide reported having driven a vehicle one or more times after drinking alcohol in the past 30 days. In the same study, 30.2% of high school students reported being a passenger in a car on one or more occasions in the past 30 days with a driver who had been drinking alcohol.[67] Heavy drinking among youth also has been linked to more sexual partners, elevated marijuana use, and poorer academic performance.[67]

The NCAA guidelines stipulate that athletic departments conduct a drug and alcohol education program once a semester to inform athletes of NCAA and institutional drug and alcohol policies.[41] The World Anti-Doping Agency (WADA) and the United States Anti-Doping Agency (USADA) prohibit alcohol during competition in several sports, including archery, soccer, gymnastics, and wrestling. It is considered ergogenic in sports such as archery, where slowed responses may be beneficial.[71,72]

ANABOLIC STEROIDS

Physical Examination Form Question

- *Have you ever taken anabolic steroids or used any other performance supplement?*

Adolescents frequently receive mixed signals about the benefits and risks of using anabolic steroids. Physicians must be familiar with incentives and disincentives for use.

Anabolic steroids are banned by every major governing body, including the International Olympic Committee, United States Olympic Committee,[73] and NCAA.[74] USA Track and Field has issued a "death penalty," or lifelong ban, from the sport for first-time steroid offenses. The NFL has strict policies against anabolic steroid use and performs random year-round testing. Major League Baseball has recently toughened its testing and penalties for anabolic steroid use. These policies now apply worldwide to most major professional sports.

Manifestations of use. A sudden increase in weight or the development of hypertension may be signs of anabolic steroid use.[75] Physical characteristics of steroid use can include gynecomastia, testicular atrophy, hirsutism, alopecia, and excessive acne. Aggressive behavior, depression, anxiety, frequent mood swings, irritability, and libido changes may also be noted.[75] Anabolic steroids can cause hypercoagulability, leading to increased incidence of life-threatening complications from pulmonary embolus, cerebrovascular accidents, sudden cardiac death, coronary thrombus, myocardial infarction and, ultimately, congestive heart failure and/or cardiomyopathy.[75,76] Anabolic steroids have been associated with premature closure of the growth plates of long bones.

Targeted counseling. Although it is unlikely the athlete will admit to steroid use, the PPE is an opportunity to inquire and counsel the athlete about peer pressure, health risks, and threat to eligibility. It is impractical to take a history to cover every abused substance or latest performance-enhancing drug, but awareness of local trends will guide counseling.

SUPPLEMENTS

Physical Examination Form Question

- *Have you ever taken any supplements to help you gain or lose weight or improve your performance?*

Nutritional or dietary supplements are a concern for 2 primary reasons: safety and eligibility. The US Food and Drug Administration (FDA) does not strictly regulate the supplement industry; therefore, purity and safety of nutritional supplements cannot be guaranteed.[77] Athletes should be informed that anabolic steroids and other banned substances have been found to contaminate some over-the-counter supplements, especially in the muscle building and weight loss categories, and coaches and parents or guardians need to understand this as well. Recent studies show that supplements may contain substances that are banned by various sports organizations that are not listed on the label, and that the amount of the substances that are listed may vary considerably.[78] Use of such banned substances, either intentionally or unintentionally, may jeopardize the athlete's eligibility. Athletes who are subject to drug testing by a sport organization are responsible for the content of any substance they ingest. A positive test that results from using a product without knowing its contents, or a product whose contents are inaccurately labeled, may nonetheless result in sanctions. With respect to drug testing, athletes should therefore be advised that those who use such products do so at their own risk. Some previously commonly used substances such as ephedrine have been banned by the FDA, but only after many reports of adverse effects and some deaths.

Ergogenic aids are drugs, techniques, substances, or devices used to enhance performance. Ergogenic substances, used for centuries by athletes trying to gain an edge on competition, have become very sophisticated, and their use is not limited to elite athletes.

Physicians should inquire about the use of any medications or supplements and advise athletes to be aware of the drug-testing policies of their sport. Athletes must be aware of the names and dosages of drugs and supplements they are taking and the policies applicable to them from their NGB. The NCAA and other NGBs place the responsibility of knowing what they are taking entirely on the athlete; however, physicians should make every effort to inform athletes of supplements and other aids known to contain banned substances. The NCAA,[74] USADA,[72] and WADA[71] all have documents listing banned substances to assist athletes and physicians.

During the PPE, physicians may often be asked questions regarding the use of medications and supplements, or they may identify athletes who have been using substances for performance enhancement. Such individuals should be counseled regarding the safety and effectiveness of such agents, as well as issues related to drug testing.

Competitors need to be aware of the names and dosages of any drugs and supplements they are taking, as well as the policies that affect them. Sports medicine physicians should be familiar with the drug testing guidelines relevant to their institution. In addition, athletes may be competing for multiple organizations with varying drug-testing regulations. Physicians should therefore be cognizant of this when counseling athletes and when prescribing medications. *Any physician prescribing medication to an athlete subject to drug testing should ensure that the medication is not a banned substance.* If a medication needed to treat a condition is on the banned list and no alternative is available, the sport organization should be contacted to determine if approval for use of the medication (therapeutic use exemption) can be obtained. Up-to-date information regarding drug testing and banned substances may be obtained from the following sources:

- NCAA Sports Medicine Handbook and Drug Testing Program Book: Can be ordered via the Web (www.ncaa.org) or by phone (888/388-9748); the Web site provides printable files of these publications, including the banned drug list.
- US Anti-Doping Agency and WADA provide prohibited drug reference lists and reference material online at www.wada-ama.org and www.usantidoping.org. US Anti-Doping Agency also has a hotline (800/233-0393) that is available if needed.

ACUTE ILLNESS

On occasion, the physician performing the PPE may encounter an athlete experiencing an acute illness. Because the PPE is performed in advance of the sports season, denial of participation because of an acute illness does not generally occur. However, the ability of the athlete to safely participate in training and conditioning may be affected until the illness has resolved.

When such a situation occurs, clearance should be based on individual assessment. Factors to consider include the risk of the illness worsening as a result of participation and the potential for spreading the disease to others. The author societies recommend restriction of participation for athletes with a febrile illness and those with ongoing fluid losses due to a gastrointestinal illnesses. Limiting activity in such patients is important in preventing complications secondary to dehydration, thermoregulatory problems, and viral infection (especially myocarditis, although this is rare).

PHYSICAL EXAMINATION

Height and Weight

Height and weight are measured and recorded. Extremely thin individuals may warrant questioning about recent weight loss, eating habits, or body image. Additional evaluation away from the PPE screening examination is indicated if an eating disorder (eg, anorexia or bulimia) or growth disturbance is suspected. Obese and overweight athletes can be referred for counseling on diet, exercise, and behavior modification for weight control.

Determination of body composition with skinfold calipers or other devices is an optional component of the PPE. It may allow estimation of an ideal weight range in sports requiring weight control, such as wrestling. Additionally, calipers may more accurately measure body composition of the thin athletes and more accurately represent muscular athletes, who frequently have a falsely high BMI and may be considered falsely obese. It is difficult, however, to predict the exact ideal percentage of body fat for a participant in a given sport. Those with abnormal BMI (verified by body composition assessment) should be counseled regarding weight loss or referred for follow-up.

Head, Eyes, Ears, Nose, and Throat (HEENT)

Visual acuity, measured with a standard Snellen eye chart, should be 20/40 or better in each eye, with or without corrective lenses. Any athlete with a difference between eyes of 2 lines or greater on the visual acuity examination chart (ie, 20/20 in one eye and 20/30 in the other) should be referred for further examination as this can indicate an undetected amblyopia. Athletes who have one eye missing or best corrected vision poorer than 20/40 in either eye will need appropriate eye protection if they wish to participate in sports that have a high risk of eye injury (see Eye Disorders and Vision on page 80).

The pupils should be examined for anisocoria (unequal size). Although many people have a slight difference in pupil size (physiologic anisocoria), a marked difference in pupil size occasionally may be noted in otherwise normal eyes. It is imperative to be aware of baseline anisocoria when evaluating a head injury. Communicating this information to the athlete's trainer and/or coach is important if the examination record is not present at all practices and games.

The remainder of the HEENT examination assesses general well-being of these areas. The clinician should be alert to

- Oral ulcers, gingival atrophy, and decreased enamel seen with disordered eating behaviors, especially bulimia
- Herpes simplex cold sores, especially in wrestlers and rugby players
- Leukoplakia seen with smokeless tobacco use
- A high-arched palate (minor diagnostic criteria)[79] in athletes with other characteristics of Marfan syndrome (see Chapter 6G: Musculoskeletal Concerns and Chapter 6A: Cardiovascular Problems for other diagnostic criteria)
- Corrective braces on the teeth that may require use of a mouth guard to prevent laceration in the event of oral trauma
- Scarring of the tympanic membrane or auditory canals related to prior tympanostomy tube or prior infection (if indicated, a hearing screen should be performed)
- Perforated tympanic membranes in athletes competing in water sports who would need protective earplugs
- Adenopathy that may suggest malignancy or infection

Nasal polyps or a deviated septum do not affect clearance but can be identified, and the patient referred for further evaluation and possible treatment.

Physical Maturity Status

Concerns may arise regarding clearance of an adolescent who is relatively delayed in physical maturation or underweight and who seeks to participate in competitive sports. There is no medical reason to exclude such an individual from sports participation unless there is a coexisting condition that warrants exclusion.

■ REFERENCES

1. Kurowski K, Chandran S. The preparticipation athletic evaluation. *Am Fam Physician.* 2000;61(9):2683–2690, 2696–2698
2. Metzl JD. Preparticipation examination of the adolescent athlete: part 1. *Pediatr Rev.* 2001;22(6):199–204
3. Ogden CL, Flegal KM, Carroll MD, Johnson CL. Prevalence and trends in overweight among US children and adolescents. *JAMA.* 2002;288(14):1728–1732
4. Fontaine KR, Redden DT, Wang C, Westfall AO, Allison DB. Years of life lost due to obesity. *JAMA.* 2003;289(2):187–193
5. Schwarz SM, Freemark M. Obesity. http://www.emedicine.com/ped/topic1699.htm#section~bibliography. Accessed January 27, 2009
6. National Institutes of Health, National Heart, Lung, and Blood Institute, NHLBI Obesity Education Initiative, North American Association for the Study of Obesity. *The Practical Guide Identification, Evaluation, and Treatment of Overweight and Obesity in Adults.* Washington, DC: National Institutes of Health; 2000. NIH Publication No. 00-4084
7. Birrer RB, Sedaghat V-D. Exercise and diabetes: optimizing performance in patients who have type 1 diabetes. *Phys Sportsmed.* 2003;31(5):29–41
8. Bhaskarabhatla KV, Birrer R. Physical activity and type 2 diabetes. Tailoring exercise to optimize fitness and glycemic control. *Phys Sportsmed.* 2009;32(1):13–17
9. American Diabetes Association. Diabetes mellitus and exercise. *Diabetes Care.* 2002;25(suppl 1):S64–S68
10. Drazin MB. Type 1 diabetes and sports participation: strategies for training and competing safely. *Phys Sportsmed.* 2000;28(12):49–56

11. Tsui EY, Chiasson JL, Tildesley H, et al. Counterregulatory hormone responses after long-term continuous subcutaneous insulin infusion with lispro insulin. *Diabetes Care*. 1998;21(1):93–96

12. Scott MJ, Scott MJ Jr. HIV infection associated with injections of anabolic steroids. *JAMA*. 1989;262(2):207–208

13. Aitken C, Delande C, Stanton K. Pumping iron, risking infection? Exposure to hepatitis C, hepatitis B and HIV among anabolic-androgenic steroid injectors in Victoria, Australia. *Drug Alcohol Depend*. 2002;65(3):303–308

14. Torre D, Sampietro C, Ferraro G, Zeroli C, Speranza F. Transmission of HIV-1 infection via sports injury. *Lancet*. 1990;335(8697):1105

15. Brown LS Jr, Drotman DP, Chu A, Brown CL Jr, Knowlan D. Bleeding injuries in professional football: estimating the risk for HIV transmission. *Ann Intern Med*. 199515;122(4):273–274

16. American Academy of Pediatrics Committee on Sports Medicine and Fitness. Human immunodeficiency virus and other blood-borne pathogens in the athletic setting. *Pediatrics*. 1999;104(6):1400–1403

17. Kashiwagi S, Hayashi J, Ikematsu H, Nishigori S, Ishiharaa K, Kaji M. An outbreak of hepatitis B in members of a high school sumo wrestling club. *JAMA*. 1982;248(2):213–214

18. Ringertz O, Zetterberg B. Serum hepatitis among Swedish track finders. An epidemiologic study. *N Engl J Med*. 1967;276(10):540–546

19. Moyer LA, Mast EE, Alter MJ. Hepatitis C: part I. Routine serologic testing and diagnosis. *Am Fam Physician*. 1999;59(1):79–88, 91–92

20. Human immundeficiency virus and other blood-borne pathogens in sports. *Clin J Sport Med*. 1995;5(3):199–204

21. Blood-borne pathogens and intercollegiate athletics. In: *2009–2010 NCAA Sports Medicine Handbook*. 20th ed. Indianapolis, IN: National Collegiate Athletic Association; 2009:66–72

22. van der Linden PD, Sturkenboom MC, Herings RM, Leufkens HM, Rowlands S, Stricker BH. Increased risk of achilles tendon rupture with quinolone antibacterial use, especially in elderly patients taking oral corticosteroids. *Arch Intern Med*. 2003;163(15):1801–1807

23. Kowatari K, Nakashima K, Ono A, Yoshihara M, Amano M, Toh S. Levofloxacin-induced bilateral achilles tendon rupture: a case report and review of the literature. *J Ortho Sci*. 2004;9(2):186–190

24. Johnson MA, Cooperburg PL, Boisvert J, Stoller JL, Winrob H. Spontaneous splenic rupture in infectious mononucleosis accessed by ultrasonic scanning. *AJR Am J Roentgenol*. 1981;136(1):111–114

25. Dommerby H, Stangerup SE, Stangerup M, Hancke S. Hepatosplenomegaly in infectious mononucleosis, assessed by ultrasonic scanning. *J Laryngol Otol*. 1986;100(5):573–579

26. Hosey RG, Kriss V, Uhl TL, et al. Ultrasonographic evaluation of splenic enlargement in athletes with acute infectious mononucleosis. *Br J Sports Med*. 2008;42:974–977

27. Barkun AN, Camus M, Green L, et al. The bedside assessment of splenic enlargement. *Am J Med*. 1991;91:512–518

28. Grover SA, Barkun AN, Sackett DL. The rational clinical examination. Does this patient have splenomegaly? *JAMA*. 1993;270:2218–2221

29. Halpern S, Coel M, Ashburn W, et al. Correlation of liver and spleen size. Determinations by nuclear medicine studies and physical examination. *Arch Intern Med*. 1974;134:123–124

30. Maki DG, Reich RM. Infectious mononucleosis in the athlete. Diagnosis, complications, and management. *Am J Sports Med*. 1982;10(3):162–173

31. Farley DR, Zuetlow SP, Bannon MP, Farnell MB. Spontaneous rupture of the spleen due to infectious mononucleosis. *Mayo Clin Proc*. 1992;67(9):846–853

32. Putukian M, O'Connor FG, Stricker P. Mononucleosis and athletic participation: an evidence-based subject review. *Clin J Sport Med*. 2008;18(4):309–315

33. Sharp DS, Ross JH, Kay R. Attitudes of pediatric urologists regarding sports participation by children with a solitary kidney. *J Urol*. 2002;168(4 Pt 2):1811–1814; discussion 1815

34. Barrow MW, Clark KA. Heat-related illnesses. *Am Fam Physician*. 1998;58(3):749–756, 759

35. Armstrong LE, De Luca JP, Hubbard RW. Time course of recovery and heat acclimation ability of prior exertional heatstroke patients. *Med Sci Sports Exerc*. 1990;22(1):36–48

36. Epstein Y. Heat intolerance: predisposing factor or residual injury? *Med Sci Sports Exerc*. 1990;22(1):29–35

37. National Athletic Trainers Association. Inter-Association Task Force on Exertional Heat Illness Consensus Statement. June 2003. http://www.nata.org/consumer/heatillness/index.htm. Accessed January 29, 2009

38. Prevention of heat illness. In: *2008–2009 NCAA Sports Medicine Handbook*. 19th ed. Indianapolis, IN: National Collegiate Athletic Association; 2008:30–32

39. American Academy of Pediatrics Committee on Sports Medicine and Fitness. Climatic heat stress and the exercising child and adolescent. *Pediatrics*. 2000;106(1 Pt 1):158–159

40. Kulka TJ, Kenney WL. Heat balance limits in football uniforms. *Phys Sportsmed*. 2002;30(7):29–39

41. Institutional alcohol, tobacco and other drug education programs. In: *2008–2009 NCAA Sports Medicine Handbook*. 19th ed. Indianapolis, IN: National Collegiate Athletic Association; 2008:22–23

42. Rice SG, American Academy of Pediatrics Council on Sports Medicine and Fitness. Medical conditions affecting sports participation. *Pediatrics*. 2008;121(4):841–848

43. Eichner ER. Sports medicine pearls and pitfalls—sickle cell trait and athletes: three clinical concerns. *Curr Sports Med Rep*. 2007;6(3):134–135

44. Pretzlaff RK. Death of an adolescent athlete with sickle cell trait caused by exertional heat stroke. *Pediatr Crit Care Med*. 2002;3(3):308–310

45. Kark JA, Poser DM, Schumacher HR, Ruehle CJ. Sickle-cell trait as a risk factor for sudden death in physical training . *N Engl J Med*. 1987;317(130):781–787

46. Drehner D, Neuhauser KM, Neuhauser TS, Blackwood GV. Death among US Air Force basic trainees, 1956 to 1996. *Mil Med*. 1999;164:841–847

47. Kerle KK, Runkle GP. Sickle cell trait and sudden death in athletes. *JAMA*. 1996;276(18):1472

48. Kerle KK, Nishimura KD. Exertional collapse and sudden death associated with sickle cell trait. *Am Fam Physician*. 1996;54(1):237–240

49. Kark JA, Ward FT. Exercise and hemoglobin S. *Semin Hematol*. 1994;31(3):181–225

50. Ramirez A, Hartley LH, Rhodes D, Abelmann WH. Morphological features of red blood cells in subjects with sickle cell trait: changes during exercise. *Ann Intern Med*. 1976;136(9):1064–1066

51. National Athletic Trainers Association. Consensus statement: sickle cell trait and the athlete. http://www.nata.org/statements/consensus/sicklecell.pdf. Accessed February 2, 2009.

52. The student-athlete with sickle cell trait. In: *2009–2010 NCAA Sports Medicine Handbook*. 20th ed. Indianapolis, IN: National Collegiate Athletic Association; 2009:86–88

53. American Academy of Pediatrics Committee on Sports Medicine and Fitness. Protective eyewear for young athletes. *Pediatrics*. 2004;113(3 Pt 1):619–622

54. US Consumer Product Safety Commission. *Sports and Recreational Eye Injuries*. Washington, DC: US Consumer Product Safety Commission; 2000

55. National Federation of State High School Associations. Protective eyewear required for girls lacrosse. July 10, 2003. www.nfhs.org/web/2003/11/protective_eyewear_required_for_girls_lacrosse.aspx. Accessed January 27, 2009

56. USA Hockey. *Rulebook and Casebook* http://www.usahockey.com//Template_Usahockey.aspx?NAV=OF_02&ID=20072

57. Jeffers JB. An on-going tragedy: pediatric sports-related eye injuries. *Semin Ophthalmol*. 1990;5:216–223

58. Larrison WI, Hersh PS, Kunzweiler T, Shingleton BJ. Sport-related ocular trauma. *Ophthalmology*. 1990;97(10):1265–1269

59. Strahlman E, Sommer A. The epidemiology of sports-related ocular trauma. *Int Ophthalmol Clin*. 1988;28(3):199–202

60. American Academy of Pediatrics Committee on Practice and Ambulatory Medicine and Section on Ophthalmology, American Association of Certified Orthoptists, American Association for Pediatric Ophthalmology and Strabismus, American Academy of Ophthalmology. Eye examination in infants, children, and young adults by pediatricians. *Pediatrics*. 2003;111(4):902–907

61. Napier SM, Baker RS, Sanford DG, Easterbrook M. Eye injuries in athletics and recreation. *Surv Ophthalmol*. 1996;41(3):229–244

62. Rodriguez JO, Lavina AM, Agarwal A. Prevention and treatment of common eye injuries in sports. *Am Fam Physician*. 2003;67(7):1481–1488

63. Smith J, Laskowski ER. The preparticipation physical examination: Mayo Clinic experience with 2,739 examinations. *Mayo Clin Proc*. 1998;73(5):419–429

64. Beck CK. Infectious diseases in sports. *Med Sci Sports Exerc*. 2000;32(7 suppl):S431–S438

65. US Department of Health and Human Services, Centers for Disease Control and Prevention. *Assessing Health Risk Behaviors Among Young People: Youth Risk Behavior Surveillance System, 2004*. http://www.cdc.gov/nccdphp/publications/aag/pdf/2006/aag_yrbss2004.pdf . Accessed October 21, 2009

66. Grunbaum JA, Kann L, Kinchen SA, et al. Youth risk behavior surveillance—United States, 2001. *MMWR Surveill Summ*. 2002;51(4):1–62

67. US Department of Health and Human Services. *Healthy People 2010: Understanding and Improving Health*. 2nd ed. Washington, DC: US Government Printing Office; 2000

68. US Department of Health and Human Services, Centers for Disease Control and Prevention. *YRBSS. National Youth Risk Behavior Survey 1991–2003. Trends in the Prevalence of Selected Risk Behaviors.* http://www.cdc.gov/yrbss. Accessed October 21, 2009

69. Escher SA, Tucker AM, Lundin TM, Grabiner MD. Smokeless tobacco, reaction time, and strength in athletes. *Med Sci Sports Exerc.* 1998;30(10):1548–1551

70. National Federation of State High School Associations Coaches Code of Ethics. http://www.wcpss.net/athletics/coaching/code-of-ethics.doc. Accessed April 1, 2009

71. World Anti-Doping Agency. http://www.wada-ama.org/en/. Accessed April 1, 2009

72. United States Anti-Doping Agency. http://www.usada.org. Accessed January 27, 2009

73. 2008 United States Olympic Committee. http://www.olympic-usa.org. Accessed January 27, 2009

74. National Collegiate Athletic Association. http://www.ncaa.org/wps/ncaa?ContentID=11

75. American Academy of Pediatrics Committee on Sports Medicine and Fitness. Adolescents and anabolic steroids: a subject review. *Pediatrics.* 1997;99(6):904–908

76. American College of Sports Medicine position stand on the use of anabolic-androgenic steroids in sports. *Med Sci Sports Exerc.* 1987;19(5):534–539

77. US Food and Drug Administration Center for Food Safety and Applied Nutrition. Dietary Supplement Health and Education Act of 1994. Dec 1,1995

78. Green GA, Catlin DH, Starcevic B. Analysis of over-the-counter dietary supplements. *Clin J Sport Med.* 2001;11(4):254–259

79. DePaepe A, Devereux RB, Dietz HC, Hennkam RC, Pyeritz RE. Revised diagnostic criteria for the Marfan syndrome. *Am J Med Genet.* 1996;62(4):417–426

D: Pulmonary System

The most common pulmonary conditions affecting athletic performance are exercise-induced asthma (EIA) and exercise-induced bronchospasm (EIB). The term *EIA* has been used to identify patients with an underlying diagnosis of asthma for whom exercise is a trigger.[1] Exercise-induced bronchospasm has been defined as airway obstruction associated with exercise, regardless of the presence of chronic asthma.[1] In athletes with EIB who have not been diagnosed with asthma, it must be considered that undiagnosed, underlying chronic asthma may be present. Respiratory infections and vocal cord dysfunction are other common diagnoses that may affect athletic participation.

■ ASTHMA AND EXERCISE ASTHMA

HISTORY FORM QUESTIONS

2. *Do you have any ongoing medical conditions? Asthma*

26. *Do you cough, wheeze, or have difficulty breathing during or after exercise?*

27. *Have you ever used an inhaler or taken asthma medicine?*

28. *Is there anyone in your family who has asthma?*

SECONDARY QUESTIONS

- Where do you keep your inhaler/puffer?
- Have you ever missed practice or games because of your asthma?
- Have you gone to the hospital because of asthma during the past year?
- Have you ever had a breathing tube passed into your lungs or been on a ventilator?
- Who is the doctor for your asthma?
- Do you smoke or have exposure to secondhand smoke?

KEY POINTS

- Most people with asthma will develop symptoms with an appropriate exercise challenge.
- Many athletes with EIB may have undiagnosed, underlying chronic asthma.
- Athletes with environmental allergies (atopy) are at increased risk for EIB.
- Vocal cord dysfunction must be considered when suspected EIB does not respond to therapy or EIB testing is negative.

BACKGROUND INFORMATION

In athletes with underlying asthma, the prevalence of EIB ranges from 50% to 90%.[1] In all athletes the prevalence ranges from 11% to 50% depending on the sport type evaluated and testing method used for diagnosis.[2-5]

Asthma is a disease of chronic airway inflammation, bronchial hyperreactivity, and reversible airflow obstruction. Exercise in combination with other possible triggers, such as environmental allergens, air pollution (smog, chlorine vapors, or nitrogen dioxide [from propane fueled Zamboni fumes][6]), or cold air, may trigger an inflammatory process in patients with EIB. In theory, exercise may trigger EIB due to an increased ventilatory rate, which overloads the ability of the airways to heat and moisturize the inhaled air before it reaches the alveoli. Relatively cold, dry air can cause dehydration of the airway, leading to increased osmolarity of the airway surface and the release of inflammatory mediators by mast and epithelial cells.[1,7,8] These inflammatory mediators cause bronchoconstriction and bronchial edema.

Athletes with environmental allergies are more likely to have EIB and may have exacerbations of their EIB symptoms during their allergic season.[4,9] Symptoms can also be triggered by airway irritants such as chlorine vapors and molds in swimming pools or pollutants from ice resurfacing machines at skating rinks.[6,10,11] Because of the role of airway cooling, winter sport athletes, especially those in endurance events, may also have increased risk for EIB symptoms.[5,7]

Other diagnoses must be considered in the athlete with respiratory complaints during exertion, especially when they do not respond as expected to treatment or provocative testing is not consistent with asthma, as there may be other or concomitant diagnoses. Vocal cord dysfunction (VCD) is a diagnosis that can cause breathing difficulties in athletes and can be mistaken for asthma.[12] Also, VCD may coexist with asthma in athletes.[12] Vocal cord dysfunction is usually associated with more acute onset, inspiratory stridor, and dyspnea. Other diagnoses to consider in the athlete with difficulty breathing during exercise include laryngeal prolapse, laryngomalacia, hyperventilation, and gastroesophageal reflux.

Athletes with rare symptoms may be treated with bronchodilators alone. Typically, the use of a bronchodilator 20 to 30 minutes prior to exercise will control symptoms well. However, athletes with EIB or chronic asthma who need to use bronchodilators more than 2 times per week independent of exercise should be placed on controller medication such as inhaled corticosteroids or leukotriene antagonists.

HISTORY

Typically, athletes with EIB will complain of coughing, wheezing, chest tightness, or shortness of breath with exercise. In athletes with EIB, cough is a more common complaint than wheezing.[13,14] Occasionally, however, more nonspecific complaints may be noted, such as feeling out of shape, excess fatigue, chest or abdominal pain, or headaches.[14] Symptoms are usually most severe 5 to 30 minutes after exercise.[12]

In athletes with a known history of asthma it is important to determine the severity of asthma and a history of current symptoms to determine current level of control. It is important to know if the athlete has ever been intubated or has been hospitalized within the last year. It is also important to know how many times in the last year the athlete has gone to their doctor, urgent care, or the emergency department for asthma symptoms and how often practices or games are missed due to asthma symptoms. The frequency of beta-agonist use and the presence of nighttime symptoms are other indicators of asthma control. Use of beta-agonist medication more than twice a week and nighttime cough with difficulty sleeping more than one time per month are indicators of suboptimal asthma control.[15] In addition, well-controlled asthma should not interfere with normal activity. The athlete with a history of asthma should have an asthma treatment action plan defining measures to take if symptoms worsen.[15] It is also important to know if the athlete has a history of atopy, as EIB is more common in athletes with environmental allergies. The list of medications currently used by the athlete should be obtained. Finally, it is useful to obtain the name and phone number of the physician who has been managing the athlete's asthma.

In athletes with no prior history of asthma who report respiratory symptoms with exercise, it is helpful to determine at what point during exercise the symptoms occur, whether they are more common during one season or sport, and if the athlete can distinguish whether symptoms occur during inspiration or expiration. The feeling of "trouble getting air in" or inspiratory stridor may be more indicative of laryngeal disorders, such as VCD, rather than EIB. Triggers for VCD may include allergic rhinitis, gastroesophageal reflux, and poorly controlled asthma, making this a challenging diagnosis in some cases.[16–18] Vocal cord dysfunction can be confirmed with inspiratory-expiratory flow loop testing or direct visualization of the vocal cords during an attack, which may be stimulated with exercise bronchoprovocation testing. Many athletes with VCD only have symptoms during the stress of competition, and the diagnosis sometimes is made clinically. A speech pathologist trained in the area of VCD can often "cure" the problem with several sessions of therapy.

PHYSICAL EXAMINATION

The pulmonary examination should reveal clear, equal breath sounds over all lung fields. Wheezing, rubs, prolonged expiratory phase, and cough with forced expiration require further evaluation. If the smell of tobacco is noted at the time of examination, smoking cessation should be discussed. A normal examination does not exclude the diagnosis of asthma or EIB, and provocative testing should be performed in athletes with a history suggestive of EIB.

TESTING

In well-trained athletes, the use of questionnaires or interviews assessing self-reported symptoms by athletes is not a good tool for diagnosing EIB,[19,20] so further testing to support the diagnosis is necessary. Because many highly trained athletes have better pulmonary function than nonathletes, baseline pulmonary function testing (PFT) is also not a reliable means for detecting EIB, particularly in athletes without underlying chronic asthma.[1,12,13,19] Some feel that an improvement in symptoms in response to beta-agonist use prior to exercise is adequate for diagnosis, especially in recreational athletes.[1] Alternatively, pre- and post-exercise spirometry performed at the physician's office after running outside or performed at the competitive site is another low-cost method of EIB screening. However, in high-level athletes, beta-agonist use may be restricted by sports governing committees, and more extensive testing is required to document EIB in order to obtain a therapeutic exemption to use beta-agonist medications.

The International Olympic Committee has identified the eucapnic voluntary hyperventilation (EVH) test as its preferred method of testing for the diagnosis of EIB; however, other provocative tests, including field and laboratory exercise challenge tests, hyperosmolar aerosols, and methacholine challenge, are also acceptable.[21] One must consider the specialized equipment needed to perform EVH testing and the difficulty some patients, especially children, may have performing the test does not necessarily make EVH the test of choice for all athletes. Laboratory treadmill challenge testing has been used extensively for the diagnosis of EIB; however, some athletes are unable to reproduce symptoms during laboratory testing and field testing during the activity that typically causes symptoms is required to document the condition.[12,22] Fortunately, PFT equipment has become quite portable, making field testing more available.[1] A drop in FEV1 (forced expiratory volume in 1 second) of 10% during free running, EVH, treadmill, or field testing is generally considered to be diagnostic for EIB.

CLEARANCE FOR PARTICIPATION

Athletes with asthma and EIB can usually be cleared to play excluding severe, acute exacerbations of asthma. Proper management of asthma and EIB symptoms will allow for safe participation. The athlete should be advised to have a rescue inhaler present at all times.

Athletes with VCD can also be cleared to play. Proper management should result in full symptom control and affected athletes being able to compete in all sports.

Athletes with current respiratory illnesses with fever should be excluded from participation until well.

■ REFERENCES

1. Weiler JM, Bonini S, Coifman R, et al. American Academy of Allergy, Asthma & Immunology Work Group Report: exercise-induced asthma. *J Allergy Clin Immunol*. 2007;119(6):1349–1358

2. Wilber RL, Rundell KW, Szmedra L, Jenkinson DM, Im J, Drake SD. Incidence of exercise-induced bronchospasm in Olympic winter sport athletes. *Med Sci Sports Exerc*. 2000; 32(4):732–737

3. Voy RO. The US Olympic Committee experience with exercise-induced bronchospasm, 1984. *Med Sci Sports Exerc*. 1984;18(3):328–330

4. Helenius IJ, Tikkanen HO, Sarna S, Haahtela T. Asthma and increased bronchial responsiveness in elite athletes: atopy and sport event as risk factors. *J Allergy Clin Immunol*. 1998;101(5):646–652

5. Pohjantähti H, Laitinen J, Parkkari J. Exercise-induced bronchospasm among healthy elite cross country skiers and non-athletic students. *Scand J Med Sci Sports*. 2005;15(5):324–328

6. Hedberg K, Hedberg CW, Iber C, et al. An outbreak of nitrogen dioxide-induced respiratory illness among ice hockey players. *JAMA*. 1989;262(21):3014–3017

7. Karjalainen EM, Laitinen A, Sue-Chu M, Altraja A, Bjermer L, Laitinen LA. Evidence of airway inflammation and remodeling in ski athletes with and without bronchial hyperresponsiveness to methacholine. *Am J Respir Crit Care Med*. 2000;161(6):2086–2091

8. Helenius I, Lumme A, Haahtela T. Asthma, airway inflammation and treatment in elite athletes. *Sports Med*. 2005;35(7):565–574

9. Helenius IJ, Tikkanen HO, Haahtela T. Occurrence of exercise induced bronchospasm in elite runners: dependence on atopy and exposure to cold air and pollen. *Br J Sports Med*. 1998;32(3):125–129

10. Helenius IJ, Haahel T. Allergy and asthma in elite summer sport athletes. *J Allergy Clin Immunol*. 2000;106(3):444–452

11. Mannix ET, Farber MO, Palange P, Galassetti P, Manfredi F. Exercise-induced asthma in figure skaters. *Chest*. 1996;109(2):312–315

12. Rundell KW, Jenkinson DM. Exercise-induced bronchospasm in the elite athlete. *Sports Med*. 2002;32(9):583–600

13. Rundell KW, Spiering BA, Evans TM, Baumann JM. Baseline lung function, exercise-induced bronchoconstriction, and asthma-like symptoms in elite women ice hockey players. *Med Sci Sports Exerc*. 2004;36(3):405–410

14. Storms WW. Review of exercise-induced asthma. *Med Sci Sports Exerc*. 2003;35(9):1464–1470

15. National Asthma Education and Prevention Program. Expert panel report 3 (EPR-3): guidelines for the diagnosis and management of asthma—summary report 2007. *J Allergy Clin Immunol*. 2007;120(5 suppl):S94–S138

16. Hicks M, Brugman SM, Katial R. Vocal cord dysfunction/paradoxical vocal fold motion. *Prim Care*. 2008;35(1):81–103, vii. Review

17. Newman KB, Mason UG III, Schmaling KB. Clinical features of vocal cord dysfunction. *Am J Respir Crit Care Med*. 1995;152(4 Pt 1):1382–1386

18. Morris MJ, Deal LE, Bean DR Grbach VX, Morgan JA. Vocal cord dysfunction in patients with exertional dyspnea. *Chest*. 1999;116(6):1676–1682

19. Rupp NT, Brudno S, Guill MF. The value of screening for risk of exercise-induced asthma in high school athletes. *Ann Allergy*. 1993;70(4):339–342

20. Rundell KW, Im J, Mayers LB, Wilber RL, Szmedra L, Schmitz HR. Self-reported symptoms and exercise-induced asthma in the elite athlete. *Med Sci Sports Exerc*. 2001;33(2):208–213

21. Ljungqvist A, Fitch KD, Sue-Chu M, et al. IOC Consensus Statement on Asthma in Elite Athletes. January 2008 http.multimedia.olympic.org/pdf/en_report_1301.pdf. Accessed September 28, 2009

22. Rundell KW, Anderson SD, Spiering BA, Judelson DA. Field exercise vs laboratory eucapnic voluntary hyperventilation to identify airway hyperresponsiveness in elite cold weather athletes. *Chest*. 2004;125(3):909–915

E: Gastrointestinal/Genitourinary

The gastrointestinal and genitourinary system screening in the preparticipation physical evaluation (PPE) does not typically address issues of a critical or life-threatening nature. However, many of the findings in the history or physical examination are important from a health maintenance or return-to-play perspective (see Table 6E-1 on page 99).

■ HISTORY FORM QUESTIONS

30. Do you have groin pain or a painful bulge or hernia in the groin area?

■ SECONDARY QUESTIONS

- Does it limit your activity?
- Does it become red, swollen, or tender to touch?

■ KEY POINTS

- Palpate the abdomen for masses (enlarged spleen or liver, enlarged kidney, gravid uterus).
- Testicular and scrotal examinations should be considered in male athletes if the practice setting allows for privacy.
- A solitary kidney may not limit participation in contact/collision sports, and each athlete should be counseled on an individual basis.[1,2]
- A solitary testicle does not limit participation in contact/collision sports, but a protective cup should be worn for high-risk sports.[1]
- The PPE is a good opportunity to teach testicular self-examination and allow the male athlete a chance to ask questions regarding his genitourinary system.

The presence of a hernia in the abdomen or groin is not a reason to limit participation. Hernias should be repaired if painful or otherwise symptomatic.

■ PHYSICAL EXAMINATION

ABDOMEN

The abdominal examination should be performed with the athlete supine. The anterior superior iliac spines should be exposed to ensure adequate inspection and palpation of all 4 quadrants. Abdominal masses, tenderness, rigidity, or enlargement of the liver or spleen requires further evaluation prior to clearance. Occasionally, an abnormal kidney may be identified by abdominal examination, again requiring further evaluation. The lower abdominal examination in the female athlete should be prefaced by a brief explanation of the reason for additional regional evaluation. This brief introduction will help establish rapport for an examination that is sensitive by nature. If necessary, a chaperone can be obtained at the athlete's discretion. The focus of the examination is to determine the presence of a palpable (gravid) uterus. If necessary, a more detailed pelvic examination should be performed by the athlete's primary care physician or a designated specialist.

GENITALIA

The male genitourinary examination should begin with a brief description and reason for the examination to establish rapport. Athletes should be asked if they would prefer to have a chaperone present. The examination should always be performed in a private setting without the possibility of interruptions (as described in Chapter 3). The focus of the examination is to determine the presence, size, and shape of both testicles. The testicular examination is commonly done with the patient standing. Testicular irregularities or masses suspicious for cancer, testicular size abnormalities (sign of steroid use if smaller), and inguinal canal hernias or pain (possible "sports hernia") may be detected. The inguinal canal should be digitally palpated if the athlete is symptomatic and need not be if asymptomatic. If the examination reveals an enlarged inguinal ring, the athlete (and parents/guardians if minor) should be educated regarding the implications of the changes in the inguinal canal.

During the examination the athlete should be taught how to do a testicular self-examination. Testicular cancer is the leading cause of cancer deaths in men 15 to 35 years of age. A family history of testicular cancer and a personal history of a previous undescended testicle increase the risk of developing testicular cancer. The PPE provides an opportunity to teach and recommend monthly testicular self-examination. The examining physician can let the athlete know that his testicles feel normal, encourage self-examination, and advise the athlete to see his physician if there are abnormal findings on the current examination or with future examinations. The PPE also affords the athlete the chance to ask questions about his genitourinary system that they may have been concerned about or afraid to ask in a non-private setting.

The genitourinary examination in female athletes is not part of the PPE. If a pelvic examination is warranted on the basis of the athlete's medical history or physical examination, it may need to be scheduled for a separate time depending on the exam setting.

Assessing physical maturity with **Tanner staging** has not been useful in determining participation except in an athlete with a history of growth or menstrual abnormalities suggestive of endocrine disease. Therefore, *the author societies continue to recommend against Tanner staging as a routine part of the PPE.*[3] However, Tanner staging should be performed at every health maintenance visit and may be useful in boys and girls 11 to 17 years old as a guide to counseling on topics of growth and development, sport safety, and steroid use. It is easy to do as part of the physical examination, and a sharp discrepancy between the athlete's age and Tanner staging should lead to a more detailed investigation. Tanner staging may also remind the physician to think about the physically immature athlete playing against more physically mature counterparts in contact/collision sports.

■ CLEARANCE FOR PARTICIPATION

ORGANOMEGALY

An enlarged liver or spleen is a cause for concern if there is increased risk of damage to the organ or malfunction of a vital organ. The underlying cause must also be determined. The spleen is discussed in detail in the general medical section in relation to the most common cause of splenomegaly in athletes: infectious mononucleosis.

Acute hepatomegaly may signal the presence of infection (eg, hepatitis, infectious mononucleosis) or malignant disease (eg, hepatocellular carcinoma, lymphoma). A liver that is enlarged beyond the bony protection of the rib cage is at risk of injury. Even though the incidence of hepatic rupture among patients with acute hepatomegaly is low, participation in all sports should be avoided. Full activity may be resumed after resolution of hepatomegaly.

TABLE 6E-1. GASTROINTESTINAL/GENITOURINARY MEDICAL CONDITIONS AND SPORTS PARTICIPATION

Condition	May Participate
Diarrhea, infectious *Explanation:* Unless symptoms are mild and athlete is fully hydrated, no participation is permitted, because diarrhea may increase risk of dehydration and heat illness (see fever in Table 5-1).	Qualified no
Gastrointestinal Malabsorption syndromes (celiac disease, cystic fibrosis) *Explanation:* Athlete needs individual assessment for general malnutrition or specific deficits resulting in coagulation or other defects; with appropriate treatment, these deficits can be adequately treated to permit normal activities. Short bowel syndrome or other disorders requiring specialized nutritional support including parenteral or enteral nutrition *Explanation:* Athlete needs individual assessment for collision, contact, or limited-contact sports. Presence of a central or peripheral indwelling venous catheter may require special considerations for activities and emergency preparedness for unexpected trauma to the device(s).	Qualified yes
Kidney, absence of one *Explanation:* Athlete needs individual assessment for contact, collision, and limited-contact sports. Protective equipment may reduce risk of injury to the remaining kidney sufficiently to allow participation in most sports, providing such equipment remains in place during activity.	Qualified yes
Liver and/or spleen, enlarged *Explanation:* If the liver or spleen is acutely enlarged, participation should be avoided because of risk or rupture. If the liver or spleen is chronically enlarged, individual assessment is needed before collision, contact, or limited-contact sports are played. Patients with chronic liver disease may have changes in liver function that may affect stamina, mental status, coagulation, or nutritional status.	Qualified yes
Ovary, absence of one *Explanation:* Risk of severe injury to the remaining ovary is minimal.	Yes
Testicle, undescended or absence of one *Explanation:* Certain sports may require a protective cup.	Yes

Adapted from Rice SG, American Academy of Pediatrics Council on Sports Medicine and Fitness. Medical conditions affecting sports participation. *Pediatrics.* 2008;121(4):841–848.

For individuals with chronic hepatomegaly, participation in sports should be assessed individually and decisions based on the degree of enlargement and the associated disease state.

INGUINAL HERNIA

An athlete with an asymptomatic inguinal hernia may participate in all sports. The athlete should be counseled regarding red flags for strangulated hernia—sudden pain, nausea, and vomiting—or change in symptoms like heaviness, swelling, and tugging or burning sensation in the area of the hernia. Males may have a swollen scrotum, and females may have a bulge in the large fold of skin (labia) surrounding the vagina. Symptomatic inguinal hernias may limit an athlete's ability to participate and may be affected by activity. Such symptomatic cases invariably require treatment at some time and should be evaluated individually.

KIDNEY ABNORMALITIES

Because of the potential for kidney injuries ranging from contusion to complete rupture, special consideration should be given when determining clearance for an athlete who has a single functioning kidney. Some, but not all, experts believe that if the kidney is pelvic, iliac, or multicystic, or shows evidence of hydronephrosis or ureteropelvic junction abnormalities, an athlete should not participate in contact/collision sports.[3–6] The consequences of the loss of a single functioning kidney (eg, transplantation or dialysis) may be severe enough to warrant disqualification from these sports, even though the risk is small.[2,4–6] The determination to restrict activities with a solitary kidney is not agreed on by all experts.[2,4–6] Evaluation by a urologist or nephrologist is recommended and the decision to play a sport made on an individualized basis.

If the athlete chooses to play in a sport that may place a solitary kidney at increased risk for damage, a full explanation should be given to the athlete, his or her parent(s) or guardian(s), and the coaches. The explanation should include the controversial use of available protection (eg, flak or shock-absorbing jacket), which has not been proven to reduce the risk of injury, potential serious long-term consequences, and treatment of injuries if they occur.[7]

TESTICULAR DISORDERS

The incidence of testicular injury in sports is extremely low.[8,9] Counseling concerning participation in contact/collision sports is required with athletes for unpaired or undescended testicles. An individual with a single testicle may be cleared for participation, with the use of a protective cup for higher-risk sports.[1] However, the athlete with a solitary testicle who wishes to participate in contact/collision sports must be informed that there is a risk of injury and loss of the remaining testicle. Although wearing a protective cup may reduce the incidence of injury, it does not guarantee complete protection. Protective cups can be cumbersome and uncomfortable, and some athletes prefer not to wear them. However, with a thorough explanation of the potential benefits and availability of more comfortable cups, many athletes will choose to wear protection to decrease their risk of injury.

If an athlete has an undescended testicle that has not been thoroughly evaluated, the examining physician should refer him for evaluation and inform him of the increased risk of testicular cancer associated with this condition. Clearance determination for an athlete who has an undescended testicle is similar to that for an athlete with a single testicle.

■ REFERENCES

1. Rice SG, American Academy of Pediatrics Council on Sports Medicine and Fitness. Medical conditions affecting sports participation. *Pediatrics.* 2008;121(4):841–848

2. Grinsell MM, Showalter S, Gordon KA, Norwood VF. Single kidney and sports participation: perception versus reality. *Pediatrics.* 2006;118(3):1019–1027

3. Carek PJ, Mainous A III. The preparticipation physical examination in athletics: a systematic review of current recommendations. *BMJ.* 2003;1327:E170–E173

4. Sharp DS, Ross JH, Kay R. Attitudes of pediatric urologists regarding sports participation by children with a solitary kidney. *J Urol.* 2002;168(4 Pt 2):1811–1814

5. Johnson B, Christensen C, Dirusso S, Choudhury M, Franco I. A need for reevaluation of sports participation recommendations for children with a solitary kidney. *J Urol.* 2005;174(2):686–689

6. Gerstenbluth RE, Spirnak JP, Elder JS. Sports participation and high grade renal injuries in children. *J Urol.* 2002;168(6):2575–2578

7. Psooy K. Sports and the solitary kidney: how to counsel parents. *Can J Urol.* 2006;13(3):3120–3126

8. McAleer IM, Kaplan GW, LoSasso BE. Renal and testis injuries in team sports. *J Urol.* 2002;168(4 Pt 2):1805–1807

9. Wan J, Corvino TF, Greenfield SP, DiScala C. Kidney and testicle injuries in team and individual sports: data from the national pediatric trauma registry. *J Urol.* 2003;170(4 Pt 2):1528–1530

F: Dermatologic Conditions

■ HISTORY FORM QUESTIONS

32. Do you have any rashes, pressure sores, or other skin problems?

33. Have you had a herpes or MRSA skin infection?

■ SECONDARY QUESTIONS

- Do you take medication for your skin problem?
- Have you ever missed practices or games because of a skin problem?

■ KEY POINTS

- Skin infections are common reasons to temporarily restrict participation in athletics.
- Herpes simplex, staphylococcal (including community-acquired methicillin-resistant *Staphylococcus aureus* [CA-MRSA]), molluscum, and tinea are common infections seen.
- Contact, collision, and shared equipment sports are of most concern.
- Proper diagnosis, documentation, and treatment are critical in determining return to play.
- A standard approach used by the NCAA for wrestling can be found in the *NCAA Sports Medicine Handbook* (accessed at www.ncaa.org/wps/ncaa?ContentID=1446).

The ability to safely compete can be compromised by various skin conditions that are common, important to correctly identify, and easily treated. Participation by athletes with active infections may lead to outbreaks among teammates and competitors. Participation must be restricted if the infections are communicable (to reduce risk to other competitors) or if the conditions increase the risk of becoming infected by blood-borne pathogens. The NCAA Injury Surveillance System indicates that skin infections are associated with at least 15% of wrestling injuries that result in lost practice time.[1] Skin infections are most easily transmitted in sports by skin-to-skin contact, but can also be spread by using shared equipment, towels, and razors and are particularly common in wrestling, martial arts, and rugby. Yard et al[2] found the incidence of skin infections to be 8% and 20% in high school and collegiate athletes respectively, with more than half of the infections involving the head, face, and neck. One study reported the likelihood of contracting herpes simplex virus (HSV) when wrestling with an infected opponent at 1 in 3.[3] These conditions and the timing of their treatment can affect whether athletes will be declared eligible by the rules of their sport at the time of practice or competition.[4] Restriction from participation due to dermatologic conditions ranges from 6% to 8%, making this one of the more common reasons to restrict participation.[5]

The examining physician needs to be alert for the signs and symptoms of skin conditions that might limit participation, whether traumatic, bacterial, parasitic, viral, or fungal. Common infectious conditions include fungal rashes such as tinea, herpes simplex, scabies and other infestations, molluscum contagiosum, warts, carbuncles, furuncles, folliculitis, and impetigo.

■ PHYSICAL EXAMINATION

A thorough skin survey should be performed with particular attention to exposed areas and those areas that might potentially come in contact with another competitor and/or equipment (wrestling mats, batting helmets). The principle objective in the dermatologic examination is to identify skin infections: bacterial, viral, fungal, and infestations. The examiner should also look for signs of trauma, acne, sun damage, rashes (contact, eczema, psoriasis, urticarial), and marks of illicit drug use.[6–8]

While a thorough search for abnormal nevi is not possible within the limits of the preparticipation physical evaluation (PPE), suspicious nevi noted during the examination should be referred for further evaluation and/or treatment. These lesions should not preclude clearance for participation.

Specific, common infections bear mention.

Herpes gladiatorum is epidemic in wrestlers. The problem can threaten individual wrestlers and even entire teams. Lesions are vesicular, generally clustered, and can progress to shallow ulcers with surrounding erythema. They are most commonly seen about the face, neck, and arms, usually on the right side because most wrestlers "lock up" on the right. During the initial outbreak, systemic symptoms may be present, including fever and adenopathy, sore throat, general malaise, and headache.

Tinea gladiatorum, fungal infection of the skin (tinea corporis) and scalp (tinea capitis), has been reported to occur in up to 42% of wrestlers.[9] Typically, these lesions will be erythematous plaques with flaking, a raised border, and central clearing. Scalp lesions may be accompanied by hair loss. Diagnosis can be confirmed with a potassium hydroxide (KOH) microscopy and/or culture.

Impetigo is a bacterial infection caused by either *Staphylococcus* or *Streptococcus* species that is highly contagious. It can appear as classic "honey"-crusted vesicles and pustules or as bullous rash that may be accompanied by adenopathy. Systemic symptoms are unusual.[10]

Molluscum contagiosum presents as flesh–colored, small (3–5 mm) papules with a central core giving the classic "umbilicated" appearance. Reportedly more common in swimmers, gymnasts, and wrestlers, these lesions are usually asymptomatic, though may develop erythema and pruritus.[11]

Warts appear as firm, skin-colored, hyperkeratotic papules and are not typically painful. They may be present anywhere on the body but typically affect the fingers and hands. Plantar warts may have a flat, skin-colored, hyperkeratotic appearance, and they may be painful. Diagnosis is typically made by simple visual inspection.[12]

Community-acquired MRSA is growing problem that seems to have a disproportionate prevalence in athletes.[13] There is no consensus as to why MRSA infection is being observed in the healthy athletic population. Carriage rates have been reported in the range of 9% to 27%. Any skin infections not responsive to standard antibiotics and all abscesses should be suspected for CA-MRSA.[10]

Methicillin-resistant *Staphylococcus aureus* manifests most commonly as a cut or abrasion that has become infected. This can be very painful and extend into adjacent soft tissue, and there seems to be a predilection for developing into an abscess.[10,14] Fever and chills may be present as bacteremia may develop.

■ CLEARANCE FOR PARTICIPATION

The presence of any open wound or infectious skin condition that cannot be protected warrants exclusion from competition. Examples include open wounds that cannot be adequately covered and infections, including herpes simplex, scabies, louse infestation, molluscum contagiosum, tinea corporis, impetigo, and furuncles or carbuncles.

Denying clearance is especially important in sports in which close physical contact occurs, such as wrestling, rugby, and martial arts, and in sports in which equipment (eg, baseball helmets) is shared. Recent studies suggest that prompt identification and treatment of infected athletes is essential to prevent the spread of the infection to teammates and opponents.[3] Participation may be resumed when the condition has been adequately treated and is no longer contagious. For athletes with recurrent herpes gladiatorum, nucleoside analogues (eg, acyclovir, famciclovir, or valcyclovir) are effective in preventing recurrence and are therefore recommended for prophylactic treatment during the season.[15]

Outbreaks of CA-MRSA skin infections have increasingly been described among competitive athletes.[16,17] Since any open skin lesion is a potential site for the development of CA-MRSA, skin wounds identified during the PPE (or at any time) should be promptly treated and covered. Athletes should be reminded to avoid sharing personal items, including towels and razors. Athletes with suspected CA-MRSA should be cultured and treated with appropriate antibiotics. Ideally, abscesses should be treated with incision and drainage. Athletes may return to play when the infection is clinically controlled as determined by the treating physician.

The specific requirements for return to participation for wrestlers with skin infections differ from high school to college, but generally require treatment and the ability to cover the lesion adequately. The requirements can be obtained through the organization Web sites for the National Federation of State High School Associations (www.nfhs.org) and the NCAA (www.ncaa.org). NCAA wrestling regulations require that HSV-infected athletes must be free of systemic symptoms, have had no new lesions for 72 hours, and have been on oral antiviral treatment for 120 hours. Questionable cases should have laboratory confirmation (herpes culture, Tzank test, or HSV polymerase chain reaction test).[18,19] Tinea corporis requires a minimum of 72 hours of a topical fungicide, while tinea capitis requires a minimum of 2 weeks with oral medication. Be aware that for tinea capitis, treatment failure is common, with one study reporting only a 70% cure.[20] Molluscum and warts require treatment (topical or surgical) and covering.[12] Bacterial dermatoses, including CA-MRSA (impetigo, furuncles, cellulitis, folliculitis, and abscesses), are grouped together and require no new lesions for 48 hours, no moist or draining lesions, and completion of at least 72 hours of oral antibiotics.[10] Detailed guidelines for return to sports with skin infections is provided in Appendix D of *NCAA Wrestling Rules and Interpretations.*[19]

Restriction of athletes with bacterial skin conditions from practice and competition is recommended until appropriate intervention, including treatment with antibiotics, and, when necessary, barrier protection has been implemented. Occlusive coverage of the lesion must be with a non-permeable membrane and a securely attached bandage or patch. Most sports require that competitors completely cover open wounds and infectious skin conditions to prevent exposure to other competitors.[4] The consequences of failure to diagnose and adequately cover skin lesions can be devastating to an athlete, who may be declared ineligible for competition after months of training, and may lead to a widespread outbreak. Standard precautions are recommended by the Centers for Disease Control and Prevention for wounds that are open or bleeding.

Early and accurate detection and quarantine from contact until the infection is eradicated with comprehensive treatment are the most effective means of containing an outbreak and minimizing the spread of the disease. The NCAA requires that wrestlers be checked by a qualified examiner prior to and during each day of a meet or tournament and that written documentation be provided regarding diagnosis, type, and time of treatment and communicability.[21]

Prevention strategies for skin infections are varied and not standardized.[3] Recommended approaches include close surveillance, elimination of organisms on mats and equipment, daily change of practice clothing, immediate showering after practices to reduce the risk of skin infection, and implementing pharmacologic intervention.[22]

Although the primary mode of transmission is through skin-to-skin contact, most support the recommendation that mats and equipment (headgear) be cleaned by using a solution of 1 part bleach in 9 parts water made daily. Season-long prophylactic treatment for HSV with antiviral agents for individuals, as well as for entire teams has been demonstrated to be effective and is increasingly being implemented to prevent widespread infection.[12,23]

Community-acquired MRSA transmission occurs through skin-to-skin contact and exposure to shared equipment. Transmission control includes hand washing, showering with soap, covering cuts and abrasions, laundering personal items such as towels and supporters, and refraining from sharing razors and towels.

Other skin conditions such as acne should be noted. While not typically a reason to restrict an athlete, it has been reported to limit participation.[24] Acne can be difficult to control, even among those athletes being treated, because sweat and constrictive uniforms and equipment may exacerbate the condition. While acne should not affect eligibility or performance, it may have adverse social and emotional consequences for the athlete.

■ REFERENCES

1. The National Collegiate Athletic. NCAA injury Surveillance System (ISS). http://www.ncaa.org/wps/ncaa?key=/ncaa/ncaa/academics+and+athletes/personal+welfare/iss/index.html. Accessed February 4, 2009

2. Yard EE, Collins CL, Dick RW, Comstock RD. An epidemiologic comparison of high school and college wrestling injuries. *Am J Sports Med.* 2008;36(1):57–64

3. Anderson BJ. The epidemiology and clinical analysis of several outbreaks of herpes gladiatorum. *Med Sci Sports Exerc.* 2003;35(11):1809–1814

4. 2008-09 NCAA Sports Medicine Handbook. http://www.ncaa.org/wps/wcm/connect/873cf8804e0db2a5ac9cfc1ad6fc8b25/SMH0708_final.pdf?MOD=AJPERES. Accessed February 5, 2009

5. Rifat S, Ruffin MT IV, Gorenflow DW. Disqualifying criteria in a preparticipation sports evaluation. *J Fam Pract.* 1995;41(1):42–50

6. Bender TW III. Cutaneous manifestations of disease in athletes. *Skinmed.* 2003;2(1):34–40

7. Brooks C, Kujawska A, Patel D. Cutaneous allergic reactions induced by sporting activities. *Sports Med.* 2003;33(9):699–708

8. Metelitsa A, Barankin B, Lin AN. Diagnosis of sport-related dermatoses. *Int J Dermatol.* 2004;43(2):113–119

9. Kohl TD, Lisney M. Tinea gladiatorum: wrestling's emerging foe. *Sports Med.* 2000;29(6):439–447

10. Sedgwick PE, Dexter WW, Smith CT. Bacterial dermatoses in sports. *Clin Sports Med.* 2007;26(3):383–396

11. Cyr PR. Preventing outbreaks in sports settings. *Phys Sportsmed.* 2004;32(7):33–38

12. Pleacher MD, Dexter WW. Cutaneous fungal and viral infections in athletes. *Clin Sports Med.* 2007;26(3):397–411

13. Benjamin HJ, Nikore V, Takagishi J. Practical management: community-associated methicillin-resistant staphylococcus aureus (CA-MRSA): the latest sports epidemic. *Clin J Sport Med.* 2007;17(5):393–397

14. Barrett TW Moran GJ. Update on emerging infections: news from the Centers for Disease Control and Prevention. Methicillin-resistant *Staphylococcus aureus* infections among competitive sports participants—Colorado, Indiana, Pennsylvania, and Los Angeles County, 2000–2003. *Ann Emerg Med.* 2004;43(1):43–45

15. Anderson BJ. The effectiveness of valcyclovir in preventing reactivation of herpes gladiatorum in wrestlers. *Clin J Sport Med.* 1999;9(2):86–90

16. Centers for Disease Control and Prevention (CDC). Methicillin-resistant staphylococcus aureus infections among competitive sports participants—Colorado, Indiana, Pennsylvania, and Los Angeles County, 2000–2003. *MMWR Morb Mortal Wkly Rep.* 2003;52(33):793–795

17. Kazakova SV, Hageman JC, Mattava M, et al. A clone of methicillin-resistant *Staphylococcus aureus* among professional football players. *N Engl J Med* 2005;352:468–475

18. NFHS Associations. Wrestling sports/rules information. Available at www.nfhs.org/sportsmed.aspx. Accessed September 25, 2009

19. 2009 NCAA Wrestling Rules and Interpretations. Appendix D: Skin infections. www.docstoc.com/docs/1848264/2009-ncaa-wrestling-rules-and-interpretations. Accessed February 5, 2009

20. Ergin S, Ergin C, Erdo an BS, Kaleli I, Evliyao lu D. An experience from an outbreak of tinea capitis gladiatorum due to *Trichophyton tonsurans. Clin Exp Dermatol.* 2006;31(2):212–214

21. NCAA Wrestling Rules and Interpretations. www.docstop.com/docs/air8264/2009-ncaa-wrestling-rules-and-interpretations. Accessed February 5, 2009

22. Adams BB. Tinea corporis gladiatorum. *J Am Acad Dermatol.* 2002;47(2):286–290

23. Howe WB. Preventing infectious disease in sports. *Phys Sportsmed.* 2003;31(2):23–29

24. Pleacher MD, Dexter WW. Acne and active patients: improving more than superficial appearances. *Phys Sportsmed.* 2005;33(9):14–26

G: Musculoskeletal Concerns

Musculoskeletal injuries and complaints are the most common problems that team physicians and health care providers see in the training room and during the preparticipation physical evaluation (PPE). During the PPE, a thorough review of the musculoskeletal history and examination pertinent for the sport and injured area may improve the outcome. This chapter will cover those areas and address the issues for clearance to play pertaining to the skeletal system.

■ HISTORY FORM QUESTIONS

17. *Have you ever had an injury to a bone, muscle, ligament, or tendon that caused you to miss a practice or a game?*

18. *Have you had any broken or fractured bones or dislocated joints?*

19. *Have you had an injury that required x-rays, MRI, CT scan, injections, therapy, a brace, a cast, or crutches?*

20. *Have you ever had a stress fracture?*

21. *Have you ever been told that you have or have you had an x-ray for neck instability or atlantoaxial instability? (Down syndrome or dwarfism)*

22. *Do you regularly use a brace, orthotics, or other assistive device?*

23. *Do you have a bone, muscle, or joint injury that bothers you?*

24. *Do any of your joints become painful, swollen, feel warm, or look red?*

25. *Do you have any history of juvenile arthritis or connective tissue disease?*

■ KEY POINTS

- Athletes with unresolved musculoskeletal pain require additional evaluation prior to sports clearance.
- Stress fractures and recurrent soft tissue injuries can be associated with nutritional deficiencies.
- A general screening examination is reasonable for asymptomatic athletes with no previous injury.

The first and most important step in the PPE for the musculoskeletal system is to take a focused musculoskeletal history.

Missed practices or games or the use of braces or other devices may be an indicator of a serious injury or condition. In such cases, inquiry should be made regarding mechanism of injury and prior medical or operative care. Documentation should include any specific rehabilitation program provided, including type and duration of exercise therapy and physical modalities. The physician should determine whether the athlete was declared fully rehabilitated by the treating physician or physical therapist and what recommendations were given to maintain strength and flexibility. In athletes with unresolved musculoskeletal pain, further workup may be warranted to exclude conditions such as occult fracture, tendinopathy, or rheumatologic disorders.

Fractures or dislocated joints are more serious orthopedic injuries. Detailed information about mechanism of injury, sport involved, treatment, and rehabilitation history should be obtained. Dislocated joints are frequently accompanied by a fracture. Such a major injury may have associated permanent neurologic deficits. In such cases, referral to a primary care sports medicine physician, orthopedic surgeon, physiatrist, neurologist, or other specialist for advice on clearance should be considered. **Stress fractures** are commonly observed in running and other sports with repetitive impact, sports specialization associated with overuse injuries (eg, figure skating, gymnastics, dance, basketball), and sports for which judging is subjective and appearance is important (eg, figure skating, gymnastics).[1] Significant risk factors for bony stress injury include training error and inadequate bone mass related to diet or hormonal factors.

Training errors usually involve either a rapid increase in the intensity and duration of training or prolonged high-level training without periodization and adequate recovery time.[2-4] The type of training schedule at the time of the stress fracture and modifications of training should be determined at the PPE. Examination for conditions that affect normal biomechanics of the lower extremity such as pes planus, pes cavus, or overpronation should be made so that corrective devices such as foot orthoses are considered.

Osteoporosis and osteopenia from inadequate caloric intake can lead to stress fractures. An athlete with a history of stress fractures should be queried about disordered eating and inadequate caloric, calcium, and vitamin D intake. Females should be asked about menstrual history due to the hormonal effects on bone health. Inadequate caloric intake leading to energy imbalance may signify a disordered eating issue and increase the risk of amenorrhea and osteoporosis or osteopenia.

A history of x-rays, magnetic resonance imaging, computed tomography, surgery, injections, rehabilitation, physical therapy, bracing, casting, or crutch use gives the physician a better idea of whether a previous injury has been serious. This inquiry may prompt an athlete to remember a procedure or workup, even if they may have forgotten the injury when answering previous questions, and provide valuable information when assessing the current status of the athlete.

Once the history form has been completed and reviewed, a screening and focused examination of the musculoskeletal system should be performed.

■ PHYSICAL EXAMINATION

The type and extent of the musculoskeletal examination appropriate for the PPE is a much-debated topic, and few studies are available to guide the clinician. Examiners need to determine which method best suits a given situation, depending on history of injury, musculoskeletal signs or symptoms, resources and time available, type of sport or activity in which the athlete will participate, and the level of expertise of the examiner.

The yield of any type of musculoskeletal examination is low in asymptomatic athletes who have no history of injury. In addition, history alone has been shown to be 92% sensitive in detecting significant musculoskeletal injuries.[5] A general screening examination (Figure 6G-1) may be a reasonable approach for asymptomatic athletes who have no previous injury, despite a sensitivity of 50%.[5] If the athlete has (1) a previous injury or (2) pain, ligamentous laxity or joint instability, locking, weakness, atrophy, or other signs or symptoms detected by the general screening examination or the history, the general screen should be supplemented with relevant elements of the joint-specific examination (see page 110), or the athlete should be referred to a specialist for further evaluation.[6] Alternatively, when time and resources permit, it is also reasonable to perform the entire joint-specific examination instead of a general screening examination, or to perform a sport-specific examination (see page 116).[6] Finally, an overview of skeletal structure may reveal the reduced upper-to-lower segment ratio or arm span–to–height ratio greater than 1.05 as 1 of the 4 major diagnostic criteria for Marfan syndrome.[7]

General screening examination. General screens may be used to quickly assess joint range of motion, gross muscle strength, and muscle asymmetry, and to identify significant injuries.[8] The general screening examination is described in Figure 6G-1.[6,8] In using the general screen, however, clinicians must be aware that it does not allow determination of a specific diagnosis or severity of musculoskeletal injury.

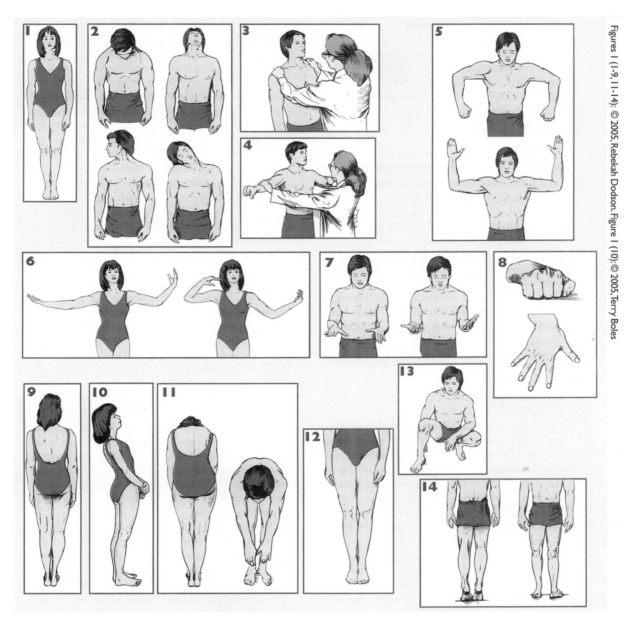

Figures 1 (1-9, 11-14): © 2005, Rebekah Dodson. Figure 1 (10): © 2005, Terry Boles

Figure 6G-1.
The general musculoskeletal screening examination consists of the following: (1) inspection, athlete standing, facing toward examiner (symmetry of trunk, upper extremities); (2) forward flexion, extension, rotation, lateral flexion of neck (range of motion, cervical spine); (3) resisted shoulder shrug (strength, trapezius); (4) resisted shoulder abduction (strength, deltoid); (5) internal and external rotation of shoulder (range of motion, glenohumeral joint); (6) extension and flexion of elbow (range of motion, elbow); (7) pronation and supination of forearm or wrist (range of motion, elbow and wrist); (8) clench fist, then spread fingers (range of motion, hand and fingers); (9) inspection, athlete facing away from examiner (symmetry of trunk, upper extremities); (10) back extension, knees straight (spondylolysis/spondylolisthesis); (11) back flexion with knees straight, facing toward and away from examiner (range of motion, thoracic and lumbosacral spine; spine curvature; hamstring flexibility); (12) inspection of lower extremities, contraction of quadriceps muscles (alignment, symmetry); (13) "duck walk" 4 steps (motion of hip, knee, and ankle; strength; balance); (14) standing on toes, then on heels (symmetry, calf; strength; balance).

For example, it does not assess the degree of instability of a shoulder with glenohumeral joint laxity, and it may not allow for detection of rotator cuff injuries. Also, if the history indicates past or current ankle injury or pain, and the patient is unable to perform the toe raise or demonstrates obvious asymmetric lateral ankle swelling, ankle instability should be evaluated by anterior drawer and talar tilt tests. Examiners should supplement any general screening examination with a thorough joint-specific examination when indicated by findings in the history or general screen. Referral to an orthopedic specialist may be considered if there is question of diagnosis, clearance, or further treatment.

Joint-specific testing. Assessing individual joints by inspection, palpation, and maneuvers well established in the literature is more definitive than the general screening examination. It may also be better suited than the sport-specific examination (see page 116) to multisport athletes. However, joint-specific examinations are more time-consuming than the general screen, may exceed the expertise of the examiner, and have a low yield in an asymptomatic athlete without a previous injury. The author societies, therefore, do not consider it necessary to perform the entire joint-specific examination for every athlete. Instead, portions of the examination are used as indicated by the history and findings on the general screen. However, because of its accuracy, some practitioners prefer to use the entire joint-specific examination as their primary evaluation tool during the musculoskeletal portion of the PPE.

The complete joint-specific screening examination includes inspection for symmetry and range-of-motion testing of the neck, spine, shoulders, elbows, wrists, fingers, hips, knees, ankles, and feet and stability assessment of the shoulders, elbows, knees, and ankles.

If the joint-specific screening examination confirms a problem, a more thorough and focused examination with relevant diagnostic testing may be indicated prior to sports clearance. If the setting and examiner expertise allow, this examination may be done at the time of screening.

Spine. The cervical spine should be inspected for posture and alignment. Forward flexion of the neck should allow the chin to touch the manubrium, extension should allow skyward gaze, rotation should let the chin almost touch the clavicle in both directions, and the ears should approach the shoulders on lateral flexion. Any asymmetric or deficient motion should be noted.

Examination of the thoracolumbar spine and back focuses on appreciating deformities. The scapulae should be level, symmetric, and flat against the thoracic cage. Presence or absence of scoliosis should be observed, as well as the degree of kyphosis at the thoracic level and lordosis at the lumbar level. Presence of rotatory deformities should be noted as the athlete bends forward at the waist (Figure 6G-2); pain or restriction of motion on forward flexion may indicate lumbar disk disease. Back extension should also be assessed; pain may increase in the presence of spondylolysis, spondylolisthesis, or a sprain/strain.

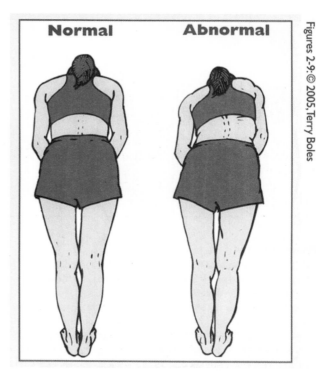

Figures 2-9. © 2005. Terry Boles

Figure 6G-2.
As part of the thoracolumbar spine examination, the athlete bends forward at the waist. The rotatory deformities of scoliosis, such as asymmetric, prominent ribs; curvature of the spine; and/or an asymmetric waist, are accentuated in this position.

Upper extremity. The shoulder examination begins with inspection for symmetry with the athlete standing. Range of motion in abduction (Figure 6G-3A), flexion (Figure 6G-3B), and internal and external rotation (Figures 6G-3C and 6G-3D) is then assessed. The condition of the rotator cuff can be tested by several maneuvers, including the "empty can test" (Figure 6G-4A), manual resistance to internal and external rotation with the arm at the side (Figure 6G-4B), and assessing for impingement symptoms (Figures 6G-4C and 6G-4D). Deltoid strength is assessed by manual resistance to straight abduction. A screen for multidirectional instability includes subluxation tests in the anterior and posterior planes in the supine athlete (Figures 6G-5A through 6G-5D), and in the inferior plane in the seated athlete (Figure 6G-5E).

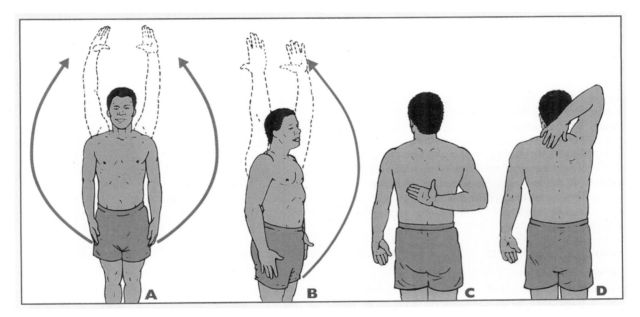

Figure 6G-3.
Shoulder range of motion is evaluated in 4 directions. In abduction (A) and forward flexion (B), the athlete should be able to reach completely overhead without excessive or asymmetric motion of the scapula; in internal rotation (C), the fingertips should reach approximately to the bottom of the opposite scapula; and in external rotation (D), the fingertips should approach the top of the opposite scapula.

The elbow is observed for swelling, discoloration, and cubital angle (Figure 6G-6A). The elbow should extend fully and then flex to allow the athlete to touch the ipsilateral shoulder with the hand. Forearm motion is assessed by having the athlete pronate and supinate the forearms with the elbows bent 90 degrees at his or her sides. The athlete should be able to turn the hand completely palm up and completely palm down.

In the throwing athlete, medial stability can be assessed by applying a valgus force to the elbow (Figure 6G-6B). The milking maneuver also assesses medial instability and is performed with the athlete's elbow flexed beyond 90 degrees and the hand supinated. The examiner reaches behind the elbow being tested and grasps the affected medial collateral ligament (MCL), applying a downward force. The test is considered positive if pain is noted over the MCL or if the joint opens medially. Direct comparison to the opposite arm is critical.

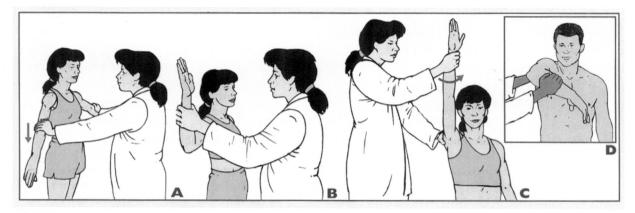

Figure 6G-4.
To assess rotator cuff function, the "empty can test" (A) can be used. The patient places both shoulders in 60 degrees to 90 degrees of abduction in the scapular plane, 30 degrees forward flexion in the sagittal plane, full elbow extension, and forearm pronation (thumbs down); the examiner resists further abduction. Comparing manual resistance to further abduction in both internal and external rotation of the entire arm (B) helps distinguish biceps tendinopathy from rotator cuff pathology. Increased pain in external rotation as opposed to internal rotation should direct the examiner to further evaluate the rotator cuff, while the reverse is true in the case of biceps tendon pathology. The Neer impingement test (C) involves fully abducting and forward flexing the shoulder and arm. An alternative examination for shoulder impingement, the Hawkin's test (D), involves forward flexion to 90 degrees and the shoulder is internally rotated. With internal shoulder rotation, the examiner notes whether there has been an exacerbation of shoulder pain. Localizing the exact site of the pain can help distinguish biceps tendinopathy or acromioclavicular pathology from rotator cuff pathology. If there is true outlet impingement, pain should localize to the anterior acromion of the shoulder and radiate laterally down the arm.

The hand and wrist are evaluated for symmetry. Wrists should palmar flex equally to about 80 degrees and dorsiflex to 70 degrees or more. There should be more ulnar deviation than radial deviation. The fingers should be able to close into a full fist, and each fingernail should point at the scaphoid bone with the fingers flexed across the palm. Intrinsic muscle function can be checked by having the athlete touch each fingertip with the thumb and spread and close the extended fingers.

Lower extremity. The hip examination begins with observation of the standing posture. Iliac crest height should be level, and the athlete should be able to stand on each foot without any tilting of the pelvis.

Hip range of motion can be assessed with the athlete lying supine. With the hip and the knee fully extended, the hip joint is rotated internally and externally (a "log roll" movement), and any asymmetry is noted. Symmetry of abduction and adduction should also be observed. Hip flexion should be beyond 90 degrees, and the knees should come straight toward the chest; any external rotation indicates an intrinsic hip deformity. With the hip and knee flexed to 90 degrees, the hip joint is rotated again (Figure 6G-7). Keeping the athlete's hip flexed 90 degrees and extending the knee checks hamstring flexibility. The popliteal angle should be 0 degrees to 10 degrees but can vary based on patient age and sex.[10,11] The popliteal angle refers to the flexion angle of the knee created by tension in the hamstring tendons as the knee is extended while the hip is flexed.

With the athlete standing, inspection should reveal a normal leg-thigh valgus angulation of 12 degrees or less in males and 18 degrees or less in females. The patella should be observed for abnormal lateral subluxation or tilt or an excessively high position (patella alta) with the athlete seated.

The remainder of the knee examination should involve both knees with the athlete supine. Each patella should be evaluated for hypermobility by translating the patella medially and laterally with the knee in approximately 20 degrees of flexion; comparison with the opposite side should be made. Joint-line tenderness may indicate a meniscal tear. Any amount of knee effusion should be noted. Knee range of

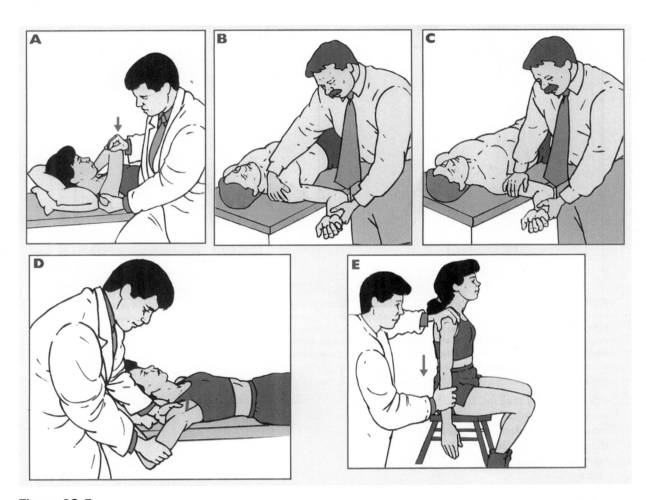

Figure 6G-5.

Multidirectional instability can be gauged by assessing glenohumeral motion in several planes. Posterior instability of the shoulder is assessed with the athlete supine by positioning the arm perpendicular to the table with the elbow bent, then applying pressure along the long axis of the arm (A). The hand supporting the posterior shoulder palpates for excessive motion. When assessing shoulder internal rotation, it is important to stabilize the scapula by placing a hand against the scapular spine in the upright patient; in the supine patient, placing the shoulder firmly against the examination table can achieve the same goal. In the apprehension test (B), which is used to assess for anterior instability, the examiner abducts the arm in the scapular plane and externally rotates the supine athlete's shoulder. It is important to look at the athlete's face while performing the maneuver to assess for visible signs of apprehension of a dislocation event. If apprehension is observed during the test, the relocation test (C) may be performed in the same position by applying a posteriorly directed force to the humeral head, reducing anterior translation of the humeral head. Relocation of the head will decrease the feeling of apprehension if instability is present. It is important to distinguish whether there is frank apprehension versus pain with this test. If the athlete experiences increasing pain with progressive internal rotation of the humeral head, this suggests that the humeral head is subluxating anteriorly; secondary (internal) impingement of the rotator cuff is occurring, causing pain.[9] The augmentation test (D) is the reverse of the relocation test. An anteriorly directed force on the posterior proximal humerus, with the arm in 90 degrees of abduction and maximal external rotation, will increase apprehension with anterior instability. The examiner's fingers should wrap around the humeral head anteriorly to prevent dislocation. When assessing the shoulder, it is important to examine the opposite arm to detect any asymmetry in degree of motion or instability between the shoulders. With the athlete seated (E), inferior subluxation is confirmed by the presence of the sulcus sign—appearance of an indentation beneath the acromion with traction along the axis of the adducted arm. In the normal shoulder, there should be some inferior laxity with the arm at the side. However, as the arm is eternally rotated with the arm maintained at the side, this laxity should correct as the rotator interval is placed in tension. Inferior subluxation that persists or is asymmetric to the opposite side suggests a tear of the rotator interval.

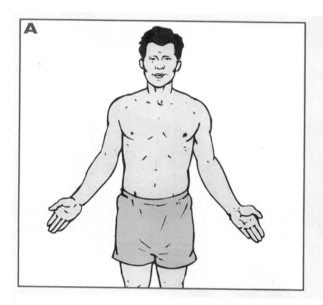

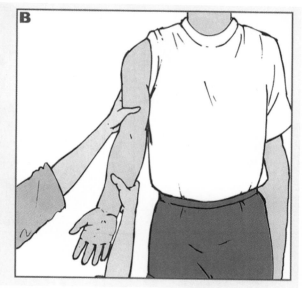

Figure 6G-6.

The normal carrying angle of the elbow is at least 15 degrees valgus with the athlete standing and the palms forward (A). An excessive valgus angle may indicate instability or a previous injury. In the throwing athlete, medial collateral ligament instability should be assessed. This is accomplished by applying a valgus force to the elbow (with forearm pronation) at 25 degrees to 30 degrees of flexion while noting laxity and endpoint (B). Placing the shoulder in maximal external rotation minimizes excessive humeral rotation, which may decrease the accuracy of medial stability testing.

motion should be from full extension to approximately 140 degrees of flexion. Knee ligament stability tests include the Lachman test for anterior cruciate ligament deficiency (Figure 6G-8A); anterior and posterior drawer tests for anterior and posterior cruciate ligament insufficiencies, respectively (Figures 6G-8B and 6G-8C); and varus and valgus stress tests for collateral ligament laxities (Figures 6G-8D and 6G-8E).

The ankles are evaluated for normal appearance with the athlete first standing, then sitting. In the seated position, active dorsiflexion to 20 degrees and plantar flexion to 40 degrees should be present. With the knee extended, tightness in the Achilles tendon can be assessed by passively dorsiflexing the seated athlete's ankle while observing the lateral aspect of the leg and ankle. The ankle should dorsiflex 15 degrees to 20 degrees past neutral. Stress testing for ligament laxity includes the anterior drawer test for anterior subluxation (Figure 6G-9A) and the talar tilt test for lateral ligament stability (Figure 6G-9B).

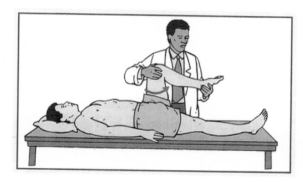

Figure 6G-7.

Hip range of motion is evaluated with the athlete supine. As part of the examination, the hip and knee are flexed to 90 degrees, and the hip joint is rotated. A rotation arc of at least 60 degrees should be observed. Pain or restriction of motion relative to the opposite side warrants further evaluation.

On inspection of the foot, cavus or rigid flatfoot deformities should be noted. A supple flatfoot does not affect the athlete's performance but may be a risk factor for lower-extremity overuse problems such as medial tibial stress syndrome or patellofemoral pain. If the flatfoot is supple, the plantar arch will increase when the athlete stands on his or her toes. Toe deformities, including bunions, contractures, and pressure

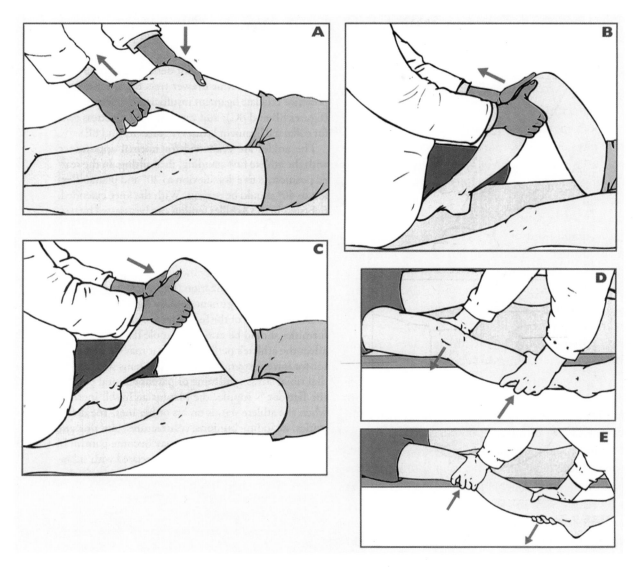

Figure 6G-8.

Several tests are used to assess ligamentous instability of the knee. For each test, the degree of excursion and the quality of the endpoint are noted and compared with the opposite side. The Lachman's test (A) is the most sensitive means to assess anterior cruciate ligament (ACL) deficiencies.[12] The patient's knee is flexed approximately 20 degrees, and the muscles are relaxed. The examiner stabilizes the femur with one hand while pulling the tibia anteriorly with the other hand. It is important to note how far the tibial tubercule translates anteriorly and whether there is a soft or firm endpoint at terminal translation. All findings should be compared with the opposite side. The anterior (B) and posterior (C) drawer tests can reveal ACL and posterior cruciate ligament (PCL) insufficiency, respectively. With the supine patient's knee bent 90 degrees, the examiner sits on the patient's foot to stabilize it and grasps the proximal tibia. The hamstrings should be palpated to ensure they are relaxed. The examiner pulls the tibia anteriorly (anterior drawer test, B) and pushes it posteriorly (posterior drawer test, C) from the neutral position. With the anterior drawer test, lack of a firm endpoint and presence of excessive anterior tibial excursion suggest ACL insufficiency. With the posterior drawer test, the presence of excessive posterior tibial sag suggests PCL insufficiency. With an intact PCL, the tibia is positioned anterior to the femur with the knee in 90 degrees of flexion. During the posterior drawer test, the examiner should palpate and quantify the change in anteromedial femoral-tibial step-off that occurs with and without a posteriorly directed force on the tibia. Varus (D) and valgus (E) stress tests gauge instability of the medial and lateral collateral ligaments of the knee. The athlete's knee is extended over the edge of the examination table and flexed to approximately 20 degrees. One of the examiner's hands stabilizes the knee at the joint line, and varus and valgus stresses are applied to the tibia. Once again, comparison with the opposite limb is essential for these tests, given the normal range of variation in joint stability.

points indicated by calluses, may become painful in athletic footwear. Abnormalities associated with subtalar, midfoot, and forefoot problems should be further assessed through a formal gait and/or running study in an exercise physiology laboratory or similar facility.

Sport-specific examinations. Some sports medicine physicians advocate sport-specific physical examinations.[13,14] Such examinations focus on areas under particular stress (and therefore at higher risk for injury) in a given sport and include strength, endurance, and flexibility testing in addition to a more general orthopedic examination. For example, for swimmers and baseball pitchers, an examiner might measure shoulder internal and external rotation strength and endurance with isokinetic testing; for running and jumping athletes, the examiner might test both knee flexion, extension, and strength and hip abductor and adductor strength with isokinetic testing and observe gait biomechanics on a treadmill.

Similarly, if there is evidence of hyperlaxity on examination, especially in the athlete engaged in overhead arm motions, growing evidence indicates that increased focus on the joint(s) at risk could be warranted.[15-17] For example, if an adolescent baseball pitcher or volleyball player comes in with limited, subtle, or frank shoulder complaints and has evidence of systemic laxity, such as hyperextension at the elbow, a thorough shoulder examination for labral pathology and shoulder subluxation should be performed. Another example is the adolescent soccer player with knee hyperextension and a history of knee problems. In this instance, a full ligamentous knee examination should be performed to assess for cruciate, collateral, and posterolateral corner knee instability. Additionally, referral may be indicated to assess for more serious conditions

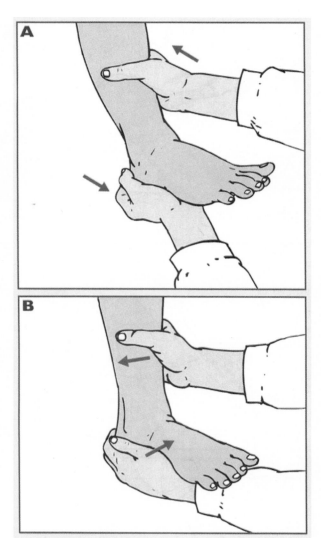

Figure 6G-9.
Two stress tests are used to assess instability of the ankle ligaments. For the anterior drawer test (A), which demonstrates anterior subluxation, the examiner pulls the heel anteriorly while pushing posteriorly on the distal tibia. For the talar tilt test (B), the examiner inverts the ankle by pushing laterally on the medial tibia and medially on the calcaneus. Excessive motion relative to the opposite edge should trigger further evaluation.

associated with generalized hypermobility such as Ehlers-Danlos or Marfan syndrome. In Ehlers-Danlos syndrome, knowledge of the Beighton scale (Carter-Wilkinson criteria) (Table 6G-1) can help to objectively make the diagnosis.[18,19] Common physical findings are hyperextension of the knees and elbows beyond 10 degrees, dorsiflexion of the metacarpalphalangeal joints beyond 90 degrees, and passive apposition of the thumb to the forearm.

TABLE 6G-1. BEIGHTON HYPERMOBILITY CRITERIA[a,b]

Physical Finding	Point value
• Passive dorsiflexion of the metacarpophalangeal joint beyond 90 degrees	1 point for each hand
• Passive apposition of the thumb to the flexor aspect of the forearm	1 point for each thumb
• Hyperextension of the elbows beyond 10 degrees	1 point for each elbow
• Hyperextension of the knees beyond 10 degrees	1 point for each knee
• Forward flexion of the trunk with knees fully extended so that the palms of the hands rest flat on the floor	1 point

[a]Adapted from Grahame R, Bird HA, Child A, et al. The British Society for Rheumatology Special Interest Group on Heritable Disorders of Connective Tissue criteria for the benign joint hypermobility syndrome. The revised (Brighton 1998) criteria for the diagnosis of BJHS. *J Rheumatol.* 2000;27:1777–1779.

[b]A total score of 5/9 or higher is generally regarded as indicating hypermobility.

Although such precisely focused tests may reveal information that can improve performance and possibly prevent injury, these examinations are time-consuming and require more in-depth knowledge of individual sports than the joint-specific or general screening examination. When time, resources, and expertise allow, however, such examinations can supplement or replace the general screening examination and/or the joint-specific examination.

■ CLEARANCE FOR PARTICIPATION

Once all of the pertinent information is gathered via the history and physical, the examining physician must decide if the patient is ready for their particular sport. Determining clearance for athletes who have musculoskeletal injuries or disorders requires assessing both short- and long-term risks and benefits with respect to the PPE findings. Some problems may exceed the capacity of the PPE venue and require additional evaluation with a repeat visit or consultation with additional specialists.

Clearance for participation must be based on the degree and type of injury, the ability of the injured athlete to compete safely, and the requirements of a given sport. Participation may be possible in activities that do not directly affect the injured site (eg, a wrist sprain might prevent a gymnast from full training, but not a runner). Therefore, the physician should also determine which strength and conditioning activities are appropriate during the recovery period so that the athlete is able to maintain some level of fitness. Protective padding, taping, or bracing may be designed to provide the athlete a safe means to compete. The types of protective splinting or bracing permitted in competition vary by the sport and the rules of the sport organization or league. If the examining physician is not certain of the rules concerning safe participation with protective devices, consultation with a sports medicine specialist is suggested. The final decision on what type of protective padding or bracing may rest with the on-site officials. In such situations, a change in the original type of protection recommended by the sports medicine staff could be deemed necessary by the official. Any alteration required by the official should be evaluated to ensure that it provides the necessary protection for the injury.

Referral to a consultant is warranted when the examiner is uncertain of the athlete's ability to participate because of the injury. In any case, physicians who initiated the treatment of an injury that was present at the time of the PPE should be included in the clearance decision. Reevaluation is required after rehabilitation. Review of every musculoskeletal problem is beyond the scope of this monograph, but selected problems deserve mention.

SPRAINS, STRAINS, SUBLUXATIONS, DISLOCATIONS, AND CONTUSIONS

Before clearance is given for either acute or overuse injuries, the athlete should be examined and the following ruled out:

- Effusion, swelling, or other signs of inflammation
- Decreased range of motion of the affected joint or joints controlled by the muscle
- Strength less than 85% to 90% of the uninjured side or insufficient for the desired activity
- Ligamentous instability of the affected joint
- Loss or alteration of sport-specific functional ability (ie, inability to complete pain-free functional activity at 80%–90% effort)

For example, a football defensive back who is rehabilitating a lateral ankle sprain could be assessed with back-pedaling and side-to-side movements. If any of these findings are abnormal, further treatment will be needed to allow for return to play. Referral, if necessary, to a physician familiar with the sport-specific requirements and injury assessment is recommended. Ultimately, the decision for clearance is based on the examiner's clinical judgment and may be withheld until further evaluation and completion of prescribed treatment or rehabilitation. Further evaluation and consultation is warranted if uncertainty about clearance persists.

FRACTURES

Clearance of an athlete with a fracture should be determined by the treating physician. The location and type of fracture, risk of reinjury or complications, and the effect of treatment should be considered. The possibility of protecting the fracture during participation with a cast or splint should be considered if the risk of worsening the injury is felt to be negligible. Also, in making clearance decisions, the physician should be aware of specific rules relevant to the athlete's sport regarding use of padded and unpadded materials on the extremities. Contacting a league representative or referral to a sports medicine specialist is warranted if the examiner or treating physician is unfamiliar with options regarding protective devices.

DEVELOPMENTAL CONDITIONS

Any history or physical finding of spinal deformity (eg, scoliosis, spondylolysis, or spondylolisthesis) requires a more thorough evaluation than is generally provided in the PPE.

Follow-up with the athlete's primary care physician, sports medicine specialist, or spine specialist is recommended should questions arise. Spondylolysis and spondylolisthesis should be evaluated individually on the basis of symptoms, physical limitations, and imaging findings. Because of the risk of progressive slippage, spondylolysis and/or spondylolisthesis may require follow-up imaging. Generally, athletes with spinal deformities need not be excluded from play. However, activities may need to be modified based on clinical symptoms and the extent of the abnormality.

Clearing athletes with apophysitis of the tibial tubercle (Osgood-Schlatter disease), calcaneus (Sever's disease), ileum, or ischium follows similar criteria as for overuse injuries and acute strains.

If there are any questions concerning clearance, consultation with a sports medicine specialist is warranted.

Following a systematic approach to history, physical examination and decisions on clearance should set the foundation for a safe sport season for the athlete.

■ REFERENCES

1. Snyder RA, Koester MC, Dunn WR. Epidemiology of stress fractures. *Clin Sports Med*. 2006;25(1):37–52

2. Kadel NJ, Teitz CC, Kronmal RA. Stress fractures in ballet dancers. *Am J Sports Med*. 1992;20:445–449

3. Brunet ME, Cook SD, Brinker MR, et al. A survey of running injuries in 1505 competitive and recreational runners. *J Sports Med Phys Fitness*. 1990;30:307–315

4. Korpelainen R, Orava S, Karpakka J, Siira P, Hulkko A. Risk factors for recurrent stress fractures in athletes. *Am J Sports Med*. 2001;29(3):304–310

5. Gomez JE, Landry GL, Bernhardt DT. Critical evaluation of the 2-minute orthopedic screening examination. *Am J Dis Child*. 1993;147(10):1109–1113

6. Garrick J. Pre-participation orthopedic screening examination. *Clin J Sports Med*. 2004;14(3):123–126

7. Jones KB, Sponseller PD, Erkula G, et al. Symposium on the musculoskeletal aspects of Marfan syndrome: meeting report and state of the science. *J Orthop Res*. 2007;25:413–422

8. American Academy of Family Physicians, American Academy of Pediatrics, American Medical Society for Sports Medicine, American Orthopaedic Society for Sports Medicine, American Osteopathic Academy of Sports Medicine. *Preparticipation Physical Evaluation*. 2nd ed. Minneapolis, MN: The Physician and Sportsmedicine; 1997.

9. Speer KP, Hannafin JA, Altchek DW, et al. An evaluation of the shoulder relocation test. *Am J Sports Med*. 1994;22(2):177–183

10. Katz K, Rosenthal A, Yosipovich Z. Normal ranges of popliteal angle in children. *J Pediatr Orthop*. 1992;12(2):229–231

11. Gajdosik R, Lusin G. Hamstring muscle tightness: reliability of an active knee-extension test. *Phys Ther*. 1983;63(7):1085–1090

12. Kim SJ, Kim HK. Reliability of the anterior drawer test, the pivot shift test, and the Lachman test. *Clin Orthop*. 1995;Aug (317):237–242

13. Kibler WB, Chandler TJ, Uhl T, et al. A musculoskeletal approach to the preparticipation physical examination: preventing injury and improving performance. *Am J Sports Med*. 1989;17(4):525–531

14. Kibler WB, Chandler TJ. Sport specific screening and testing. In: Renstrom P, ed. *Sports Injuries: Basic Principles of Prevention and Care: Olympic Encyclopedia of Sports Medicine*. Vol 4. Boston, MA: Blackwell Scientific Pubs; 1993

15. Amir D, Frankl U, Pogrund H. Pulled elbow and hypermobility of joints. *Clin Orthop*. 1990;Aug(257):94–99

16. Decoster LC, Vailas JC, Lindsay RH, et al. Prevalence and features of joint hypermobility among adolescent athletes. *Arch Pediatr Adolesc Med*. 1997;151(10):989–992

17. Didia BC, Dapper DV, Boboye SB. Joint hypermobility syndrome among undergraduate students. *East Afr Med J*. 2002;79(2):80–81

18. Beighton PH. The Ehler-Danlos syndromes. In: Beighton PH, ed. *Heritable Disorders of Connective Tissue*. 5th ed. St Louis, MO: Mosby; 1983:189–251

19. Gedalia A, Brewer EJ Jr. Joint hypermobility in pediatric practice—a review. *J Rheumatol*. 1993;20:371–374

H: The Female Athlete

The basics of the preparticipation physical evaluation (PPE) are the same for both sexes; however, there are specific medical and musculoskeletal concerns that should be considered when evaluating the female athlete.

■ MEDICAL HISTORY

The medical history is the most crucial component of the PPE when approaching female issues.

MUSCULOSKELETAL INJURY

History Form Questions

17. *Have you ever had an injury to a bone, muscle, ligament, or tendon that caused you to miss a practice or game?*

18. *Have you had any broken or fractured bones or dislocated joints?*

20. *Have you ever had a stress fracture?*

Key Points

- Eating disorders and energy imbalance may be associated with persistent injury, recurrent injury, or stress fractures.
- Female athletes with musculoskeletal injuries and menstrual dysfunction have a longer interruption of training than those with regular cycles.
- The PPE is an opportunity to discuss the quality and quantity of calories needed to participate in sport.
- Vitamin D deficiency is becoming increasingly common due to inadequate vitamin D dietary intake and/or reduced exposure to sunlight.

Most athletes have experienced a musculoskeletal injury, but the answers to these questions can be an indicator of not only the severity, but also the chronicity or recurrence of the injury or condition. In female athletes with unresolved musculoskeletal pain, further questioning and workup are warranted to exclude conditions such as occult fracture and tendinopathy and to explore comorbid conditions such as menstrual irregularities and disordered eating patterns. Female athletes with menstrual dysfunction have been found to have a longer interruption of training due to musculoskeletal injuries than those with regular cycles,[1] and female collegiate athletes in the aesthetic sports, like gymnastics, versus endurance and team sports, like cross-country running and basketball, experienced more muscle and bone injuries.[2]

Female athletes are also at higher risk for certain musculoskeletal conditions such as non-contact anterior cruciate ligament injuries, recurrent dislocation of the patella, patellofemoral pain syndrome, and adolescent idiopathic scoliosis.[3] A significant increase in distal forearm fractures in children and adolescents in the past 2 decades has been noted in several studies, with some showing a greater increase in girls compared to boys.[4] While this increased incidence could be due to overall increased physical activity in this population, another cause could be the decreased acquisition of bone mass during this pubertal longitudinal bone growth and time of greater calcium demand. Low bone density has been found to be more common throughout the skeleton in girls with forearm fractures than in those who have never broken a bone, and those girls aged 11 to 15 years reported lower current calcium intakes than their controls.[5] In 1996, among children aged 12 to 19 years, daily calcium intake was 771 mg/d for girls and 1,145 mg/d for boys.[6] While soft drink consumption has increased dramatically, only the 2- to 8-year-old age group has an adequate intake of calcium to meet nutritional standards for age. (The adequate intake is the average amount needed to maintain a nutritional state of adequacy in nearly all members of a specific age and sex group). The lowest intakes of vitamin D from food are also in our female teens and female adults.

Previous stress fractures should prompt inquiries into menstrual history, nutritional status, bone health, and the possibility of disordered eating patterns, in addition to possible training errors and biomechanical evaluation of specific movement patterns particular to their sport. Stress fractures are commonly observed in running sports and sports for which judging is subjective and appearance is important (eg, figure skating, gymnastics).[7,8] Undernutrition impairs skeletal health, and both menstrual irregularities and low bone mineral density (BMD) increase stress fracture risk in women.[9]

An athlete with a history of stress fractures should also be queried about inadequate caloric, calcium, and vitamin D intake. The adequate intake for calcium is 1,300 mg/day for those males and females 9 to 18 years of age.[6] The recommended daily intake of vitamin D for children and adolescents was recently increased by the American Academy of Pediatrics to 400 IU/day.[10] Females should be asked about menstrual history, because inadequate caloric intake and body mass index (BMI) less than 18.5 kg/m^2 (underweight for adults >20 years old as defined by the World Health Organization [WHO]) may indicate disordered eating or the female athlete triad of disordered eating, osteoporosis or osteopenia, and amenorrhea.

Excessive training volume is a major cause of stress fractures, and the type of training schedule at the time of the stress fracture should be determined at the PPE.[11] Some athletes with eating disorders participate in excessive and addictive exercise in an attempt to control or lose weight. They may use extreme training as one way to expend calories in an attempt to improve performance or achieve a desired body shape or weight. Many compulsive exercisers will suffer from overuse injuries (with frequent muscle strains and tendonitis) and sometimes develop overtraining syndrome.

NEUROLOGIC CONDITIONS

History Form Questions

34. *Have you ever had a head injury or concussion?*

35. *Have you ever had a hit or blow to the head that caused confusion, prolonged headache, or memory problems?*

Key Points

• Female athletes have higher rates of concussion.

This topic is addressed in much greater detail in the central nervous system section (see page 58), but it is important to note that recent studies have shown that in sports played by both sexes, high school and college female athletes had higher rates of concussion than male athletes.[12]

NUTRITIONAL CONCERNS

History Form Questions

47. *Do you worry about your weight?*

48. *Are you trying to or has anyone recommended you gain or lose weight?*

49. *Are you on a special diet or do you avoid certain types of foods?*

50. *Have you ever had an eating disorder?*

Secondary Questions

- How much would you like to weigh?
- In the last year, what was your highest weight? Lowest weight?
- Have you ever tried diet pills, sitting in a sauna, diuretics, laxatives, vomiting, or similar techniques to lose weight?
- What exercises do you do in addition to training for your sport?*

*This final secondary question may elicit a response indicating the athlete might be training excessively, which may lead to overuse injuries and also excessive weight loss and menstrual disorders.[13]

Key Points

- Disordered eating is relatively common in female athletes.
- Eating disorders and energy imbalance may be associated with amenorrhea, persistent or recurrent injury, or stress fractures.
- Body mass index percentiles are age and sex specific below age 20.

Nutrition is very important in optimizing performance for the female athlete. It is well documented that some athletes, especially those in sports in which "making weight" is important and those with subjective judging, as in the aesthetic sports of gymnastics and diving, do not have adequate caloric intake. Even 5- to 7-year-old girls participating in these appearance-oriented sports reported higher weight concerns than girls involved in nonaesthetic (soccer, volleyball, tennis) and no sport groups.[14] The underweight and undernourished athlete is a concern, and the PPE is an opportune time to engage in a discussion about nutrition and weight.[15]

Athletes may falsify information about nutrition to mask weight-loss techniques. Fears of restricted athletic participation, loss of self-control, and uncovering of underlying personal stressors may make athletes leery of providing accurate information, so a useful history may be difficult to obtain. Asking gender-neutral questions is important in order to identify both male and female athletes with body weight issues. More subtle questions are also recommended so that athletes don't become defensive or deny certain conditions.[16] As more preadolescents become involved in organized sports, they are increasingly exposed to coaching and parent/guardian demands and expectations, some of which can have a negative influence on young athletes. A common type of verbal abuse in sports includes comments regarding weight and performance, including real or perceived threats to keep athletes from participating unless weight expectations are met. Identifying any external pressures on athletes to alter their weight is essential, as weight loss recommendations without proper guidance are a risk factor for the development of maladaptive weight loss behaviors.[17]

Asking about special diets or the avoidance of any food groups is another subtle way to discern whether a female athlete is at risk for disordered eating behaviors or nutritional deficiencies.[18] The extent of vegetarianism among young people with eating disorders is higher than in any other age group,[19] while college-aged women who are self-reported vegetarian are more likely to display disordered eating attitudes and behaviors than nonvegetarians.[20] Dietary fat avoidance, or the low-fat diet, may also be a predictor of eating pathology and psychosocial problems such as low self-esteem.[21] Detecting that an athlete is vegetarian or lactose intolerant also provides the opportunity to discuss iron and calcium intake. Note that several symptoms pertaining to the cardiovascular system, such as syncope or near-syncope, chest pain, or tachycardia during exercise, can also be symptoms of anemia. Iron deficiency anemia is much more common in female athletes, especially those of menstruating age. The recommended daily allowance (RDA) for elemental iron for girls aged 9 to 13 is 8 mg/day, aged 14 to 18 is 15 mg/day, and aged 19 to 50 is 18 mg/day. The RDA is increased to 33 mg/day if vegetarian. The average US diet only provides 5 to 7 mg of iron per 1,000 Kcal.[22]

Asking about a history of an eating disorder in the past tense may be a transparent question, but this question is important nonetheless, as some may not admit to any problems now, but are quite proud to indicate that they are "fully recovered" and have "beat it." However, although body fat content and overall psychosocial adjustment may be normal, most patients who recover from eating disorders still have a restricted eating pattern with nutritional intake below energy requirements.[23] Long-term studies following those diagnosed with anorexia nervosa found that almost 25% continued to have amenorrhea and almost 50% had *Diagnostic and Statistical Manual of Mental Disorders, Fourth Edition, Text Revision (DSM-IV-TR)* diagnostic criteria for an eating disorder. Bulimia nervosa had a more favorable outcome, with 23% showing a *DSM-IV-TR* eating disorder.[24,25]

Disordered eating in the adolescent and athletic population is increasing.[26] This includes a spectrum of unhealthy nutritional behaviors from inadvertent (ie, poor nutritional habits) or calculated calorie deprivation, self-induced vomiting, laxative use, diuretic use, anorexia nervosa, and bulimia nervosa to overeating. Disordered eating with calorie deprivation is most prevalent in athletes participating in sports with weight classes (eg, wrestling, rowing [crew], and judo), sports in which judging may be influenced by appearance (eg, gymnastics, figure skating, diving, dancing, and cheerleading), and sports emphasizing leanness for optimal performance (eg, track and field, distance running, and Nordic skiing).[9] However, the index of suspicion for disordered eating should be high for all types of sports, as the intensified pressure to achieve an ideal body weight or physique may not be inherent in the sport itself but rather be in the athlete's perception of what is necessary for optimal performance.[27]

The prevalence of eating disorders in elite athletes is higher than in the general population and higher in female athletes than male athletes.[8] At any given time, 10% or more of college-aged women report symptoms of eating disorders. Although these symptoms may not satisfy full diagnostic criteria, they do often cause distress. Interventions with these individuals may be helpful and may prevent the development of more serious disorders.

Body mass index is the most commonly used screening tool for obesity and correlates with percentage of body fat in most people. The relation between fatness and BMI differs with age and sex.[27] In children and teens, BMI is referred to as "BMI-for-age," and is both sex and age specific. BMI-for-age is plotted on sex-specific growth charts for children and teens aged 2 to 20 years (http://www.cdc.gov/growthcharts). Straight-calculated BMI is used to determine the weight status for adults older than 20 years, without regard to sex or age.

Body mass index for age at less than the fifth percentile is considered underweight for children and teens, and BMI less than 18.5 is classified as underweight for adults older than 20 years by the Centers for Disease Control and Prevention and the WHO.[27] Athletes below this value should undergo a thorough medical evaluation and must be counseled about proper weight and nutrition and asked about emotions related to food. All underweight athletes should be referred to a nutritionist, and strong consideration should be made for referral to a psychologist or psychiatrist for a workup and specific diagnosis. These are best made by clinicians on the basis of specific criteria from the *DSM-IV-TR*.

MENSTRUAL HISTORY

History Form Questions

52. *Have you ever had a menstrual period?*

53. *How old were you when you had your first menstrual period?*

54. *How many periods have you had in the last 12 months?*

Secondary Questions

- How much time do you usually have from the start of one period to the start of another?
- What was the longest time between periods in the last year?
- Do you frequently miss school or practices due to menstrual cramps?*
- Are you currently taking oral contraceptives?**

*Menstrual cramps or dysmenorrhea is a common problem among adolescent girls and can affect not only school attendance but sports performance. The PPE is an ideal opportunity to provide relevant information on treatment options.

**Oral contraceptives may be overlooked by athletes when answering the medication question on the medical history form. Oral contraceptives are used not only for birth control, but are also frequently used for management of irregular menstrual cycles, hypermenorrhea, or dysmenorrhea. However, their usage may actually mask the signs and symptoms of menstrual dysfunction.

Key Points

- Disordered eating is associated with menstrual dysfunction.
- Eating disorders and energy imbalance may be associated with amenorrhea, persistent or recurrent injury, or stress fractures.
- Anemia is associated with heavy or frequent menstrual cycles.

Menstrual history is important for female athletes, because menstrual cycle abnormalities may be a sign of disordered eating, pregnancy, or other gynecologic or medical conditions. A detailed menstrual history is important if answers to any of the first primary questions indicate a possible menstrual problem.

Amenorrhea, both primary and secondary, should be detected by history. Primary amenorrhea is defined as the absence of menarche at age 16. In addition, the absence of pubertal development by 14 years of age or the delay in progression of pubertal development including menarche within 2 years of starting puberty should be cause for concern. Secondary amenorrhea refers to missing at least 3 to 6 consecutive menstrual periods in a previously menstruating female; among the most common causes in athletes is pregnancy, and this should be considered as a possible cause early in the evaluation.

Athletes who are underweight should be assessed for nutritional status. Low body fat can be a factor in the development of amenorrhea and oligomenorrhea (ie, periods that occur at intervals greater than every 35 days). In the athlete, menstrual dysfunction is at least 2 to 3 times more common than in the nonathlete, and 10% to 15% of athletes have amenorrhea or oligomenorrhea.[28] Amenorrhea occurs more frequently in sports that emphasize leanness, such as running, gymnastics, and figure skating.[9]

Athletes with amenorrhea or oligomenorrhea need further evaluation. A thorough workup for other causes of menstrual disturbance should be undertaken before attributing amenorrhea to the female athlete triad or to excessive exercise. Problems that may accompany exercise-associated amenorrhea include poor nutrition, inadequate bone mineralization, and stress fractures.

Hypermenorrhea (or menorrhagia) and polymenorrhea may lead to blood loss and iron deficiency, resulting in anemia, fatigue, and poor athletic performance. Hypermenorrhea is menstruation at regular cycle intervals but with excessive flow and duration. Polymenorrhea is having menstrual cycles of greater than usual frequency. If these conditions are present, coordination of care for further workup to determine the underlying cause and investigate for possible anemia is strongly recommended. Deteriorating performance may be accompanied by physical signs such as pale conjunctiva, rapid pulse, and high-output flow murmur.

The physician should inquire about any gynecologic examinations and Pap tests, especially in females who are sexually active, and advise the athlete to follow up for health maintenance, Pap testing if sexually active for 3 or more years, and instruction in breast self-examination.

LOW IRON AND ANEMIA

Key Points

- Anemia is associated with heavy or frequent menstrual cycles and nutritional energy deficit.
- There is limited evidence to support iron supplementation for low serum ferritin levels without an associated anemia.

If an athlete presents clinically with symptoms of exertional fatigue, tachycardia, dyspnea, and headache, it may be due to iron deficiency anemia. It is clear that both endurance and performance will be impaired until the anemia is corrected, usually with oral iron supplementation over 2 to 3 months. Activity level and training should be adjusted as symptoms resolve and exercise tolerance improves. However, even after the anemia is corrected, the iron stores will still be low, and supplementation is recommended for an additional 6 months. The actual prevalence of iron deficiency anemia is 3% and is similar in athletes and nonathletes.[29]

It is commonly believed by athletes and coaches that low ferritin may adversely affect athletic performance, and there is current debate in the medical community as to whether screening tests of complete blood count and ferritin should be performed on all female athletes during their PPE. Ferritin levels of 12 ng/mL or lower correlate with lack of bone marrow iron stores, although up-regulated absorption rates have been found even with ferritin values as high as 60 ng/mL.[30] The assessment of iron status with serum ferritin levels can be falsely elevated due to variations in the ferritin levels associated with infection, inflammation, and other diseases.[31] Endurance athletes especially have a high prevalence of non-anemic iron deficiency, based on ferritin cutoff values of 12 to 20 ng/mL. Recent double-blind, placebo-controlled studies have shown that iron supplementation in iron-depleted (ferritin <16–20 ng/mL) yet non-anemic women resulted in improved performance parameters independent of an increase in hemoglobin.[29]

There are still questions regarding the appropriate ferritin level to begin iron supplementation, but most reports use a ferritin level of 30 to 35 ng/mL, with an aim to continue empirically for 6 months or until ferritin reaches 50 ng/mL.[32] Iron is best obtained through the diet as heme iron found in meat or nonheme iron from vegetables and grains. Heme iron is better absorbed than nonheme iron, but ascorbic acid and meat proteins can enhance the absorption of the latter. However, tannins (from tea), calcium, antacids, and phytates (legumes and whole grains) can decrease absorption of the nonheme iron. Ferrous iron supplements are better absorbed than the ferric iron supplements, with ferrous fumarate, ferrous sulfate, and ferrous gluconate averaging 33%, 20%, and 12% absorption, respectively. The amount absorbed is labeled as elemental iron, and supplementation above 45 mg/day of elemental iron increases the risk of gastrointestinal side effects.

■ PHYSICAL EXAMINATION

The physical examination in the PPE is a screening tool emphasizing the areas of greatest concern in the female athlete's sports participation and areas identified as problems in the female athlete's medical history. After the PPE, those athletes who have health problems and need further evaluation should follow up with the team physician performing the PPE or be referred to their primary care physician or to a specialist as indicated. While complications of eating disorders can affect every organ system, it is important to note that many female athletes who are suffering from an eating disorder may have a completely normal physical examination, especially in the early stages.

GENERAL ASSESSMENT

Ideally the female athlete should be dressed in shorts, T-shirt, and tank top or sports bra to facilitate an adequate examination. Observation of nutritional status, body fat, and clinical evidence for an eating disorder or other medical conditions should be made.

HEIGHT AND WEIGHT

Height and weight are measured and recorded in a private area, ideally with the athlete in shorts and sports bra or lightweight tank top. Some athletes will put heavy keys or coins in their pockets and wear layers of bulky clothing in order to avoid revealing their true weight. If a female athlete is noted to be extremely thin, yet the medical history yielded no positive answers, it may warrant additional questioning about recent weight loss, eating habits, or body image. Further evaluation is indicated if an eating disorder (eg, anorexia or bulimia) or growth disturbance is suspected.

Determination of body composition with skinfold calipers or other body fat measurement devices is an optional component of the PPE. It may allow estimation of an ideal weight range in sports requiring weight control, such as wrestling or lightweight crew. Additionally, calipers may more accurately measure body composition of thin athletes and more accurately represent muscular athletes, who frequently have a falsely high BMI and may inadvertently be considered obese. It is difficult, however, to predict the exact ideal percentage of body fat for a participant in a given sport. Those with abnormal BMI (verified by body composition assessment) should be further evaluated.

HEAD, EYES, EARS, NOSE, AND THROAT

Parotid gland enlargement resulting in "chipmunk cheeks" and erosion of dental enamel or excessive dental caries are signs of purging behavior. Complaints of a dry sore throat (from vomiting) can also alert the physician to bulimic behavior.

CARDIOVASCULAR SYSTEM

Athletes with significant or long-standing anorexia nervosa will be hypotensive and bradycardic (suspect if <50 bpm). Ipecac use can cause cardiomegaly. Resting heart rate may be elevated with anemia. With chronic anemia, auscultation of the hyperdynamic heart will reveal a prominent point of maximal impulse, a systolic ejection flow murmur, and occasionally an S_3 heart sound. An electrocardiogram may reveal a prolonged QT interval and/or T-wave abnormalities related to electrolyte abnormalities in bulimic individuals.

LUNGS

Pulmonary examination should reveal clear breath sounds. An athlete undergoing refeeding after a period of severe caloric restriction may experience pulmonary edema. While rare, vomiting can cause a pneumomediastinum.

ABDOMEN

In addition to the general abdominal assessment, if there is a high index of suspicion for an eating disorder, the gastrointestinal system can be more closely evaluated. Abdominal distention can result from decreased bowel motility, and stool may also be palpable in the left lower quadrant if constipated.

Epigastric pain from gastritis and gastroesophageal reflux may be present. The lower abdominal examination in the female athlete should be prefaced by a brief explanation of the reason for additional regional evaluation. This brief introduction will help establish rapport for an examination that is sensitive by nature. If necessary, a chaperone can be obtained at the athlete's discretion.

GENITALIA

The genitourinary examination in female athletes is usually not part of the PPE, unless the PPE is part of the health maintenance examination. If a pelvic examination is warranted on the basis of the athlete's medical history or physical examination, it should be scheduled for a separate time. Breast examinations are also not usually performed as part of the PPE, but it is an opportune time to educate the female athlete about the importance of routine breast self-examination.

SKIN

Abnormal skin findings may include sallow skin discoloration, dry skin and mucous membranes, loss of subcutaneous fat, cold hands and feet, and the presence of lanugo (or fine body hair). A callus on the knuckles of the dominant hand (Russell sign), from the induction of vomiting, is a physical sign associated with purging behavior.

MUSCULOSKELETAL SYSTEM

It is essential that the physician performing the musculoskeletal evaluation during a PPE has a good working knowledge of those musculoskeletal injuries for which female athletes are at increased risk.

■ DETERMINING CLEARANCE

DISORDERED EATING AND THE FEMALE ATHLETE TRIAD

When disordered eating alone or the female athlete triad (interrelated disordered eating, amenorrhea, and osteopenia or osteoporosis) is suspected, evaluation and treatment, using a multidisciplinary approach, is warranted.[9] Athletes may often be reluctant to undergo treatment, but their cooperation is imperative. Once the athlete is "cleared" for her sport, it may become even more difficult to motivate her to comply with treatment recommendations. Depending on the individual situation, clearance may be withheld until the athlete has undergone more extensive medical, psychiatric, and/or nutritional assessment. It must be stressed to the athletes, parents or guardians, and coaches that inadequate caloric intake or disordered eating behaviors may impair athletic performance and predispose the athlete to injury, particularly stress fractures.[33]

Athletic participation should be restricted when there is evidence of compromised performance or when disordered eating or the female athlete triad has threatened the athlete's health in such a way that continued participation could cause injury or deterioration of the athlete's health status. Level-of-care criteria for patients with eating disorders are outlined by the American Psychiatric Association, and include clear criteria for inpatient hospitalization (eg, vital sign criteria of temperature <36.1°C [97°F] and heart rate <40 bpm for adults and <50 bpm for children and adolescents).[34] However, if medically stable, temporary restrictions or limitations from athletic participation are often made on an individualized basis, dependent on the athlete and demands of the sport, and whether the athlete's physical or emotional health is at risk. An athlete in treatment for an eating disorder or disordered eating may be asked to sign a contract stipulating the minimum criteria to meet in order to continue participating in her sport.

Examples would include compliance with treatment, regular visits with the health care team, and modification of training. If the contract is broken, or weight or eating behavior does not improve, the athlete could be restricted from athletic participation.

Certainly the treatment goal for those athletes with disordered eating is to optimize overall nutritional status, normalize eating behavior, attain and maintain a healthy weight, manage any physical complications, modify unhealthy thought processes that maintain the disorder, treat possible emotional issues that may create a need for the disorder, and prevent the possibility of relapse.

In addition, research has emphasized the role of inadequate energy availability in the development of oligomenorrhea or amenorrhea and osteopenia or osteoporosis in athletes.[33,35] Individuals who do not display disordered eating behavior of psychological origin may develop oligomenorrhea or amenorrhea or have lower BMD simply due to inadequate caloric intake. Modifying diet and exercise in order to increase energy availability, and therefore increase body weight, may be necessary to increase BMD.[36] This increase in energy availability and subsequent increase in body weight may also restore menstrual cycles.[37,38] However, restoration of normal menstrual cycles with oral contraceptive pills (OCP) is unlikely to fully reverse the low BMD,[39] and attempts to show a reduction in fractures in women on OCP have been inconclusive.[40]

Further tests can be ordered following the initial evaluation at the PPE. While laboratory results are usually normal and should not lead to false reassurance, findings of hypokalemia from purging, diuretic use, and laxative use or hyponatremia from excessive water intake are reasons to restrict all activity and initiate immediate medical treatment. However, there is no blood test for functional hypothalamic amenorrhea; this condition can only be diagnosed by excluding other causes of amenorrhea.[9]

Vitamin D is becoming increasingly recognized for its critical role in bone health and the management of osteoporosis, although the evidence for fracture reduction is inconsistent.[41] Levels of serum 25-hydroxyvitamin D [25(OH)D] of less than 20 ng/mL are considered to be deficient, and 21 to 29 ng/mL insufficient.[42] There is also a growing consensus that the daily vitamin D intake should be increased in children to 400 IU/day [43] and in adults to 1,000 to 2,000 IU/day. Lastly, improved vitamin K status has been associated with a lower rate of bone turnover and increased bone mass in children and adults.[44]

Bone mineral density assessment by dual energy x-ray absorptiometry is warranted if there is a recurrent history of fractures or stress fractures, or history of hypoestrogenism (amenorrhea or oligomenorrhea) and disordered eating for at least 6 months.[45] The diagnosis of low BMD is based on the lowest Z-score of either the posterior-anterior (PA) spine or hip (femoral neck or total hip).[46] For those younger than 20 years, PA spine and whole body are the preferred sites of measurement.[47]

GYNECOLOGIC DISORDERS AND PREGNANCY

Because ovarian injury is so unlikely in sports, there are no restrictions for female athletes with only one ovary. Athletes with menstrual disorders should receive a complete evaluation by a physician. Such individuals should also be screened for signs of disordered eating and a history of stress fractures. A nutritional evaluation to assess the adequacy of caloric intake relative to the athlete's energy expenditure should be considered.[33,35] Athletes with oligomenorrhea or amenorrhea may usually be cleared for participation while undergoing further evaluation, but it should be emphasized to them that menstrual irregularities and low BMD increase stress fracture risk,[9] and they should be diligent to report any symptoms that appear during training. If pregnancy is suspected, a pregnancy test should be obtained. If pregnancy is documented, clearance should be determined by the clinician who is following the pregnancy. The need for routine gynecologic care in an asymptomatic individual (eg, Pap smear) is not a reason to deny or delay clearance.

■ REFERENCES

1. Beckvid Henriksson G, Schnell C, Lindén Hirschberg A. Women endurance runners with menstrual dysfunction have prolonged interruption of training due to injury. *Gynecol Obstet Invest* 2000;49(1):41–46

2. Beals KA, Manore MM. Disorders of the female athlete triad among collegiate athletes. *Int J Sport Nutr Exerc Metab.* 2002;12(3):281–293

3. Loud KJ, Micheli LJ. Common athletic injuries in adolescent girls. *Curr Opin Pediatr.* 2001;13(4):317–322

4. Khosla S, Melton LJ, Dekutoski MB, Achenbach SJ, Oberg AL, Riggs BL. Incidence of childhood distal forearm fractures over 30 years: a population-based study. *JAMA.* 2003;290(11):1479–1485

5. Goulding A, Cannan R, Williams SM, Gold EJ, Taylor RW, Lewis-Barned NJ. Bone mineral density in girls with forearm fractures. *J Bone Miner Res* 1998;13(1):143–148

6. Standing Committee on the Scientific Evaluation of Dietary Reference Intakes, Food and Nutrition Board, Institute of Medicine. *Dietary Reference Intakes for Calcium, Phosphorus, Magnesium, Vitamin D and Fluoride.* Washington, DC: The National Academies Press; 1997

7. Marx RG, Saint-Phard D, Callahan LR, Chu J, Hannafin JA. Stress fracture sites related to underlying bone health in athletic females. *Clin J Sports Med.* 2001;11(2):73–76

8. Sundgot-Borgen J, Torstveit MK. Prevalence of eating disorders in elite athletes is higher than in the general population. *Clin J Sport Med.* 2004;14(1):25–32

9. Nattiv A, Loucks AB, Manore MM, et al. American College of Sports Medicine position stand. The female athlete triad. *Med Sci Sports Exerc.* 2007;39(10):1867–1882

10. Wagner CL, Greer FR, American Academy of Pediatrics Section on Breastfeeding, American Academy of Pediatrics Committee on Nutrition. Prevention of rickets and vitamin D deficiency in infants, children and adolescents. *Pediatrics.* 2008;122(5):1142–1152

11. Harmon KG. Lower extremity stress fractures. *Clin J Sport Med.* 2003;13(6):358–364

12. Gessel LM, Fields SK, Collins CL, Dick RW, Comstock RD. Concussions among United States high school and collegiate athletes. *J Athl Train.* 2007;42(4):495–503

13. American Academy of Pediatrics Committee on Sports Medicine and Fitness. Medical concerns in the female athlete. *Pediatrics.* 2000;106(3):610–613

14. Davison KK, Earnest MB, Birch LL. Participation in aesthetic sports and girls' weight concerns at ages 5 and 7 years. *Int J Eat Disord.* 2002;31(3):312–317

15. Tanner SM. Preparticipation examination targeted for the female athlete. *Clin Sports Med.* 1994;13(2):337–353

16. Rumball JS, Lebrun CM. Preparticipation physical examination: selected issues for the female athlete. *Clin J Sport Med.* 2004;14(3):153–160

17. Sundgot-Borgen J. Risk and trigger factors for the development of eating disorders in female elite athletes. *Med Sci Sports Exerc.* 1994;26(4):414–419

18. Gonzalez VM, Vitousek KM. Feared food in dieting and non-dieting young women: a preliminary validation of the Food Phobia Survey. *Appetite.* 2004;43(2):155–173

19. Aloufy A, Latzer Y. Diet or health—the linkage between vegetarianism and anorexia nervosa [in Hebrew]. *Harefuah.* 2006;145(7):526–531, 549. Review

20. Klopp SA, Heiss CJ, Smith HS. Self-reported vegetarianism may be a marker for college women at risk for disordered eating. *J Am Diet Assoc.* 2003;103(6):745–747

21. Liebman M, Cameron BA, Carson DK, Brown DM, Meyer SS. Dietary fat reduction behaviors in college students: relationship to dieting status, gender and key psychosocial variables. *Appetite.* 2001;36(1):51–56

22. Food and Nutrition Board, Institute of Medicine. *Dietary Reference Intakes for Vitamin A, Vitamin K, Arsenic, Boron, Chromium, Copper, Iodine, Iron, Manganese, Molybdenum, Nickel, Silicon, Vanadium and Zinc.* Washington, DC: National Academy Press; 2001

23. Windauer U, Lennerts W, Talbot P, Touyz SW, Beumont PJ. How well are 'cured' anorexia nervosa patients? An investigation of 16 weight-recovered anorexic patients. *Br J Psychiatry.* 1993;163:195–200

24. Fichter MM, Quadflieg N. Twelve-year course and outcome of bulimia nervosa. *Psychol Med.* 2004;34(8):1395–1406

25. Fichter MM, Quadflieg N, Hedlund S. Twelve-year course and outcome predictors of anorexia nervosa. *Int J Eat Disord.* 2006;39(2):87–10026.

26. Grunbaum JA, Kann L, Kinchen SA, et al. Youth risk behavior surveillance—United States, 2001. *MMWR Surveill Summ.* 2002;51(4):1–62

27. Bonci CM, Bonci LJ, Granger LR, et al. National athletic trainers' association position statement: preventing, detecting, and managing disordered eating in athletes. *J Athl Train.* 2008;43(1):80–108

28. American Academy of Family Physicians, American Academy of Orthopedic Surgeons, American College of Sports Medicine, American Medical Society for Sports Medicine, American Orthopedic Society for Sports Medicine, American Osteopathic Academy of Sports Medicine. Female athlete issues for the team physician: a consensus statement. *Med Sci Sports Exerc.* 2003;35(10):1785–1793

29. Fallon KE. Utility of hematological and iron-related screening in elite athletes. *Clin J Sport Med.* 2004;14(3):145–152

30. Neilsen P, Nachtigall D. Iron supplementation in athletes. *Sports Med.* 1998;26(4):207–216

31. Suedekum NA, Dimeff RJ. Iron and the athlete. *Curr Sports Med Rep.* 2005;4(4):199–202

32. Rodenberg RE, Gustafson S. Iron as an ergogenic aid: ironclad evidence? *Curr Sports Med Rep.* 2007;6(4):258–264

33. De Souza MJ, Williams NI. Physiological aspects and clinical sequelae of energy deficiency and hypoestrogenism in exercising women. *Hum Reprod Update.* 2004;10(5):433–448

34. American Psychiatric Association. Treatment of patients with eating disorders, third edition. *Am J Psychiatry.* 2006;163(7 suppl):4–54

35. Loucks AB, Verdun M, Heath EM. Low energy availability, not stress of exercise, alters LH pulsatility in exercising women. *J Appl Physiol.* 1998;84(1):37–46

36. Dominguez J, Goodman L, Sen Gupta S, et al. Treatment of anorexia nervosa is associated with increases in bone mineral density, and recovery is a biphasic process involving both nutrition and return of menses. *Am J Clin Nutr.* 2007;86(1):92–99

37. Warren MP, Brooks-Gunn J, Fox RP, Holderness CC, Hyle EP, Hamilton WG. Osteopenia in exercise-associated amenorrhea using ballet dancers as a model: a longitudinal study. *J Clin Endocrinol Metab.* 2002;87(7):3162–3168

38. Zanker CL, Cooke CB, Truscott JG, Oldroyd B, Jacobs HS. Annual changes of bone density over 12 years in an amenorrheic athlete. *Med Sci Sports Exerc.* 2004;36(1):137–142

39. Warren MP, Brooks-Gunn J, Fox RP, et al. Persistent osteopenia in ballet dancers with amenorrhea and delayed menarche despite hormone therapy: a longitudinal study. *Fertil Steril.* 2003;80(2):398–404

40. Lopez LM, Grimes DA, Schulz KF, Curtis KM. Steroidal contraceptives: effect on bone fractures in women. *Cochrane Database Syst Rev.* 2006;4:CD006033

41. Cranney A, Horsley T, O'Donnell S, et al. Effectiveness and safety of vitamin D in relation to bone health. *Evid Rep Technol Assess (Full Rep).* 2007;158:1–235

42. Holick MF. Vitamin D status: measurement, interpretation, and clinical application. *Ann Epidemiol.* 2009;19(2):73–78

43. Roux C, Bischoff-Ferrari HA, Papapoulos SE, de Papp AE, West JA, Bouillon R. New insights into the role of vitamin D and calcium in osteoporosis management: an expert roundtable discussion. *Curr Med Res Opin.* 2008;24(5):1363–1370

44. van Summeren MJ, van Coeverden SC, Schurgers LJ, et al. Vitamin K status is associated with childhood bone mineral content. *Br J Nutr.* 2008;100(4):852–858

45. Khan AA, Hanley DA, Bilezikian JP, et al. Standards for performing DXA in individuals with secondary causes of osteoporosis. *J Clin Densitom.* 2006;9(1):47–57

46. Hans D, Downs RW Jr, Duboeuf F, et al. Skeletal sites for osteoporosis diagnosis: the 2005 ISCD Official Positions. *J Clin Densitom.* 2006;9(1):15–21

47. Khan AA, Bachrach L, Brown JP, et al. Standards and guidelines for performing central dual-energy x-ray absorptiometry in premenopausal women, men, and children. *J Clin Densitom.* 2004;7(1):51–64

CHAPTER 7

The Athlete With Special Needs

Athletes with special needs (physical and cognitive disabilities) represent a growing population of sports participants. Federal legislation mandating equal access and equal opportunity to physical education and sports for persons with special needs as well as extraordinary accomplishments by athletes with special needs have ignited this growth.[1]

The Americans with Disabilities Act defines a disability as impairment that limits a major life activity.[2] Types of disabilities include cerebral palsy, blindness, deafness, paralysis, intellectual disabilities, and amputation, as well as other disabilities that affect multiple systems such as autoimmune-mediated arthritis, muscular dystrophy, and multiple sclerosis.

Today there are more than 21 million Americans with a physical disability. During the past several years thousands of military personnel have sustained serious injuries resulting in disabilities. These and all individuals at the secondary school and college level with special needs should have the opportunity to participate and compete in sports activities.

■ BENEFITS OF SPORTS

Sports participation for athletes with special needs provides the same benefits as for athletes without special needs: increased exercise endurance, muscle strength, and flexibility; improved cardiovascular function, balance, and motor skills; and psychological benefits including increased self-esteem, reduced anxiety and depression, and the satisfaction derived from participation and competition. In addition, some benefits from sports participation are unique to the athlete with special needs (Box 7-1).[3]

Box 7-1. Benefits of Sports Participation Unique to Those With Special Needs (Compared With Inactive Counterparts)

Athletes With Paraplegia	Athletes With Amputations
Fewer pressure ulcers Fewer infections Lower likelihood of hospitalization	Improved proprioception Increased proficiency using prosthetic devices

■ Preparticipation Physical Evaluation (PPE) for Special Needs

The PPE for the athlete with special needs should be similar to that of an athlete without a physical or cognitive disability. In addition, the PPE should address the particular concerns of the athlete with special needs. The health care provider should be aware of common problems associated with different disabilities and be able to diagnose abnormalities that may endanger the athlete. Just as important, the health care provider should provide support and encourage physical activity.

Athletes with special needs are classified according to the severity of their disability. To promote fairness in competition, athletes with similar degrees of disability compete against one another.

■ Competitions for the Physically or Cognitively Impaired

Several states have physically impaired (PI) and cognitively impaired (CI) competition groupings at the high school level. The criteria for inclusion in these groups are defined by each state and are reviewed below. The fairness of the competitions requires that the qualification criteria are strictly defined and enforced, because individuals who are more qualified than the inclusion criteria allow upset the balance of competition and raise the risk of injury to the other competitors.

Physically impaired. Physically impaired competition criteria require that there is an actual physical functional limitation that interferes with participation in regular competition, such as a neuromuscular, postural, skeletal, traumatic, growth, or neurologic impairment or loss of limb that significantly impairs physical functioning, modifies gait patterns, or requires mobility devices. Physically impaired competition is not for those who do not qualify for CI competition or cannot make the cut for regular competition without some form of physical limitation. In Minnesota, high school PI competition specifically excludes asthma, diabetes mellitus, seizure disorder, attention-deficit disorder, Tourette syndrome, autistic spectrum disorders, deafness, blindness, obesity, and similar maladies that may interfere with regular competition but do not involve an actual physical impairment unless physical impairment can be demonstrated in sports settings.

Cognitively impaired. Cognitively impaired competition is for individuals with lower IQ levels, commonly less than 70. A physical handicap is not a prerequisite for CI competition, and participants with higher IQ levels than the prescribed cutoff could dominate the events. These athletes enjoy the competition and social nature of the events and deserve to participate on a "level playing field" with others of similar cognitive ability.

Special Olympics and Paralympics. The Special Olympics and the United States Paralympics, a division of the United States Olympic Committee, have organized sports events for athletes with special needs. In the community setting, athletes participate in Special Olympics and Paralympics competitions. Each organization has its own set of governing rules and inclusion criteria for competition.

Special Olympics is an international organization dedicated to empowering individuals aged 8 years and older with intellectual disabilities to become physically fit through sports training and competition.[4] Special Olympics offers year-round training and competition in 30 summer and winter sports. The Special Olympics has requirements for PPE assessment that include radiographic imaging for atlantoaxial instability (AAI) in asymptomatic Down syndrome (trisomy 21) competitors.

The Special Olympics currently serves more than 2.5 million people who have intellectual disabilities in more than 200 programs in more than 180 countries. Since 2000, Special Olympics has had tremendous growth and has transformed itself into a more global organization. This means that more physicians will encounter increasing numbers of Special Olympians who will seek PPEs and sports-related medical and surgical care.

The Special Olympics are arranged at local, state, national, and international levels, and participation requires a PPE.[5] Depending on the state or level of competition, the PPE needs to be performed every 1 to 3 years. Special Olympics World Games, for example, requires a PPE to be performed within 12 months of a competition.

International Paralympics assigns numerical rank to the level of disability. Teams need to stay within a defined sum of the grades to compete. If a 2-person sailboat can have a team total of 8; a 2 can pair with a 6, a 3 can pair with a 5, and a 4 can pair with a 4. Again, this provides fair participation. Accurate assessment of ability is critical to fair competition.

United States Paralympics features competition in more than 20 sports and provides funding and facilities for athletes with physical disabilities.[6] The Paralympic Games are held every Olympic year and provide competitions in Summer and Winter Games. The 2008 Beijing Summer Paralympics Games had more than 4,000 athletes from 150 countries and regions competing in 20 sports. New technology applied to prosthetic and assistive devices allows increasingly more physically impaired athletes to participate at higher levels of competition.

■ METHODS OF EVALUATION

The office-based PPE is preferred to the station-based or mass screening examination. The decreased mobility of some athletes with special needs makes the station method less practical. The PPE should be performed by a health care provider involved in the longitudinal care of the athlete as described in Chapter 3. Specialty consultations are sometimes necessary.

■ THE PPE MEDICAL HISTORY

As in the general PPE guidelines, a thorough medical history is essential for the provider to develop an informed participation recommendation (see sample PPE history form for athletes with special needs on page 154). The history form should be completed by the athlete (if possible) and parents or guardians familiar with the athlete's medical history. In addition, a parent or guardian may need to be present at the time of the PPE in order to obtain the most accurate answers to questions. This is especially true for athletes participating in the Special Olympics.

The history should include a detailed summary of previous injuries and illnesses, risk factors for injuries and illnesses, and current medications.

Questions. In addition to the questions asked of an athlete without a physical or cognitive disability (see Chapter 5 and the history form on page 153), questions in the history of an athlete with special needs should be individualized and address the particular disability. The questions that follow emphasize areas of greatest concern for sports participation.

1. *Does the athlete have a history of seizures? Are the seizures controlled?* These are common abnormalities seen in Special Olympics and Paralympics athletes.[7] Uncontrolled seizures often require a consultation with a neurologist and a delay in clearing the athlete for sports participation.

2. *Does the athlete have a history of hearing loss?*

3. *Does the athlete have a history of vision loss?*

4. *Does the athlete have a history of cardiopulmonary disease?* Congenital cardiac disorders, including heart murmurs, ventricular septal defects, and endocardial cushion defects, are more common in persons with Down syndrome and may limit participation.

5. *Does the athlete have a history of renal disease or unilateral kidney?* Various renal anomalies, such as hypoplasia, dysplasia, and obstruction, are common in people with Down syndrome,[8] and many athletes with disabilities may have other congenital or acquired renal abnormalities such as diabetic nephropathy.

6. *Does the athlete have a history of atlantoaxial instability?* Spontaneous or traumatic subluxation of the cervical spine is a potential risk in athletes with Down syndrome.[9]

7. *Has the athlete had heatstroke or heat exhaustion?* Thermoregulation in athletes with spinal cord injuries is impaired because of skeletal muscular paralysis and a loss of autonomic nervous system control.[10] Medications used for pain and bladder dysfunction can interfere with the normal sweat response. Also, athletes who have had a history of heat illness are more prone to redevelop the condition.

8. *Has the athlete had any fractures or dislocations?* Ligamentous laxity and joint hypermobility are prominent features in athletes with Down syndrome and Ehlers-Danlos syndrome. Wheelchair athletes can have premature osteoporosis.[11]

9. *What prosthetic devices or special equipment does the athlete use during sports participation?* Health care providers need to be aware of an athlete's need for adaptive equipment and regulations concerning their use in different sports.

10. *Does the athlete use an indwelling urinary catheter or require intermittent catheterization of the bladder?* Athletes with spinal cord injuries or other neurologic disorders often have bladder dysfunction or neurogenic bladders and may suffer from frequent urinary tract infections.

11. *Does the athlete have a history of pressure sores or ulcers?* Athletes who use wheelchairs are prone to pressure ulcers at the sacrum and ischial tuberosities, and athletes who use prostheses are prone to pressure ulcers at prosthesis sites.

12. *At what levels of competition has the athlete previously participated?*

13. *What is the athlete's level of independence for mobility and self-care?*

14. *What medication(s) is the athlete taking?*

15. *Is the athlete on a special diet?*

16. *Does the athlete have a history of autonomic dysreflexia?* This is an acute, potentially life-threatening syndrome of excessive, uncontrolled sympathetic output that can occur in athletes with spinal cord injuries at or above the sixth thoracic spinal cord level.[12] This reflex may happen spontaneously or may be self-induced ("boosting") by an athlete in an attempt to improve performance.[13] Triggers for autonomic dysreflexia include bowel or bladder distention, infections (especially of the urinary tract), sunburn, ingrown toenails, and wearing tight garments. Signs and symptoms of autonomic dysreflexia include excessively high blood pressure, a pounding headache, sweating above the level of spinal injury, flushed face, and bradycardia.

Boosting is a dangerous performance-enhancing technique that is strictly forbidden by all sports governing bodies. Athletes with spinal cord injuries at T-6 or above sometimes use this technique in an effort to improve cardiopulmonary performance, oxygen utilization, and noradrenaline release.[3] Methods of boosting include occluding one's own urinary catheter, ingesting large amounts of fluids prior to an event to extend the bladder, use of tight leg straps, and sitting on sharp objects.[3,5]

■ THE PPE PHYSICAL EXAMINATION

The PPE physical examination for the athlete with a special need should include all parts of the examination as for the athlete without a physical or intellectual disability (see Chapter 5 and the physical examination form on page 155). Particular attention should be given to the visual, cardiovascular, musculoskeletal, neurologic, and dermatologic systems (Box 7-2).

Box 7-2. Findings to Screen for When Performing Physical Examinations on Athletes With Special Needs

Vision Poor visual acuity Refractive errors Astigmatism Strabismus
Cardiovascular System Congenital heart disease

Neurologic System
Peripheral nerve entrapment
    Carpal tunnel syndrome
    Ulnar neuropathy (cubital tunnel, Guyon canal)
Inadequate motor control
Inadequate coordination and balance
Impaired hand-eye coordination
Ataxia
Muscle weakness
Fatigue
Spasticity
Sensory dysfunction
Atlantoaxial instability
Hyperreflexia
Clonus
Upper motor neuron and posterior column signs and symptoms

Dermatologic System Abrasions Lacerations Blisters Pressure ulcers Rashes
Musculoskeletal System Limited neck range of motion Torticollis Decreased flexibility, often with contractures, decreased strength, and muscle strength imbalance Pelvic dysfunction due to lower extremity prosthetic use (unequal leg lengths) Rotator cuff tendonitis and impingement in wheelchair athletes Wrist extensor tendonitis in wheelchair athletes

In addition to examining the athlete, health care providers or the athlete's prosthetist should thoroughly inspect all prostheses, orthoses, and assistive or adaptive devices to ensure adequate construction for sports participation and proper fit.[14]

Vision. Eye examinations of Special Olympics athletes reveal a high prevalence of vision abnormalities. A study of Special Olympics athletes at the 1995 International Summer Games revealed that almost one-third of the athletes had ocular problems.[15] The most common problems identified were poor visual acuity, refractive errors, astigmatism, and strabismus.

Cardiovascular system. Congenital heart disease is present in as many as 50% of athletes with Down syndrome.[16] Many of these athletes may require further testing (eg, electrocardiogram, echocardiogram) or clearance from a cardiologist before participating in sports. Decisions for further testing or consultation should follow the same guidelines as for the athlete without a disability.

Neurologic system. Since many athletes with special needs have some form of neurologic deficit, a complete neurologic evaluation should be performed.

Peripheral nerve entrapment syndromes of the upper extremities are common in wheelchair athletes. Two of the most common entrapment syndromes are carpal tunnel syndrome and ulnar neuropathy at the wrist (Guyon tunnel syndrome). The examiner should look for signs of muscle atrophy and weakness in the hand, test for sensory deficits following a specific nerve distribution, and perform provocative tests such as Tinel's sign over the median and ulnar nerves in the wrist.

Athletes with autism spectrum disorders often have motor clumsiness and apraxia, placing them at increased risk for injuries.[17]

Athletes with cerebral palsy frequently have inadequate motor control and lack adequate coordination and balance for participation in certain sports. Hand-eye coordination can also be impaired. Evaluating these functions will reveal whether sports requiring catching, throwing, and controlling equipment such as floor hockey sticks, rackets, and bats will be difficult or even dangerous to the athlete or other competitors.

Athletes with multiple sclerosis have varying degrees of disability. The examiner should check for ataxia, muscle weakness, fatigue, spasticity, and sensory dysfunction.

Approximately 15% of children with Down syndrome have AAI,[9] almost all of whom are asymptomatic. A very small number of these children develop signs and symptoms of cervical cord myelopathy. The neurologic manifestations of symptomatic AAI include easy fatigue, abnormal gait, incoordination and clumsiness, sensory deficits, spasticity, hyperreflexia, clonus, and other upper motor neuron and posterior column signs and symptoms. Other conditions at increased risk for AAI include rheumatoid arthritis, achondroplastic dwarfism (skeletal dysplasia), and Klippel-Feil syndrome. Children with skeletal dysplasias often have associated cervical spine instability with serious danger of spinal cord compression.[18] General screening must include a history and physical examination with a focus on the neurologic assessment. Radiographic screening (generally lateral cervical spine with flexion and extension views) for AAI in asymptomatic athletes is controversial, because there is little evidence to suggest it is a significant risk factor for symptomatic AAI. The condition appears as a space larger than 5 mm between the posterior aspect of the anterior arch of the atlas and the odontoid. Neurologic signs and symptoms (Box 7-3)[9] may be more predictive of risk of injury progression than are radiographic abnormalities in asymptomatic patients.

Dermatologic system. Athletes in wheelchairs are especially prone to skin injuries. The upper extremities should be examined for abrasions and blisters caused by friction, shear, and irritation from repeated contact with the wheelchair push rim. Skin wounds can also result from contact with other chairs, wheelchair brakes, or sharp edges of the wheelchair.

Box 7-3. Common Signs and Symptoms of Symptomatic Atlantoaxial Instability

Easy fatigability	Sensory deficits
Difficulty in walking	Spasticity
Abnormal gait	Hyperreflexia
Neck pain	Clonus
Limited neck mobility	Extensor-plantar reflex
Torticollis	Upper motor neuron signs and symptoms
Incoordination	Posterior column signs and symptoms

The skin over the sacrum and ischial tuberosities should be inspected for pressure ulcers. Athletes in wheelchairs have elevated skin pressures in these regions for prolonged periods during training, competition, and normal daily activity. Sports wheelchairs are designed so that the athlete's knees are at a higher level than the buttocks, a position that leads to increased pressure over the sacrum and ischial tuberosities.[1] During sports participation, the combination of skin pressure, shear, and moisture increases the risk for pressure ulcers. Athletes in wheelchairs who have a pressure ulcer should not be cleared for sports participation until there is complete healing of the wound. The chair seat should be modified to decrease the risk of future skin trauma.

Prostheses can cause skin trauma; the prosthesis site should be inspected for abrasions, blisters, rashes, and pressure ulcers. The presence of pressure ulcers usually precludes participation in sports until the condition has resolved. The prosthesis should be evaluated for proper fit and reconditioned to decrease the risk of future problems. In the skeletally immature athlete, overgrowth of the stump can be a problem leading to breakdown of the overlying skin and soft tissues.[14]

Genitourinary system. Examination should involve the same evaluation as for athletes without a disability, as well as any external devices used for bladder drainage.

Musculoskeletal system. The musculoskeletal examination of an athlete who uses a wheelchair should include evaluation of the stability, flexibility, and strength of commonly injured sites (eg, shoulder, hand, and wrist) and the trunk.[3]

Athletes with lower limb amputation and prostheses require a full assessment of the lower back, pelvis, and lower extremities. These are common areas of injury resulting from abnormal forces and motions placed during sports activities.

Musculoskeletal manifestations of AAI in athletes with Down syndrome include limited range of motion of the neck and torticollis or head tilt. Because of hypermobility and ligamentous laxity, athletes with Down syndrome have an increased incidence of hip and knee injuries.[16] Examination may reveal signs of instability and weakness.

As many as 78% of people with spinal cord injuries who are wheelchair users report having shoulder pain at some time. Shoulder pain has been reported more commonly in nonathletic wheelchair users compared to wheelchair athletes.[19]

Athletes with cerebral palsy have decreased musculotendinous flexibility, often with contractures, decreased strength, and muscle strength imbalances, especially of the lower extremities, that vary in severity from mild and nearly imperceptible to very severe and wheelchair bound.[1] Overuse injuries, strains, and sprains are common, especially at the hips, knees, ankles, and feet. The PPE should include a thorough examination of these regions.

■ FUNCTIONAL ASSESSMENT

An individualized functional assessment of all athletes with special needs should be part of the PPE. An athlete's overall mobility while using prosthetic, orthotic, assistive, or adaptive devices should be evaluated. Sport-specific tasks should also be incorporated into the evaluation. A physical therapist or occupational therapist with expertise in the area can assist with this portion of the evaluation.

■ DIAGNOSTIC IMAGING

Athletes with symptomatic AAI should have cervical spine radiographic imaging to assess the extent of the problem. Radiographs of the lateral cervical spine with adequate flexion and extension views assess the space between the posterior aspect of the anterior arch of the atlas and the odontoid.[20]

Despite the lack of evidence confirming the value of these radiographs in asymptomatic athletes with Down syndrome and AAI, the Special Olympics requires that athletes with Down syndrome competing in certain sports and events have a radiologic evaluation for AAI. The Special Olympics has chosen an atlanto-dens interval (ADI) of greater than 4.5 mm for the diagnosis of atlantoaxial subluxation in children. An ADI greater than 2.5 mm is consistent with atlantoaxial subluxation in adults. The events for which such a radiologic examination is required are listed in Box 7-4.[21]

Box 7-4. High-Risk Sports in Patients With Atlantoaxial Instability[a]

Judo	High jump
Equestrian sports	Alpine skiing
Gymnastics	Snowboarding
Diving	Squat lift
Pentathalon	Soccer
Butterfly stroke and diving starts in swimming	

[a]From: Special Olympics General Rules (Section 6.02, page 50). Special Olympics, 2004. http://www.specialolympics.org/uploadedFiles/2003%20General%20Rules.pdf. Accessed September 25, 2009.

■ DETERMINING CLEARANCE

Clearance for sports participation should follow the same principles as for athletes without physical or intellectual disabilities (see Chapter 5). Many of the abnormalities identified by history and physical examination will not preclude the athlete from participating in sports. Instead, conditions identified may need further evaluation, treatment, or rehabilitation before final clearance is granted similar to the athlete without special needs. The PPE for children with special needs will rarely be completed in a single office visit. A multidisciplinary approach involving subspecialists, physical and occupational therapists, and an adaptive physical education specialist may be needed to determine clearance and safe participation. The multidisciplinary team needs to assess the safety of a given sport for an athlete with special needs. The athlete's medical condition, functional abilities, and the demands of the sport need to be considered in the decision.

Athletes with AAI should be restricted from sports that require excessive neck flexion or extension.[9] See Box 7-4 for a list of those sports.

Pressure sores are common occurrences in athletes using prostheses or wheelchairs.[22] Athletes with pressure sores should not be cleared for sports participation until there is complete healing at the involved sites.

■ REFERENCES

1. Halpern BC, Cardone DA. The athlete with a disability. In: Safran MR, McKeag DB, Van Camp SP, eds. *Manual of Sports Medicine*. Philadelphia, PA: Lippincott-Raven; 1998:190–198

2. Nichols AW. Sports medicine and the Americans with Disabilities Act. *Clin J Sport Med*. 1996;6(3):190–195

3. Malanga GA, Bloomgarden J, Filart R, Cheng J. Athletes with disabilities. http://www.eMedicine.com/sports/topic144.htm. Accessed February 3, 2009

4. Special Olympics. http://www.specialolympics.org. Accessed February 3, 2009

5. Klenck C, Gebke K. Practical management: common medical problems in disabled athletes. *Clin J Sport Med*. 2007;17(1):55–60

6. US Paralympics. http://www.usparalympics.org. Accessed February 3, 2009

7. McCormick DP, Ivey FM Jr, Gold DM, Zimmerman DM, Gemma S, Owen MJ. The preparticipation sports examination in Special Olympics athletes. *Tex Med*. 1988;84(4):39–43

8. Mercer ES, Broecker B, Smith EA, Kirsch AJ, Scherz HC, Massad C. Urological manifestations of Down syndrome. *J Urol*. 2004;171(3):1250–1253

9. American Academy of Pediatrics Committee on Sports Medicine and Fitness. Atlantoaxial instability in Down syndrome. *Pediatrics*. 1995;96(1 pt 1):151–154

10. Price MJ, Campbell IG. Effects of spinal cord lesion level upon thermoregulation during exercise in the heat. *Med Sci Sports Exerc*. 2003;35(7):1100–1107

11. Jiang SD, Jiang LS, Dai LY. Mechanisms of osteoporosis in spinal cord injury. *Clin Endocrinol*. 2006;65(5):555–565

12. Blackmer J. Rehabilitation medicine: 1. Autonomic dysreflexia. *CMAJ*. 2003;169(9):931–935

13. Boosting and autonomic dysreflexia. In: *International Paralympic Committee Handbook*. Bonn, Germany: 2002; section II, Chapter 8. http://servicios.conade.gob.mx/DOCS_NORMATECA/259_5B8E149330684AAC98DA93ED3262C185.pdf. Accessed February 4, 2009

14. Patel DR, Greydanus DE. The pediatric athlete with disabilities. *Pediatr Clin North Am*. 2002;49(4):803–827

15. Block SS, Beckerman SA, Berman PE. Vision profile of the athletes of the 1995 Special Olympics World Summer Games. *J Am Optom Assoc*. 1997;68(11):699–708

16. Winell J, Burke SW. Sports participation of children with Down syndrome. *Orthop Clin North Am*. 2003;34(3):439–443

17. Ramirez M, Yang J, Bourque L, et al. Sports injuries to high school athletes with disabilities. *Pediatrics*. 2009;123(2):690–696

18. Svensson O, Aaro S. Cervical instability in skeletal dysplasia. Report of 6 surgically fused cases. *Acta Orthop Scand*. 1988;59(1):66–70

19. Fullerton HD, Borckardt JJ, Alfano AP. Shoulder pain: a comparison of wheelchair athletes and nonathletic wheelchair users. *Med Sci Sports Exerc*. 2003;35(12):1958–1961

20. Tassone JC, Duey-Holtz A. Spine concerns in the Special Olympian with Down syndrome. *Sports Med Arthrosc*. 2008;16(1):55–60

21. Special Olympics General Rules (Section 6.02, page 50). Special Olympics, 2004. http://www.specialolympics.org/uploaded-Files/2003%20General%20Rules.pdf. Accessed September 25, 2009.

22. Dec KL, Sparrow KJ, McKeag DB. The physically-challenged athlete: medical issues and assessment. *Sports Med*. 2000;29(4):245–258

CHAPTER 8

Research

It is important to recognize that the evidence base for the preparticipation physical evaluation (PPE) is limited. While there has been progress in our understanding of the PPE, much work is needed to develop a sound knowledge base to improve the PPE content and process. The purpose of this chapter is to present questions, rather than recommendations. It is intended to highlight some areas where further investigation is needed and to stimulate more thought about how to improve the PPE.

■ HISTORY

As discussed previously, studies of preparticipation screening consistently demonstrate the essential role of the history. Between 65% to 77% of medical and musculoskeletal conditions identified during the PPE are elicited from the history[1-4] (level of evidence=B; see Table 1-1 on page 4). This is true despite limitations due to recall bias and other issues that may affect the accuracy of the history.[2,5]

The questionnaire put forth in this monograph represents the best attempt of the author societies to incorporate the available medical evidence and consensus opinion; however, few of the individual questions have been studied or scientifically validated.

Thus, although the history in its current and previous forms has proven to be quite valuable, there is a great need to refine the questionnaire. Systematic study of the questionnaire to describe which questions most frequently elicit positive or negative responses, the sensitivity and specificity of the questions for evaluating the issue of concern, and which questions may be simply misinterpreted is needed. Because such findings likely will vary depending on the group being examined (children, high school students, college students, or professional athletes), research in one athlete population may not be applicable to others. In addition, developing questions for the PPE that are of acceptable sensitivity for areas of concern for the athlete (eg, concussion, cardiovascular conditions, exercise-induced bronchospasm [EIB], disordered eating, musculoskeletal injuries) would be ideal. Finally, studying these issues among specific groups of athletes will be helpful in developing features of the history that might be tailored to individual sports or populations, including adolescents and female athletes.[6,7]

■ PHYSICAL EXAMINATION

The physical examination remains an integral part of the PPE. Research has clearly shown that blood pressure and visual acuity are among the most common abnormalities identified during the PPE[1-3,8-11] (level of evidence=B). The yield of other components of the physical examination is less well established. Recording of body mass index (BMI) should be considered during PPE screening. While it is clear that an elevated BMI may indicate the presence of comorbidities and increases the risk for the development of several clinical conditions such as hypertension and diabetes mellitus type 2, few data address these issues in young athletes. Further, recent data have shown that waist circumference and measures of abdominal adiposity are independent predictors of morbidity and mortality in the general population, and should be considered in addition to the measurement of BMI.[12] Thus research of the effects of BMI and waist circumference in this population is needed. Furthermore, the potential interactive effects of body composition, BMI, and waist circumference have not been well studied in young athletes. Research evaluating the role of BMI and waist circumference with respect to the risk of musculoskeletal injury and heat illness, for example, may allow the physician to provide specific recommendations for prevention and monitoring of these conditions.

The components of the screening medical examination are much the same as that traditionally performed as part of a well-child check or complete physical examination for an adult. The cardiovascular examination is the most pertinent to the PPE. The American Heart Association (AHA) has published guidelines for the screening of competitive athletes that lists recommended components of the cardiovascular examination[13] (see Cardiovascular Problems section of Chapter 6 on page 39). Further research that establishes the efficacy of the cardiovascular history, examination, and screening studies in the US population is needed (see below).

The value of the musculoskeletal screening examination deserves further analysis. This examination, originally described by Garrick and Reque,[14] is designed primarily to identify asymmetries that may indicate an underlying injury or an imbalance that might predispose to injury. Current research reveals that most musculoskeletal conditions can be identified from the questionnaire[1-4,15] (level of evidence=B). However, the overall sensitivity of the musculoskeletal screening physical *examination* has been reported to be low (50%).[15,16] The effectiveness of this aspect of the PPE may be highly dependent on age of the participant, level of competition, and the sport involved. Perhaps more importantly, there is little evidence that findings identified in an asymptomatic individual on the musculoskeletal screening examination predict injury susceptibility.[16] Ideally, research in this area would lead to physical examination findings that would predict injury risk and interventions such as specific training programs that would decrease the injury risk.

■ SCREENING STUDIES

The implementation of screening studies as part of the PPE remains controversial. Various measures, including laboratory tests (sickle cell trait, hemoglobin, and others), pulmonary evaluation for EIB, and cardiac screening, have been proposed. Part of the controversy centers on whether the studies are used truly for "screening" or as diagnostic (case finding) tests. The value of a screening test or procedure depends on 2 variables: (1) the predictive value of the proposed screen, which is in turn affected by the prevalence of the condition in the population being screened, and (2) the ability to reduce morbidity and mortality once a condition has been identified with the screening method. The screening test must also be acceptable in terms of cost and potential side effects, including false-positive tests, which may temporarily or indefinitely remove the athlete from participation. The value of a diagnostic test, on the other hand, is in its ability to pinpoint a condition for which suspicion already exists based on history or physical examination.

When evaluating screening tests with the aforementioned criteria, studies have not supported general screening with tests such as urinalysis, complete blood count, chemistry profile, or lipid profile in the PPE.[17-21]

Exertional sickling leading to acute rhabdomyolysis has caused several deaths in competitive athletes.[22] This has led to discussion regarding screening for sickle cell trait during the PPE. At this time, evidence that screening for sickle cell trait prevents death from exertional sickling is not available.[22] Nonetheless, when documented newborn screening results are not known, some institutions have chosen to perform laboratory screening in order to confirm sickle cell trait status despite the current lack of data regarding its effectiveness. In addition, recent publications from organizations including the NCAA recommend screening for sickle cell trait if sickle cell trait status is not already known.[22,23] While further research is needed, institutions should educate staff, coaches, and athletes concerning recognition of this condition and prevention of possible complications.[22] Institutions should carefully consider screening when sickle cell trait status is not known.[22,23]

Another area of interest with respect to laboratory screening concerns iron deficiency. While it is well established that iron deficiency with accompanying anemia impairs athletic performance, the effects of iron deficiency in the absence of anemia is less clear.[24,25] Recent studies, however, have suggested that iron deficiency may indicate a "relative anemia" in some athletes, as evidenced by improvements in performance parameters among those receiving iron supplementation.[26-30] While more research is needed to clarify this question, this is of particular interest among female athletes, among whom the prevalence of iron deficiency is higher.[31] In one recent study, 19% of elite female athletes were found to have a serum ferritin of less than 30.[32] Nonetheless, the same study found that in most circumstances iron deficiency is accompanied by clinical findings that can be detected with a preparticipation history and examination.[32] Thus the value of ferritin screening in the absence of clinical symptoms or findings seems to be of low yield.

Cardiac screening beyond the essential components of the history and physical examination remains controversial. As discussed in the preceding chapters, there are significant limitations to the current literature involving the routine use of electrocardiogram and/or echocardiography in the screening of athletes. Some of these limitations involve the low prevalence of cardiac conditions that can result in sudden death and genetic variations among populations at risk. Other important issues include the cost of screening on a national basis, the number and outcomes of false-positive tests, and perhaps even sport-specific issues. These areas all deserve further attention.

Exercise-induced bronchospasm has a relatively high prevalence among athletes that varies by sport. For example, recent screens of elite runners revealed 10% of the men and 26% of the women had EIB.[33] Studies of athletes competing in winter sports have demonstrated positive tests for approximately 50% of figure skaters[34,35] and 79% of cross-country skiers.[36] The prevalence of EIB in Olympic athletes is estimated as high as 20%, with a significant number of these athletes undiagnosed.[37]

Although the condition is prevalent, a screening method that is sensitive and specific is lacking. Exercise challenge testing in the competition environment or eucapneic hyperventilation testing, both of which are more sensitive than the history and physical examination alone, may be necessary to identify the disorder.[38] However, unless large studies indicate that these tests can efficiently and inexpensively be incorporated into the PPE, they are not likely to be recommended. Studies that focus on specific populations at greatest risk, such as cross-country skiing, are needed to further develop screening options for EIB.

■ STANDARDIZATION OF THE PPE

The success of performing the PPE lies not only in how effective the components of the evaluation are in achieving the goals of the PPE, but also in ensuring that it is consistently implemented. Although nearly all states have an approved form for the PPE, the content of the forms used continues to vary.[39]

The cardiovascular screening portion of the PPE has been the most frequently studied. Since the initial AHA recommendations for cardiovascular screening were published in 1996, the number of states incorporating these guidelines has increased.[40] The status of the other aspects of PPE is less established. As the content of the PPE is evaluated and updated, the extent of the implementation of these recommendations among adolescent, collegiate, and elite/professional athletes warrants further study.

■ ELECTRONIC PPE

Web-based electronic versions of the PPE have been proposed as a means to improve not only the efficiency of screening athletes, but also as a method to provide a more extensive questionnaire that can be used to identify conditions that require further evaluation.[41,42] Preparticipation physical evaluation screening performed in this manner will also allow for the development of databases that can be used to prospectively analyze the effectiveness of each component of the questionnaire. In addition, this technique has the potential to facilitate the standardization of the PPE. Establishing electronic databases holds much promise in not only improving and standardizing the PPE process, but also in optimizing the follow-up and ongoing medical care for athletes who have had a condition identified during the PPE.

■ CONCLUSION

Research that substantiates the value of the content and format of the PPE remains limited. In order to provide an evidenced-based approach for the PPE and to standardize the examination, more research is clearly needed. The issues cited in this chapter are intended to generate further discussion that will hopefully lead to studies that expand the scientific basis for the PPE. This, coupled with the clinical skill and experience of the physicians who implement it, will serve to improve the PPE and ultimately enhance the health and safety of the millions of adolescents and young adults participating in athletic activities in the United States.

■ REFERENCES

1. Goldberg B, Saraniti A, Witman P, Gavin M, Nicholas JA. Pre-participation sports assessment: an objective evaluation. *Pediatrics*. 1980;66(5):736–745
2. Risser WL, Hoffman HM, Bellah GG Jr. Frequency of preparticipation sports examinations in secondary school athletes: are the University Interscholastic League guidelines appropriate? *Tex Med*. 1985;81(7):35–39
3. Lively MW. Preparticipation physical examinations: a collegiate experience. *Clin J Sport Med*. 1999;9(1):3–8
4. Chun J, Haney S, DiFiori JP. The relative contributions of the history and physical examination in the preparticipation evaluation of collegiate student-athletes. *Clin J Sport Med*. 2006;16(5):437–438
5. Carek PJ, Futrell M, Hueston WJ. The preparticipation physical examination history: who has the correct answers? *Clin J Sport Med*. 1999;9(3):124–128
6. Batt ME, Jaques R, Stone M. Preparticipation examination (screening): practical issues as determined by sport. A United Kingdom perspective. *Clin J Sport Med*. 2004;14(3):178–182
7. Rumball JS, Lebrun CM. Preparticipation physical examination. Selected issues for the female athlete. *Clin J Sport Med*. 2004;14(3):153–160
8. Tennant FS Jr, Sorenson K, Day CM. Benefits of preparticipation sports examinations. *J Fam Pract*. 1981;13(2):287–288
9. Thompson TR, Andrish JT, Bergfeld JA. A prospective study of preparticipation sports examinations of 2670 young athletes: method and results. *Cleve Clin Q*. 1982 Winter;49(4):225–233
10. Magnes SA, Henderson JM, Hunter SC. What conditions limit sports participation: experience with 10,540 athletes. *Phys Sportsmed*. 1992;20(3):143–158

11. Dixit S, DiFiori JP. Prevalence of hypertension and prehypertension among collegiate student-athletes. *Clin J Sport Med.* 2006;16(5):440

12. Pischon T, Boeing H, Hoffmann K, et al. General and abdominal adiposity and risk of death in Europe. *N Engl J Med.* 2008;359(20):2105–2120

13. Maron BJ, Thompson PD, Ackerman MJ, et al. Recommendations and considerations related to preparticipation screening for cardiovascular abnormalities in competitive athletes: 2007 update: a scientific statement from the American Heart Association Council on Nutrition, Physical Activity, and Metabolism: endorsed by the American College of Cardiology Foundation. *Circulation.* 2007;115(12):1643–1655

14. Garrick JG, Requa RK. Injuries in high school sports. *Pediatrics.* 1978;61(3):465–469

15. Gomez JE, Landry GL, Bernhardt DT. Critical evaluation of the 2-minute orthopedic screening examination. *Am J Dis Child.* 1993;147:1109–1113

16. Garrick JG. Preparticipation orthopedic screening evaluation. *Clin J Sport Med.* 2004;14(3):123–126

17. Dodge WF, West EF, Smith EH, Bruce H III. Proteinuria and hematuria in schoolchildren: epidemiology and early natural history. *J Pediatr.* 1976;88(2):327–347

18. Peggs JF, Reinhardt RW, O'Brien JM. Proteinuria in adolescent sports physical examinations. *J Fam Pract.* 1986;22(1):80–81

19. Taylor WC III, Lombardo JA. Preparticipation screening of college athletes: value of the complete blood cell count. *Phys Sportsmed.* 1990;18(6):106–118

20. Vehaskari VM, Rapola J. Isolated proteinuria: analysis of a school-age population. *J Pediatr.* 1982;101(5):661–668

21. Fallon KE. The clinical utility of screening of biochemical parameters in elite athletes: analysis of 100 cases. *Br J Sports Med.* 2008;42(5):334–337

22. National Athletic Trainers Association. Consensus statement: sickle cell trait and the athete. http://www.nata.org/statements/consensus/sicklecell.pdf. Accessed February 2, 2009

23. The student-athlete with sickle cell trait. In: *NCAA Sports Medicine Handbook.* http://www.ncaapublications.com/Uploads/PDF/Sports_Medicine_Handbookc8cd2dbe-6aa9-4d9a-bbee-2e426d0759a2.pdf

24. Haas JD, Brownlie T IV. Iron deficiency and reduced work capacity: a critical review of the research to determine a causal relationship. *J Nutr.* 2001;131(2S-2):676S–688S

25. Garza D, Shrier I, Kohl HW III, Ford P, Brown M, Matheson GO. The clinical value of serum ferritin tests in endurance athletes. *Clin J Sport Med.* 1997;7(1):46–53

26. LaManca JJ, Haymes EM. Effects of iron repletion on VO2max, endurance, and blood lactate in women. *Med Sci Sports Exerc.* 1993;25(12):1386–1392

27. Hinton PS, Giordano C, Brownlie T, Haas JD. Iron supplementation improves endurance after training in iron-depleted, non-anemic women. *J Appl Physiol.* 2000;88(3):1103–1111

28. Friedman B, Weller E, Mairbauri H, Bärtsch P. Effects of iron repletion on blood volume and performance capacity in young athletes. *Med Sci Sports Exerc.* 2001;33(5):741–746

29. Brownlie T IV, Utermohlen V, Hinton PS, Giordano C, Haas JD. Marginal iron deficiency without anemia impairs aerobic adaptation among previously untrained women. *Am J Clin Nutr.* 2002;75(4):734–742

30. Brutsaert TD, Hernandez-Cordero S, Rivera J, Viola T, Hughes G, Haas JD. Iron supplementation improves progressive fatigue resistance during dynamic knee extensor exercise in iron-depleted, non-anaemic women. *Am J Clin Nutr.* 2003;77(2):411–418

31. Fogelholm M. Indicators of vitamin and mineral status in athletes' blood. *Int J Sport Nutr.* 1995;5(4):267–284

32. Fallon KE. Screening for haematological and iron-related abnormalities in elite athletes—analysis of 576 cases. *J Sci Med Sport.* 2008;11(3):329–336

33. Schoene RB, Giboney K, Schimmel C, et al. Spirometry and airway reactivity in elite track and field athletes. *Clin J Sport Med.* 1997;7(4):257–261

34. Mannix ET, Manfredi F, Farber MO. A comparison of two challenge tests for identifying exercise-induced bronchospasm in figure skaters. *Chest.* 1999;115(3):649–653

35. Provost-Craig MA, Arbour KS, Sestili DC, Chabalko JJ, Ekinci E. The incidence of exercise-induced bronchospasm in competitive figure skaters. *J Asthma.* 1996;33(1):67–71

36. Mannix ET, Farber MO, Palange P, Galassetti P, Manfredi F. Exercise-induced asthma in figure skaters. *Chest.* 1996;109(2):312–315

37. Wilber RL, Rundell KW, Szmedra L, Jenkinson DM, Im J, Drake SD. Incidence of exercise-induced bronchospasm in Olympic winter sport athletes. *Med Sci Sports Exerc.* 2000;32(4);732–737

38. Corrigan B, Kazlauskas R. Medication use in athletes selected for doping control at the Sydney Olympics (2000). *Clin J Sport Med.* 2003;13(1):33–40

39. Holzer K, Bruckner P. Screening of athletes for exercise-induced bronchoconstriction. *Clin J Sport Med.* 2004;14(3):134–138

40. Glover DW, Glover DW, Maron BJ. Evolution in the process of screening United States high school student-athletes for cardio-vascular disease. *Am J Cardiol.* 2007;100(11):1709–1712

41. Peltz JE, Haskell WL, Matheson GO. A comprehensive and cost-effective preparticipation exam implemented on the World Wide Web. *Med Sci Sports Exerc.* 1999;31(12):1727–1740

42. Flore RD. The development and implementation of a Web-based participation athletics health questionnaire. *J Ath Training. NATA News.* 2003;09-03:49–58

CHAPTER 9

Conclusion

The preparticipation physical evaluation (PPE) is ideally done as a part of routine health screening examinations by an athlete's primary physician and should be considered a part of the preventive health examination for all children and adolescents to encourage safe physical activity of any kind on a regular basis. If integrating the examination into periodic health screening is not possible, a PPE involving multiple examiners in private screening areas can be employed. The group examination format can be optimized by using one physician to do the entire history review, examination, and clearance statement for each athlete. When the provider staffing mix does not allow a single physician approach, the station-based format can be tailored to optimize the available specialty mix.

With one-third of young athletes discontinuing organized sports by age 13,[1] and many youth sports leagues not requiring a PPE for participation, young patients should be asked, as a part of their health screening examinations, if they participate in or intend to participate in youth sports or any physical activity. It is important to note that young patients who play a sport recreationally (ie, not as part of a high school or club sport that requires a PPE) are not at any lower risk for some of the conditions discussed. The PPE should become an integral part of the health screening examinations for any active patient. If the patient does not intend to participate in any regular physical activity, every well-child, adolescent, or adult preventive health encounter should be used to encourage physical activity, and the same questions critical to the PPE (especially as it pertains to the cardiovascular and central nervous systems) should be addressed.

Although the PPE should be done about 6 weeks prior to the onset of the season, in reality, many of the examinations are done on a more urgent basis. This does not leave adequate time for evaluation of suspicious or abnormal findings prior to the start of practices and training. Physicians must be resolute in completing the full evaluation of any positive findings from the screening prior to allowing an athlete to participate in either practices or competitions. Athletes and their parents or guardians need to be educated to have the examinations conducted in a timely manner to avoid loss of practice time in the early season. State high school sports leagues and colleges vary in their preparticipation examination requirements from full physicals done yearly to those done every 2 to 3 years, most often with some form of health questionnaire in the "off" year or years.

The physician-athlete interaction associated with the PPE should serve as the foundation for a trusting relationship and help optimize the athlete's long-term health. For many healthy adolescent athletes, the PPE may be their only contact with the health care system. It is important to emphasize the need for regular preventive examinations to ensure full immunization status and address other health maintenance issues for each athlete who is examined inside or outside the medical home. Young athletes should know that the examination is in their best interest and will be conducted with full confidentiality.

With a thorough evaluation and knowledgeable counseling, physicians and other health care professionals can use the PPE as an opportunity to enhance safe sports participation and promote healthy lifestyles. The PPE can provide a teachable moment that is not always available to teenaged athletes who are often involved in high-risk activities away from the playing field. As a whole, the examination should promote safe, cost-effective athletic participation while guiding the athlete toward healthy behaviors during the risky adolescent years and throughout life.

The PPE continues to evolve, especially in the areas of cardiovascular risk reduction and syncope. From 2001 to 2006, 50 to 75 athletes in the age range of 13 to 25 years have died each year in the United States,[2] and the estimated frequency of sudden cardiac death (SCD) during sports activity is 0.6 deaths per 100,000 person-years. [2] This compares to the SCD rate of 0.87 deaths per 100,000 person-years from the Italian data (Veneto region) over 11 years[3] where 12 lead electrocardiograms (ECGs) are required and the SCD rate of 0.93 deaths per 100,000 person-years from the state of Minnesota where an every 3-year history and physical examination without mandatory ECG screening is required.[4]

This fourth edition of the monograph has made some valuable changes to the SCD screening by including unexplained or undiagnosed seizure activity, drowning, unexplained car accidents, and sudden infant death syndrome (SIDS) in the personal and family history of athletes. The syncope issue spans not just athletes, but drives at identifying any child at risk for sudden death, which is why these questions should be included in routine preventive health discussions with athletes and their parents or guardians. How many athletes with underlying heart disease have non–exercise-related syncope? It's simply not known. But it is known that some youngsters who ultimately suffer SCD have a history of recurrent syncope (ie, long QT syndrome, catecholaminergic polymorphic ventricular tachycardia) that is not necessarily exercise related. Therefore, a positive answer pertaining to the issue of syncope should alert the provider to perform a more detailed investigation. Questions pertaining to undiagnosed seizure activity, unexplained car accidents and drowning, and SIDS are attempting to identify this relatively rare subset of diseases.

The recommendations for the use of ECG and echocardiography may change to global screening for all athletes and active people from our current use to pursue abnormal findings found on history and physical examination as our understanding of this area becomes more clearly defined. As technology improves to reduce both false-positive and false-negative results, the recommendations of the American Heart Association regarding ECG screening may change. It will be important for the users of this monograph to stay abreast of current recommendations.

The issues pertaining to screening, the accuracy of the screening questions in predicting who may be at risk for certain conditions (sudden death, concussions, specific cardiac questions), and the predictability of examination findings continues to be ripe for further investigation. Further research in this area will help standardize this challenging process, improve the identification of at-risk athlete (and nonathlete), and risk-stratify those who are detected with certain conditions in terms of continued sport participation. Research in this area may or may not result in a more costly screening process. It is imperative that the PPE screening not create unnecessary financial or logistical roadblocks to athlete participation. As physicians and as a society, we must accept the imperfection of any screening tool and that participation in athletics will always carry some risk.

Finally, the physician performing the PPE should not be a technician rushing through the clinic appointment or group examination stations to determine the athlete's eligibility to participate in a sport. Rather, the physician should be an educator and advocate for the healthy active lifestyle of every patient participating in an organized sport, recreational play, or fitness activity.

■ REFERENCES

1. Wolff A. The American athlete, age 10: time of their lives or too much too soon? *Sports Illustrated.* 2003;99(14):59–67
2. Maron BJ, Doerer JJ, Haas TS, Tierney DM, Mueller FO. Sudden deaths in young competitive athletes: analysis of 1866 deaths in the United States, 1980–2006. *Circulation.* 2009;119:1085–1092
3. Corrado D, Basso C, Pavei A, Michieli P, Schiavon M, Thiene G. Trends in sudden cardiovascular death in young competitive athletes after implementation of a preparticipation screening program. *JAMA.* 2006;296:1593–1601
4. Maron BJ, Haas TS, Doerer JJ, Thompson PD, Hodges JS. Comparison of cardiovascular disease mortality in young US and Italian competitive athletes: which preparticipation screening strategy is really more effective [abstract]? *Circulation.* 2008;118:S1083

Forms

History Form
The Athlete With Special Needs: Supplemental History Form
Physical Examination Form
Clearance Form

■ PREPARTICIPATION PHYSICAL EVALUATION
HISTORY FORM

(Note: This form is to be filled out by the patient and parent prior to seeing the physician. The physician should keep this form in the chart.)

Date of Exam _____

Name _____ Date of birth _____

Sex _____ Age _____ Grade _____ School _____ Sport(s) _____

Medicines and Allergies: Please list all of the prescription and over-the-counter medicines and supplements (herbal and nutritional) that you are currently taking

_____

_____

_____

Do you have any allergies? ☐ Yes ☐ No   If yes, please identify specific allergy below.
☐ Medicines   ☐ Pollens   ☐ Food   ☐ Stinging Insects

Explain "Yes" answers below. Circle questions you don't know the answers to.

GENERAL QUESTIONS	Yes	No
1. Has a doctor ever denied or restricted your participation in sports for any reason?		
2. Do you have any ongoing medical conditions? If so, please identify below: ☐ Asthma ☐ Anemia ☐ Diabetes ☐ Infections Other: _____		
3. Have you ever spent the night in the hospital?		
4. Have you ever had surgery?		

HEART HEALTH QUESTIONS ABOUT YOU	Yes	No
5. Have you ever passed out or nearly passed out DURING or AFTER exercise?		
6. Have you ever had discomfort, pain, tightness, or pressure in your chest during exercise?		
7. Does your heart ever race or skip beats (irregular beats) during exercise?		
8. Has a doctor ever told you that you have any heart problems? If so, check all that apply: ☐ High blood pressure ☐ A heart murmur ☐ High cholesterol ☐ A heart infection ☐ Kawasaki disease Other: _____		
9. Has a doctor ever ordered a test for your heart? (For example, ECG/EKG, echocardiogram)		
10. Do you get lightheaded or feel more short of breath than expected during exercise?		
11. Have you ever had an unexplained seizure?		
12. Do you get more tired or short of breath more quickly than your friends during exercise?		

HEART HEALTH QUESTIONS ABOUT YOUR FAMILY	Yes	No
13. Has any family member or relative died of heart problems or had an unexpected or unexplained sudden death before age 50 (including drowning, unexplained car accident, or sudden infant death syndrome)?		
14. Does anyone in your family have hypertrophic cardiomyopathy, Marfan syndrome, arrhythmogenic right ventricular cardiomyopathy, long QT syndrome, short QT syndrome, Brugada syndrome, or catecholaminergic polymorphic ventricular tachycardia?		
15. Does anyone in your family have a heart problem, pacemaker, or implanted defibrillator?		
16. Has anyone in your family had unexplained fainting, unexplained seizures, or near drowning?		

BONE AND JOINT QUESTIONS	Yes	No
17. Have you ever had an injury to a bone, muscle, ligament, or tendon that caused you to miss a practice or a game?		
18. Have you ever had any broken or fractured bones or dislocated joints?		
19. Have you ever had an injury that required x-rays, MRI, CT scan, injections, therapy, a brace, a cast, or crutches?		
20. Have you ever had a stress fracture?		
21. Have you ever been told that you have or have you had an x-ray for neck instability or atlantoaxial instability? (Down syndrome or dwarfism)		
22. Do you regularly use a brace, orthotics, or other assistive device?		
23. Do you have a bone, muscle, or joint injury that bothers you?		
24. Do any of your joints become painful, swollen, feel warm, or look red?		
25. Do you have any history of juvenile arthritis or connective tissue disease?		

MEDICAL QUESTIONS	Yes	No
26. Do you cough, wheeze, or have difficulty breathing during or after exercise?		
27. Have you ever used an inhaler or taken asthma medicine?		
28. Is there anyone in your family who has asthma?		
29. Were you born without or are you missing a kidney, an eye, a testicle (males), your spleen, or any other organ?		
30. Do you have groin pain or a painful bulge or hernia in the groin area?		
31. Have you had infectious mononucleosis (mono) within the last month?		
32. Do you have any rashes, pressure sores, or other skin problems?		
33. Have you had a herpes or MRSA skin infection?		
34. Have you ever had a head injury or concussion?		
35. Have you ever had a hit or blow to the head that caused confusion, prolonged headache, or memory problems?		
36. Do you have a history of seizure disorder?		
37. Do you have headaches with exercise?		
38. Have you ever had numbness, tingling, or weakness in your arms or legs after being hit or falling?		
39. Have you ever been unable to move your arms or legs after being hit or falling?		
40. Have you ever become ill while exercising in the heat?		
41. Do you get frequent muscle cramps when exercising?		
42. Do you or someone in your family have sickle cell trait or disease?		
43. Have you had any problems with your eyes or vision?		
44. Have you had any eye injuries?		
45. Do you wear glasses or contact lenses?		
46. Do you wear protective eyewear, such as goggles or a face shield?		
47. Do you worry about your weight?		
48. Are you trying to or has anyone recommended that you gain or lose weight?		
49. Are you on a special diet or do you avoid certain types of foods?		
50. Have you ever had an eating disorder?		
51. Do you have any concerns that you would like to discuss with a doctor?		

FEMALES ONLY		
52. Have you ever had a menstrual period?		
53. How old were you when you had your first menstrual period?		
54. How many periods have you had in the last 12 months?		

Explain "yes" answers here

_____

_____

_____

_____

_____

_____

_____

I hereby state that, to the best of my knowledge, my answers to the above questions are complete and correct.

Signature of athlete _____ Signature of parent/guardian _____ Date _____

THE ATHLETE WITH SPECIAL NEEDS: SUPPLEMENTAL HISTORY FORM

Date of Exam _____

Name _____ Date of birth _____

Sex _____ Age _____ Grade _____ School _____ Sport(s) _____

	Yes	No
1. Type of disability		
2. Date of disability		
3. Classification (if available)		
4. Cause of disability (birth, disease, accident/trauma, other)		
5. List the sports you are interested in playing		
6. Do you regularly use a brace, assistive device, or prosthetic?		
7. Do you use any special brace or assistive device for sports?		
8. Do you have any rashes, pressure sores, or any other skin problems?		
9. Do you have a hearing loss? Do you use a hearing aid?		
10. Do you have a visual impairment?		
11. Do you use any special devices for bowel or bladder function?		
12. Do you have burning or discomfort when urinating?		
13. Have you had autonomic dysreflexia?		
14. Have you ever been diagnosed with a heat-related (hyperthermia) or cold-related (hypothermia) illness?		
15. Do you have muscle spasticity?		
16. Do you have frequent seizures that cannot be controlled by medication?		

Explain "yes" answers here

_____

_____

_____

_____

_____

Please indicate if you have ever had any of the following.

	Yes	No
Atlantoaxial instability		
X-ray evaluation for atlantoaxial instability		
Dislocated joints (more than one)		
Easy bleeding		
Enlarged spleen		
Hepatitis		
Osteopenia or osteoporosis		
Difficulty controlling bowel		
Difficulty controlling bladder		
Numbness or tingling in arms or hands		
Numbness or tingling in legs or feet		
Weakness in arms or hands		
Weakness in legs or feet		
Recent change in coordination		
Recent change in ability to walk		
Spina bifida		
Latex allergy		

Explain "yes" answers here

_____

_____

_____

_____

I hereby state that, to the best of my knowledge, my answers to the above questions are complete and correct.

Signature of athlete _____ Signature of parent/guardian _____ Date _____

PHYSICAL EXAMINATION FORM

Name _____ Date of birth _____

PHYSICIAN REMINDERS

1. Consider additional questions on more sensitive issues
   - Do you feel stressed out or under a lot of pressure?
   - Do you ever feel sad, hopeless, depressed, or anxious?
   - Do you feel safe at your home or residence?
   - Have you ever tried cigarettes, chewing tobacco, snuff, or dip?
   - During the past 30 days, did you use chewing tobacco, snuff, or dip?
   - Do you drink alcohol or use any other drugs?
   - Have you ever taken anabolic steroids or used any other performance supplement?
   - Have you ever taken any supplements to help you gain or lose weight or improve your performance?
   - Do you wear a seat belt, use a helmet, and use condoms?
2. Consider reviewing questions on cardiovascular symptoms (questions 5–14).

EXAMINATION					
Height		Weight		☐ Male ☐ Female	
BP / (/) Pulse			Vision R 20/	L 20/	Corrected ☐ Y ☐ N

MEDICAL	NORMAL	ABNORMAL FINDINGS
Appearance • Marfan stigmata (kyphoscoliosis, high-arched palate, pectus excavatum, arachnodactyly, arm span > height, hyperlaxity, myopia, MVP, aortic insufficiency)		
Eyes/ears/nose/throat • Pupils equal • Hearing		
Lymph nodes		
Heart[a] • Murmurs (auscultation standing, supine, +/- Valsalva) • Location of point of maximal impulse (PMI)		
Pulses • Simultaneous femoral and radial pulses		
Lungs		
Abdomen		
Genitourinary (males only)[b]		
Skin • HSV, lesions suggestive of MRSA, tinea corporis		
Neurologic[c]		
MUSCULOSKELETAL		
Neck		
Back		
Shoulder/arm		
Elbow/forearm		
Wrist/hand/fingers		
Hip/thigh		
Knee		
Leg/ankle		
Foot/toes		
Functional • Duck-walk, single leg hop		

[a]Consider ECG, echocardiogram, and referral to cardiology for abnormal cardiac history or exam.
[b]Consider GU exam if in private setting. Having third party present is recommended.
[c]Consider cognitive evaluation or baseline neuropsychiatric testing if a history of significant concussion.

☐ Cleared for all sports without restriction

☐ Cleared for all sports without restriction with recommendations for further evaluation or treatment for _____

_____

☐ Not cleared

      ☐ Pending further evaluation

      ☐ For any sports

      ☐ For certain sports _____

         Reason _____

Recommendations _____

_____

I have examined the above-named student and completed the preparticipation physical evaluation. The athlete does not present apparent clinical contraindications to practice and participate in the sport(s) as outlined above. A copy of the physical exam is on record in my office and can be made available to the school at the request of the parents. If conditions arise after the athlete has been cleared for participation, the physician may rescind the clearance until the problem is resolved and the potential consequences are completely explained to the athlete (and parents/guardians).

Name of physician (print/type) _____ Date _____

Address _____ Phone _____

Signature of physician _____ , MD or DO

■ PREPARTICIPATION PHYSICAL EVALUATION
CLEARANCE FORM

Name _____ Sex ☐ M ☐ F Age _____ Date of birth _____

☐ Cleared for all sports without restriction

☐ Cleared for all sports without restriction with recommendations for further evaluation or treatment for _____

_____

☐ Not cleared

    ☐ Pending further evaluation

    ☐ For any sports

    ☐ For certain sports _____

    Reason _____

Recommendations _____

_____
_____
_____
_____
_____
_____

I have examined the above-named student and completed the preparticipation physical evaluation. The athlete does not present apparent clinical contraindications to practice and participate in the sport(s) as outlined above. A copy of the physical exam is on record in my office and can be made available to the school at the request of the parents. If conditions arise after the athlete has been cleared for participation, the physician may rescind the clearance until the problem is resolved and the potential consequences are completely explained to the athlete (and parents/guardians).

Name of physician (print/type) _____ Date _____

Address _____ Phone _____

Signature of physician _____, MD or DO

EMERGENCY INFORMATION

Allergies _____

_____
_____
_____
_____

Other information _____

_____
_____
_____
_____
_____
_____
_____
_____
_____
_____
_____

Appendices

■ APPENDIX A
EXAMPLE OF A COLLEGE PPE CONSENT FORM

CONSENT TO PARTICIPATE IN VARSITY ATHLETICS

Student Information

Student Name _____

Address _____ City, State_____

Phone _____ Birth date _____ Sex _____

Medical Insurance Company _____ Policy number _____

Parent/Guardian and Student Consent

I consent to the participation of the above-named student in varsity athletics, including practice sessions and travel to and from athletic contests. If the medical status of the student changes in any significant manner after passing the physical examination, I will notify the university immediately. I also consent to the use of the data collected in the health questionnaire for research purposes, the results of which will be restricted to sports participation health risk assessment. Release of any information for research purposes, including published results, will not in any way identify the student.

Signature of Parent/Guardian (if student under 18 years) _____ Date _____

Signature of Student _____ Date _____

Physician Clearance

I certify that I have on this date examined this student and that, on the basis of the examination requested by the NCAA and the student's medical history as furnished to me, this student is

CLEARED TO PARTICIPATE WITH
☐ No restrictions
☐ The following restrictions (explain below)

NOT CLEARED TO PARTICIPATE
☐ Deferred—may be reconsidered after further evaluation (explain below)
☐ Not fit (give reason below)

Explanations

_____

_____

_____

_____

_____

_____

_____

_____

_____

Examiner's Signature _____ Date _____

Name _____ Address _____ Phone _____

■ APPENDIX B
EXAMPLE OF A TEEN SCREEN USED IN MINNESOTA

SCREEN FOR TEENS (12 YEARS OLD)–YOUNG ADULTS (20 YEARS OLD)

In order to help you the best we can, we would like you to answer the questions below. We ask all teenagers these questions because we feel they are things that affect your health and well-being. All of the questions may not fit you. You may leave those that do not apply blank. Please answer the questions alone, away from your parents or friends, so you can be as honest as possible. The questionnaire is not mandatory and if there is any disagreement with some of the questions asked, feel free to discuss these with the physician.

Your answers are a confidential/private part of your medical record. However, for your safety, we are required by law to share information involving physical/sexual abuse and suicide. Every situation is individual and our staff will always talk with you before sharing any of this information.

1. Do you get some exercise at least 3 times a week? ☐ Yes ☐ Sometimes ☐ No

2. Do you wear a seat belt in a car/truck? ☐ Yes ☐ Sometimes ☐ No

3. Do you wear a helmet when you skateboard, bicycle, motorcycle, snowmobile, or use an ATV? ☐ Yes ☐ Sometimes ☐ No

4. How often do you eat a well-balanced diet?
   A well-balanced diet includes selections from each of these groups

Fruits and vegetables	☐ Every day	☐ Most days	☐ Some days	☐ Rarely or never
Bread/cereal/rice/pasta	☐ Every day	☐ Most days	☐ Some days	☐ Rarely or never
Milk/yogurt/cheese	☐ Every day	☐ Most days	☐ Some days	☐ Rarely or never
Meat/poultry/fish/dry beans	☐ Every day	☐ Most days	☐ Some days	☐ Rarely or never

5. Do you use sun block at SPF 15 or greater to protect skin from the sun? ☐ Always ☐ Most of the time ☐ Sometimes ☐ Rarely or never

6. In general, are you happy with the way things are going for you? ☐ Yes ☐ Sometimes ☐ No

7. Do you get along with your family? ☐ Yes ☐ Sometimes ☐ No

8. Do you go to school regularly? ☐ Yes ☐ Sometimes ☐ No

9. Have your grades gotten worse than they used to be? ☐ No ☐ Yes

10. Do you have at least one adult you can really talk to? ☐ Yes ☐ Sometimes ☐ No

11. Do you feel you are about the right weight for your height? ☐ Yes ☐ Sometimes ☐ No

12. Do you ever use laxatives or throw up on purpose after eating? ☐ No ☐ Sometimes ☐ Yes

13. Do you smoke cigarettes or chew tobacco? ☐ No ☐ Sometimes ☐ Yes

14. Do you drink alcohol? ☐ No ☐ Sometimes ☐ Yes

15. Have you tried any drugs (pot, crack, cocaine, heroin, acid, speed, etc)? ☐ No ☐ Sometimes ☐ Yes

16. Do you—or does anyone you live with—have a gun or carry a gun around? ☐ No ☐ Sometimes ☐ Yes

17. Are you—or have you been—in a gang? ☐ No ☐ Sometimes ☐ Yes

18. Are you worried about money, a place to live, or having enough food to eat? ☐ No ☐ Sometimes ☐ Yes

19. Have you ever had sex (with women, men, or both)? ☐ No ☐ Yes

20. Have you ever been tested for or diagnosed with a sexually transmitted disease (VD)? (herpes, gonorrhea, chlamydia, genital warts, PID, syphilis) ☐ No ☐ Yes

21. Are you—or do you ever wonder if you are—gay, lesbian, bisexual, or transgender? ☐ No ☐ Sometimes ☐ Yes

22. How often are you using birth control (such as birth control pills, condoms, diaphragms, or Depo-Provera)? ☐ Does not apply ☐ Always ☐ Sometimes ☐ Never

23. Are you planning a pregnancy or at risk for becoming pregnant? ☐ No ☐ Uncertain ☐ Yes

Please re-read the italicized paragraph at the top before answering the following questions.

24. Have you ever thought about killing yourself? ☐ No ☐ Yes

25. Do you feel afraid in any of your relationships? ☐ No ☐ Yes

26. Have you ever been physically or sexually abused or mistreated by anyone (kicked, hit, pushed, forced or tricked into having sex, touched on your private parts)? ☐ No ☐ Yes

Adapted with permission from Ramsey Family Physicians Clinic Teen Screen.

SCAT2

Sport Concussion Assessment Tool 2

Name _____

Sport/team _____

Date/time of injury _____

Date/time of assessment _____

Age _____ Gender ☐ M ☐ F

Years of education completed _____

Examiner _____

What is the SCAT2?[1]

This tool represents a standardized method of evaluating injured athletes for concussion and can be used in athletes aged from 10 years and older. It supersedes the original SCAT published in 2005[2]. This tool also enables the calculation of the Standardized Assessment of Concussion (SAC)[3,4] score and the Maddocks questions[5] for sideline concussion assessment.

Instructions for using the SCAT2

The SCAT2 is designed for the use of medical and health professionals. Preseason baseline testing with the SCAT2 can be helpful for interpreting post-injury test scores. Words in Italics throughout the SCAT2 are the instructions given to the athlete by the tester.

This tool may be freely copied for distribtion to individuals, teams, groups and organizations.

What is a concussion?

A concussion is a disturbance in brain function caused by a direct or indirect force to the head. It results in a variety of non-specific symptoms (like those listed below) and often does not involve loss of consciousness. Concussion should be suspected in the presence of **any one or more** of the following:
- Symptoms (such as headache), or
- Physical signs (such as unsteadiness), or
- Impaired brain function (e.g. confusion) or
- Abnormal behaviour.

Any athlete with a suspected concussion should be REMOVED FROM PLAY, medically assessed, monitored for deterioration (i.e., should not be left alone) and should not drive a motor vehicle.

Symptom Evaluation

How do you feel?

You should score yourself on the following symptoms, based on how you feel now.

	none	mild		moderate		severe	
Headache	0	1	2	3	4	5	6
"Pressure in head"	0	1	2	3	4	5	6
Neck Pain	0	1	2	3	4	5	6
Nausea or vomiting	0	1	2	3	4	5	6
Dizziness	0	1	2	3	4	5	6
Blurred vision	0	1	2	3	4	5	6
Balance problems	0	1	2	3	4	5	6
Sensitivity to light	0	1	2	3	4	5	6
Sensitivity to noise	0	1	2	3	4	5	6
Feeling slowed down	0	1	2	3	4	5	6
Feeling like "in a fog"	0	1	2	3	4	5	6
"Don't feel right"	0	1	2	3	4	5	6
Difficulty concentrating	0	1	2	3	4	5	6
Difficulty remembering	0	1	2	3	4	5	6
Fatigue or low energy	0	1	2	3	4	5	6
Confusion	0	1	2	3	4	5	6
Drowsiness	0	1	2	3	4	5	6
Trouble falling asleep (if applicable)	0	1	2	3	4	5	6
More emotional	0	1	2	3	4	5	6
Irritability	0	1	2	3	4	5	6
Sadness	0	1	2	3	4	5	6
Nervous or Anxious	0	1	2	3	4	5	6

Total number of symptoms (Maximum possible 22) ▢

Symptom severity score
(Add all scores in table, maximum possible: 22 x 6 = 132) ▢

Do the symptoms get worse with physical activity? ☐ Y ☐ N
Do the symptoms get worse with mental activity? ☐ Y ☐ N

Overall rating
If you know the athlete well prior to the injury, how different is the athlete acting compared to his / her usual self? Please circle one response.

no different	very different	unsure

Reprinted with permission from: McCrory P, Meeuwisse W, Johnston K, et al. Consensus statement on concussion in sport: 3rd International conference on concussion in sport held in Zurich, November 2008. *Clin J Sport Med.* 2008;19(3):185–200.

SPORT CONCUSSION ASSESSMENT TOOL 2 (SCAT2), CONTINUED

Cognitive & Physical Evaluation

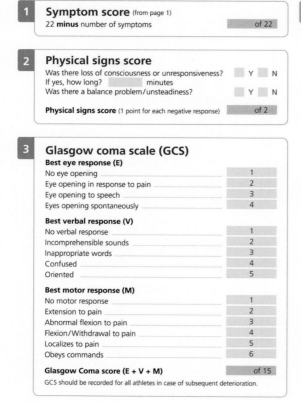

1 **Symptom score** (from page 1)

22 **minus** number of symptoms   ☐ of 22

2 **Physical signs score**

Was there loss of consciousness or unresponsiveness?   ☐ Y   ☐ N
If yes, how long? ☐ minutes
Was there a balance problem/unsteadiness?   ☐ Y   ☐ N

Physical signs score (1 point for each negative response)   ☐ of 2

3 **Glasgow coma scale (GCS)**

Best eye response (E)

No eye opening	1
Eye opening in response to pain	2
Eye opening to speech	3
Eyes opening spontaneously	4

Best verbal response (V)

No verbal response	1
Incomprehensible sounds	2
Inappropriate words	3
Confused	4
Oriented	5

Best motor response (M)

No motor response	1
Extension to pain	2
Abnormal flexion to pain	3
Flexion/Withdrawal to pain	4
Localizes to pain	5
Obeys commands	6

Glasgow Coma score (E + V + M)   ☐ of 15

GCS should be recorded for all athletes in case of subsequent deterioration.

4 **Sideline Assessment – Maddocks Score**

"I am going to ask you a few questions, please listen carefully and give your best effort."

Modified Maddocks questions (1 point for each correct answer)

	0	1
At what venue are we at today?	0	1
Which half is it now?	0	1
Who scored last in this match?	0	1
What team did you play last week/game?	0	1
Did your team win the last game?	0	1

Maddocks score   ☐ of 5

Maddocks score is validated for sideline diagnosis of concussion only and is not included in SCAT 2 summary score for serial testing.

5 **Cognitive assessment**

Standardized Assessment of Concussion (SAC)

Orientation (1 point for each correct answer)

	0	1
What month is it?	0	1
What is the date today?	0	1
What is the day of the week?	0	1
What year is it?	0	1
What time is it right now? (within 1 hour)	0	1

Orientation score   ☐ of 5

Immediate memory

"I am going to test your memory. I will read you a list of words and when I am done, repeat back as many words as you can remember, in any order."

Trials 2 & 3:

"I am going to repeat the same list again. Repeat back as many words as you can remember in any order, even if you said the word before."

Complete all 3 trials regardless of score on trial 1 & 2. Read the words at a rate of one per second. Score 1 pt. for each correct response. Total score equals sum across all 3 trials. Do not inform the athlete that delayed recall will be tested.

List	Trial 1	Trial 2	Trial 3	Alternative word list		
elbow	0 1	0 1	0 1	candle	baby	finger
apple	0 1	0 1	0 1	paper	monkey	penny
carpet	0 1	0 1	0 1	sugar	perfume	blanket
saddle	0 1	0 1	0 1	sandwich	sunset	lemon
bubble	0 1	0 1	0 1	wagon	iron	insect
Total						

Immediate memory score   ☐ of 15

Concentration

Digits Backward:

"I am going to read you a string of numbers and when I am done, you repeat them back to me backwards, in reverse order of how I read them to you. For example, if I say 7-1-9, you would say 9-1-7."

If correct, go to next string length. If incorrect, read trial 2. One point possible for each string length. Stop after incorrect on both trials. The digits should be read at the rate of one per second.

			Alternative digit lists		
4-9-3	0 1		6-2-9	5-2-6	4-1-5
3-8-1-4	0 1		3-2-7-9	1-7-9-5	4-9-6-8
6-2-9-7-1	0 1		1-5-2-8-6	3-8-5-2-7	6-1-8-4-3
7-1-8-4-6-2	0 1		5-3-9-1-4-8	8-3-1-9-6-4	7-2-4-8-5-6

Months in Reverse Order:

"Now tell me the months of the year in reverse order. Start with the last month and go backward. So you'll say December, November ... Go ahead"

1 pt. for entire sequence correct

Dec-Nov-Oct-Sept-Aug-Jul-Jun-May-Apr-Mar-Feb-Jan   0 1

Concentration score   ☐ of 5

[1] This tool has been developed by a group of international experts at the 3rd International Consensus meeting on Concussion in Sport held in Zurich, Switzerland in November 2008. The full details of the conference outcomes and the authors of the tool are published in British Journal of Sports Medicine, 2009, volume 43, supplement 1.
The outcome paper will also be simultaneously co-published in the May 2009 issues of Clinical Journal of Sports Medicine, Physical Medicine & Rehabilitation, Journal of Athletic Training, Journal of Clinical Neuroscience, Journal of Science & Medicine in Sport, Neurosurgery, Scandinavian Journal of Science & Medicine in Sport and the Journal of Clinical Sports Medicine.

[2] McCrory P et al. Summary and agreement statement of the 2nd International Conference on Concussion in Sport, Prague 2004. British Journal of Sports Medicine. 2005; 39: 196-204

[3] McCrea M. Standardized mental status testing of acute concussion. Clinical Journal of Sports Medicine. 2001; 11: 176-181

[4] McCrea M, Randolph C, Kelly J. Standardized Assessment of Concussion: Manual for administration, scoring and interpretation. Waukesha, Wisconsin, USA.

[5] Maddocks, DL; Dicker, GD; Saling, MM. The assessment of orientation following concussion in athletes. Clin J Sport Med. 1995;5(1):32–3

[6] Guskiewicz KM. Assessment of postural stability following sport-related concussion. Current Sports Medicine Reports. 2003; 2: 24-30

6 Balance examination

This balance testing is based on a modified version of the Balance Error Scoring System (BESS)[6]. A stopwatch or watch with a second hand is required for this testing.

Balance testing

"I am now going to test your balance. Please take your shoes off, roll up your pant legs above ankle (if applicable), and remove any ankle taping (if applicable). This test will consist of three twenty second tests with different stances."

(a) Double leg stance:
"The first stance is standing with your feet together with your hands on your hips and with your eyes closed. You should try to maintain stability in that position for 20 seconds. I will be counting the number of times you move out of this position. I will start timing when you are set and have closed your eyes."

(b) Single leg stance:
"If you were to kick a ball, which foot would you use? [This will be the dominant foot] Now stand on your non-dominant foot. The dominant leg should be held in approximately 30 degrees of hip flexion and 45 degrees of knee flexion. Again, you should try to maintain stability for 20 seconds with your hands on your hips and your eyes closed. I will be counting the number of times you move out of this position. If you stumble out of this position, open your eyes and return to the start position and continue balancing. I will start timing when you are set and have closed your eyes."

(c) Tandem stance:
*"Now stand heel-to-toe with your **non-dominant** foot in back. Your weight should be evenly distributed across both feet. Again, you should try to maintain stability for 20 seconds with your hands on your hips and your eyes closed. I will be counting the number of times you move out of this position. If you stumble out of this position, open your eyes and return to the start position and continue balancing. I will start timing when you are set and have closed your eyes."*

Balance testing – types of errors
1. Hands lifted off iliac crest
2. Opening eyes
3. Step, stumble, or fall
4. Moving hip into > 30 degrees abduction
5. Lifting forefoot or heel
6. Remaining out of test position > 5 sec

Each of the 20-second trials is scored by counting the errors, or deviations from the proper stance, accumulated by the athlete. The examiner will begin counting errors only after the individual has assumed the proper start position. **The modified BESS is calculated by adding one error point for each error during the three 20-second tests. The maximum total number of errors for any single condition is 10.** If an athlete commits multiple errors simultaneously, only one error is recorded but the athlete should quickly return to the testing position, and counting should resume once subject is set. Subjects that are unable to maintain the testing procedure for a minimum of **five seconds** at the start are assigned the highest possible score, ten, for that testing condition.

Which foot was tested: ☐ Left ☐ Right
(i.e. which is the **non-dominant** foot)

Condition	Total errors
Double Leg Stance (feet together)	of 10
Single leg stance (non-dominant foot)	of 10
Tandem stance (non-dominant foot at back)	of 10
Balance examination score (30 **minus** total errors)	of 30

7 Coordination examination

Upper limb coordination
Finger-to-nose (FTN) task: *"I am going to test your coordination now. Please sit comfortably on the chair with your eyes open and your arm (either right or left) outstretched (shoulder flexed to 90 degrees and elbow and fingers extended). When I give a start signal, I would like you to perform five successive finger to nose repetitions using your index finger to touch the tip of the nose as quickly and as accurately as possible."*

Which arm was tested: ☐ Left ☐ Right

Scoring: 5 correct repetitions in < 4 seconds = 1

Note for testers: Athletes fail the test if they do not touch their nose, do not fully extend their elbow or do not perform five repetitions. Failure should be scored as 0.

Coordination score	of 1

8 Cognitive assessment

Standardized Assessment of Concussion (SAC)

Delayed recall
"Do you remember that list of words I read a few times earlier? Tell me as many words from the list as you can remember in any order."

Circle each word correctly recalled. Total score equals number of words recalled.

List	Alternative word list		
elbow	candle	baby	finger
apple	paper	monkey	penny
carpet	sugar	perfume	blanket
saddle	sandwich	sunset	lemon
bubble	wagon	iron	insect

Delayed recall score	of 5

Overall score

Test domain	Score
Symptom score	of 22
Physical signs score	of 2
Glasgow Coma score (E + V + M)	of 15
Balance examination score	of 30
Coordination score	of 1
Subtotal	**of 70**
Orientation score	of 5
Immediate memory score	of 5
Concentration score	of 15
Delayed recall score	of 5
SAC subtotal	**of 30**
SCAT2 total	**of 100**
Maddocks Score	**of 5**

Definitive normative data for a SCAT2 "cut-off" score is not available at this time and will be developed in prospective studies. Embedded within the SCAT2 is the SAC score that can be utilized separately in concussion management. The scoring system also takes on particular clinical significance during serial assessment where it can be used to document either a decline or an improvement in neurological functioning.

Scoring data from the SCAT2 or SAC should not be used as a stand alone method to diagnose concussion, measure recovery or make decisions about an athlete's readiness to return to competition after concussion.

SPORT CONCUSSION ASSESSMENT TOOL 2 (SCAT2), CONTINUED

Athlete Information

Any athlete suspected of having a concussion should be removed from play, and then seek medical evaluation.

Signs to watch for

Problems could arise over the first 24-48 hours. You should not be left alone and must go to a hospital at once if you:
- Have a headache that gets worse
- Are very drowsy or can't be awakened (woken up)
- Can't recognize people or places
- Have repeated vomiting
- Behave unusually or seem confused; are very irritable
- Have seizures (arms and legs jerk uncontrollably)
- Have weak or numb arms or legs
- Are unsteady on your feet; have slurred speech

Remember, it is better to be safe.
Consult your doctor after a suspected concussion.

Return to play

Athletes should not be returned to play the same day of injury. When returning athletes to play, they should follow a stepwise symptom-limited program, with stages of progression. For example:
1. rest until asymptomatic (physical and mental rest)
2. light aerobic exercise (e.g. stationary cycle)
3. sport-specific exercise
4. non-contact training drills (start light resistance training)
5. full contact training after medical clearance
6. return to competition (game play)

There should be approximately 24 hours (or longer) for each stage and the athlete should return to stage 1 if symptoms recur. Resistance training should only be added in the later stages.
Medical clearance should be given before return to play.

Tool	Test domain	Time	Score			
		Date tested				
		Days post injury				
SCAT2	Symptom score					
	Physical signs score					
	Glasgow Coma score (E + V + M)					
	Balance examination score					
	Coordination score					
SAC	Orientation score					
	Immediate memory score					
	Concentration score					
	Delayed recall score					
	SAC Score					
Total	SCAT2					
Symptom severity score (max possible 132)						
Return to play			☐ Y ☐ N	☐ Y ☐ N	☐ Y ☐ N	☐ Y ☐ N

Additional comments

_____

_____

✂ -

Concussion injury advice (To be given to concussed athlete)

This patient has received an injury to the head. A careful medical examination has been carried out and no sign of any serious complications has been found. It is expected that recovery will be rapid, but the patient will need monitoring for a further period by a responsible adult. Your treating physician will provide guidance as to this timeframe.

If you notice any change in behaviour, vomiting, dizziness, worsening headache, double vision or excessive drowsiness, please telephone the clinic or the nearest hospital emergency department immediately.

Other important points:
- **Rest and avoid strenuous activity for at least 24 hours**
- **No alcohol**
- **No sleeping tablets**
- **Use paracetamol or codeine for headache. Do not use aspirin or anti-inflammatory medication**
- **Do not drive until medically cleared**
- **Do not train or play sport until medically cleared**

Clinic phone number _____

Patient's name

_____

Date/time of injury

_____

Date/time of medical review

_____

Treating physician

_____

```
┌─────────────────────────────────┐
│                                 │
│                                 │
│                                 │
│                                 │
│                                 │
│                 Contact details or stamp │
└─────────────────────────────────┘
```

SPORT CONCUSSION ASSESSMENT TOOL 2 (SCAT2), CONTINUED

Pocket SCAT2

Concussion should be suspected in the presence of **any one or more** of the following: symptoms (such as headache), or physical signs (such as unsteadiness), or impaired brain function (e.g. confusion) or abnormal behaviour.

1. Symptoms
Presence of any of the following signs & symptoms may suggest a concussion.

- Loss of consciousness
- Seizure or convulsion
- Amnesia
- Headache
- "Pressure in head"
- Neck Pain
- Nausea or vomiting
- Dizziness
- Blurred vision
- Balance problems
- Sensitivity to light
- Sensitivity to noise
- Feeling slowed down
- Feeling like "in a fog"
- "Don't feel right"
- Difficulty concentrating
- Difficulty remembering
- Fatigue or low energy
- Confusion
- Drowsiness
- More emotional
- Irritability
- Sadness
- Nervous or anxious

2. Memory function
Failure to answer all questions correctly may suggest a concussion.

"At what venue are we at today?"
"Which half is it now?"
"Who scored last in this game?"
"What team did you play last week / game?"
"Did your team win the last game?"

3. Balance testing
Instructions for tandem stance
*"Now stand heel-to-toe with your **non-dominant** foot in back. Your weight should be evenly distributed across both feet. You should try to maintain stability for 20 seconds with your hands on your hips and your eyes closed. I will be counting the number of times you move out of this position. If you stumble out of this position, open your eyes and return to the start position and continue balancing. I will start timing when you are set and have closed your eyes."*

Observe the athlete for 20 seconds. If they make more than 5 errors (such as lift their hands off their hips; open their eyes; lift their forefoot or heel; step, stumble, or fall; or remain out of the start position for more that 5 seconds) then this may suggest a concussion.

Any athlete with a suspected concussion should be IMMEDIATELY REMOVED FROM PLAY, urgently assessed medically, should not be left alone and should not drive a motor vehicle.

■ APPENDIX D
CODING FOR THE PREPARTICIPATION PHYSICAL EVALUATION

Coding and payment for preparticipation physical evaluation examinations can be challenging. There are options, but they are not always the best options that will optimize payment for the work that is done. Each option will require proactive effort on the part of your office staff to determine what the patient's health plan covers and how best to report the service.

The ideal option is to perform a full preventive medicine service and bill the patient's health plan. Most payers pay for one preventive medicine examination annually or provide a fixed-dollar benefit allocated for preventive medicine services provided during a calendar year. With this type of coverage, using the benefit for a limited sports physical may not be advantageous to you or the patient. Therefore, if the patient has not had a full preventive medicine service within the past 12 months, the scheduler should inform the parent when he/she calls for an appointment that a full preventive medicine service is recommended and that the sports physical form can be incorporated into the exam and completed in conjunction with the preventive visit. It may be beneficial to develop a patient handout to emphasize the importance of a well-child examination.

However, in situations where the patient has already come in for his/her well-child examination yet returns at a later date for a sports physical, it may be appropriate to report the office or other outpatient services codes **(99201–99215)**. If the requirements for a comprehensive preventive medicine service are not met, codes **99201– 99215** or **99241–99245** may be alternatively reported. While these codes are usually viewed as "sick visit" codes, their *Current Procedural Terminology (CPT®)* definition is really broader than that. Carriers may balk at paying for such codes, particularly when they are linked to "V" diagnosis codes (eg, **V70.3**). However, such denials may be overcome through payer education and persistent claims appeals.

There may be an option to perform the sports physical and bill the patient directly. For cases where the patient's preventive service benefit has been exhausted by a full preventive medicine examination in the last year or the patient's health plan won't pay for a sports physical under any circumstances, your practice should set a fee and instruct your scheduler to inform anyone wishing to schedule a sports physical that it must be paid for at the time of service. Most computerized billing systems allow you to set up codes for services that are not billed to the carrier. These are often alphabetical codes so as to avoid confusion with *CPT* codes (eg, "sport"). This enables the practice to track utilization data and to generate itemized statements. You should ensure that the statement provides a detailed description of the service for the benefit of parents with health care reimbursement accounts and those who track medical expenses for tax purposes.

You and your staff should make every effort to understand the reporting requirements of your most common payers. You should also work with families to better understand their benefit coverage for preventive medicine services. If the sports physical is a noncovered service and cannot be provided within the context of a full preventive medicine service, you should have policies in place to bill patients directly.

QUICK REFERENCE TO USEFUL CODES FOR THE PREPARTICIPATION PHYSICAL EVALUATION

Procedural Services	CPT Codes
Preventive medicine service (New Pt)	99383–99385
Preventive medicine service (Est Pt)	99393–99395
Office or other outpatient service (New Pt)	99201–99205
Office or other outpatient service (Est Pt)	99211–99215
Unlisted preventive medicine service	99429
Complete blood count (CBC) w/ diff, automated	85025
Complete CBC, automated (no white blood count diff)	85027
Lipid profile	80061
Urinalysis—nonautomated w/ micro	81000
Urinalysis automated w/ micro	81001
Urinalysis—nonautomated w/o micro	81002
Routine venipuncture	36415
Specimen handling	99000[a]

[a] Payment for this code is subject to contractual issues and currently most plans do not routinely reimburse for this service.

Diagnosis	ICD-9-CM Code
Sports examination	V70.3
Routine child health check	V20.2[b]
Other nutritional deficiency	269.8
Hyperlipidemia, other and unspecified	272.4
Anemia, unspecified	285.9
Obesity, unspecified	278.00
Overweight	278.02
Hypertension, malignant	401.0
Hypertension, unspecified	401.9
Asthma, extrinsic	493.0x
Asthma, intrinsic	493.1x
Asthma, exercise induced bronchospasm	493.81
Asthma, unspecified	493.9x
Hematuria, unspecified	599.70
Hematuria, gross	599.71
Hematuria, microscopic	599.72
Amenorrhea	626.0
Excessive or frequent menstruation	626.2
Irregular menstrual cycle	626.4
Scoliosis (and kyphoscoliosis), idiopathic	737.30
Scoliosis, other	737.39
Scoliosis, congenital	754.2
Other fatigue	780.79
Pallor	782.61
Heart murmur	785.2
Dysuria	788.1
Proteinuria	791.0
Elevated blood pressure reading w/o hypertension	796.2
Family history of atherosclerotic premature heart disease	V17.49
Family history of dyslipidemia	V18.19
Family history of polycystic kidney disease	V18.61
Family history of other kidney disease	V18.69

[b] Report V20.2 in conjunction with the V70.3 when a PPE is provided during an age-appropriate preventive medicine service.

x—These ICD-9-CM codes require a 5th digit. 0—unspecified; 1—with status asthmaticus; 3—with (acute) exacerbation

Differentiated Small-Group Reading Lessons

Margo Southall

W9-BMP-312

■SCHOLASTIC

New York • Toronto • London • Sydney
Mexico City • New Delhi • Hong Kong • Buenos Aires

This book is dedicated to my mother, Barbara Lea Taylor,
who has continuously encouraged me to put my ideas
in writing.

I would like to thank the following reading specialists
and teachers from the Metropolitan Nashville
Public Schools who graciously offered to provide
the photographs for this book: Susan Porter at
Maxwell Elementary, Jacqueline Jones and
Pennie Pulley at Goodlettsville Elementary, and
Judith Jones and Barbara Edwards at Andrew
Jackson Elementary.

To my editor, Joanna Davis-Swing, your insight into
differentiated instruction and ability to transform an
author's thinking into a visual teaching tool are valued
and appreciated.

Editor: Joanna Davis-Swing
Cover and Icon design: Jorge J. Namerow
Cover Photo Credit: Maria Lilja © Scholastic
Interior design: Kelli Thompson

ISBN-13: 978-0-439-83920-4
ISBN-10: 0-439-83920-3

Contents

Introduction

The Purpose of This Book

The process of planning and teaching lessons for diverse groups of students can be an overwhelming task, even for the most experienced teacher. The purpose of this book is to increase the effectiveness of your small-group reading instruction with lesson formats that are designed to meet the needs of specific profiles of readers.

In the following chapters, I share a menu of classroom-tested lessons for word solving, fluency, and comprehension that target typical challenges and difficulties students experience during the process of learning to read. Each skill and strategy-based lesson is designed to increase the rate of student progress by closely aligning instruction with demonstrated student need.

How to Use This Book

The lessons in Chapters 4 through 6 will complement your whole-class teaching, or core program, by providing students with the opportunity to review and extend their understanding of skills and strategies in a small-group setting. In each lesson, you will find practical suggestions for scaffolding instruction to support students who do not demonstrate adequate progress in a specific skill or strategy. For each skill area, I provide guidelines for monitoring student progress along with the recommended responsive instruction, enabling you to adjust the frequency, intensity, and pace of instruction to ensure success for every student.

A differentiated reading program requires planning and teaching skill-focused lessons for multiple reading groups, adjusting instruction to meet changes in student need, and selecting supporting reading materials. Let's examine how to put this all together in a workable framework.

Chapter 1 describes how to structure your reading group program to more effectively differentiate instruction and increase the rate of student achievement. Here you will find the criteria for grouping students and guidelines for varying the lesson content, structure, and reading material.

Chapter 2 provides a four-step process for linking the information from your assessment data to the formation of differentiated reading groups and the selection of lessons that target their reading goals. When/Then charts are provided, which list student profiles of need (When) aligned with the corresponding lesson(s) in word solving, fluency, and comprehension (Then) found in Chapters 4 through 6. This information is recorded on the Student Reading Goals and Observations Form, Planning for Group Instruction Form, and Tracking Class Reading Goals Form so that the status of individual students and of class is easily accessible.

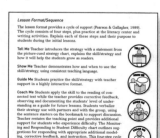

Lesson Format/Sequence

The lesson format provides a cycle of support (Pearson & Gallagher, 1989). The cycle consists of four steps, plus practice at the literacy center and writing activities. Explain each of these steps and their purpose to students during the initial lessons.

Tell Me Teacher introduces the strategy with a statement from the picture-cued strategy chart, explains the skill/strategy and how it will help the students grow as readers.

Show Me Teacher demonstrates how and when to use the skill/strategy, using consistent teaching language.

Guide Me Students practice the skill/strategy with teacher support in a highly interactive format.

Coach Me Students apply the skill to the reading of connected text while the teacher provides corrective feedback, observing and documenting the students' level of understanding as a guide for future lessons. Students verbalize their strategy use with partners and with the group, using the sentence starters on the bookmark to support discussion. Teacher restates the teaching point and provides additional support for students who experience difficulty. The Monitoring and Responding to Student Difficulty chart outlines suggestions for responding with appropriate additional modeling, corrective feedback, and instruction. This four-step cycle is bolstered by the following.

Reading-Writing Connection Students complete an independent writing activity that reinforces the skill/strategy in their reading response journal or a graphic organizer.

Practice at the Literacy Center Students link the comprehension, fluency, or word-solving skill or strategy to independent and collaborative tasks at the literacy centers.

See Page 12

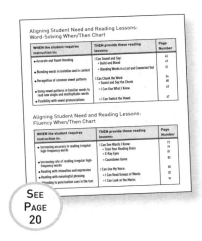

SEE PAGE 20

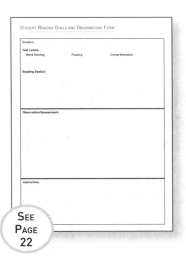

SEE PAGE 22

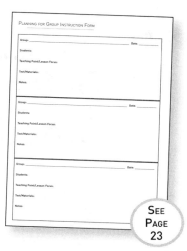

SEE PAGE 23

Chapter 3 answers common questions that arise regarding the daily management of small-group instruction in the classroom, including scheduling issues. A discussion of how to design and stock your small-group teaching space includes suggestions for organizing your planning notebook, using strategy charts, student bookmarks, and other interactive learning tools to ensure that students are engaged and that every-pupil responses (EPR) are incorporated throughout the lesson.

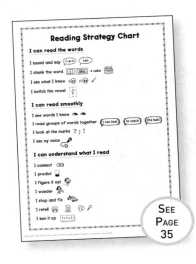

SEE PAGE 35

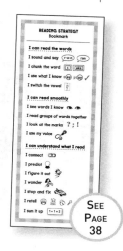

SEE PAGE 38

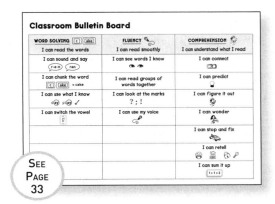

SEE PAGE 33

Chapters 4 through 6 provide ready-to-go, research-based lessons in word solving, fluency, and comprehension. These lessons are designed to be used with any reading series. Each lesson can be used over a series of multiple small-group sessions by varying the text, while keeping the format consistent. This will enable you to implement a unit of study on a specific skill or strategy to achieve student reading goals.

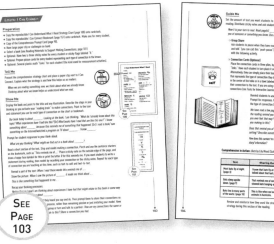

SEE PAGE 103

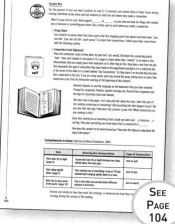

SEE PAGE 104

Differentiating Our Small-Group Reading Instruction

SWIMMING IN A SEA OF GROUPS, SKILLS, AND BOOKS: A GUIDED READING SCENARIO

It's time for Kaylie's group to come to the teacher table for guided reading. I have selected the book *Henry and Mudge in Puddle Trouble* by Cynthia Rylant (1990) based on the rate of accuracy students have achieved with this level of text and the supports the series offers. After the book introduction and modeling of a useful strategy, the group members read at their own pace while I listen to individual students read, reinforcing their use of effective strategies and coaching for strategies they neglect to apply.

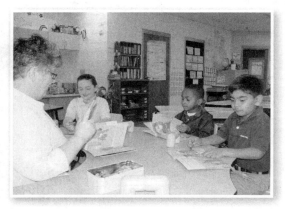

Small-group lessons are the heart of a differentiated reading program.

Ben is having difficulty recognizing familiar chunks in words. He tries to decode the word *glory* by analyzing the word phoneme by phoneme. I prompt him to find a part of the word he knows (such as *gl_* and *_or_*), a part he can say, then blend the parts together. He hesitates. I use masking cards from my reading toolbox to isolate *_or_* and model blending the parts to pronounce the whole word. Together we repeat the process and read the word in context, discussing how it is used to name a type of flower in the story.

Mikhela hesitates at the same sight word, *would*, on two successive pages. It's on our word wall, and the class has practiced reading and spelling this word over multiple multisensory practice sessions, but it is evident that she does not have a complete picture of this word in her visual memory. I write the word on an index card and ask her to read it, say the letters in sequence, say the word again, then reread the word in the text, as I place the card under it in the book to support this transfer process.

Will is reading as fast as he can in a monotone voice, skipping over commas and periods in an effort to beat the clock (or be finished first!), it seems. I point to a section of dialogue and ask him to think about how the character might say that part. I ask him to make an inference using what he already knows about dogs together with clues the author has provided in the dialogue (such as *shouted*, words in italics, and punctuation marks). I prompt Will to read that part again, as if he were Henry, so that he can gain insight into how the character responded to a problem in the story.

Kaylie runs her eyes across the pages, skimming the text. She looks at me blankly when I ask her to generate a "teacher" question about what she has just read to ask the rest of the group. I point to a place in the text and ask her to reread and retell what has happened in that part of the story. I model how to turn that information into a question.

Time is up and the next group is on its way. Phew! These students are able to read this text at instructional level, but each one demonstrates a very different profile of strengths and needs. I feel scattered, and I know each student requires a different instructional focus at this point in their reading development. There has to be a more efficient way to address this range of needs before me; at this rate, I am going to be coaching each student for the same neglected strategy for many more guided reading sessions. How, I wonder, can I find more time to give them the targeted instruction that they require to develop an understanding of reading strategies and a mastery of foundational skills? Not in our whole-class reading mini-lessons; we have already gone beyond some of these skills and strategies in our core reading program. Not during guided reading, either. I have used the guided reading format for over a decade and work hard to protect this small-group time in my schedule. But I know that to effectively meet the needs of these readers, I will need more flexibility in lesson structure, scheduling, and materials than our current "traditional" guided reading format allows.

How Does Differentiation Work With Small-Group Reading Instruction?

Building upon my experience as a reading specialist and special education resource teacher, and drawing on the principles of differentiated instruction, I set out to rethink and restructure my small-group reading program. The culmination of this process was the insight to differentiate small-group instruction based on student need. I would form reading groups strategically by common need for instruction in a skill or strategy, and I would teach each group a series of lessons that targeted the specific skill or strategy intensively over consecutive lessons. These changes to my program were made in response to two key questions:

1. *What are the alternatives to grouping students by reading levels?*
2. *How can I make my small-group instruction more responsive to the differing needs and reading goals of my students?*

We can group students by their demonstrated needs, and we can tailor the lessons we offer to those needs. I explore each of these questions further in the following pages.

Comparing Guided Reading and Differentiated Reading Groups

The following chart summarizes the similarities and differences between guided reading lessons and differentiated reading lessons.

Guided Reading Group Lessons	Both	Differentiated Reading Group Lessons
• Focus on integrated strategy use • Instructional level text is selected for each group. Students progress through a leveled set of materials • Students in the group are all at the same reading level • Same lesson structure is used for each session: ∗ Teacher introduces the text and any important or challenging vocabulary ∗ Students read the text while teacher coaches for integrated strategy use ∗ Teacher and students discuss the text ∗ Teacher may extend the lesson with a strategy mini-lesson using examples from the book	• Teacher-directed • Practice of skills/strategies with connected text • Teacher prompting for strategy use during reading • Informal assessment and documentation of student progress during each session • Interactive format • Student-student dialogue structures (partner activities sometimes incorporated in guided reading)	• Focus on one to two skills/strategies • Level of text varies according to skill/strategy focus. Both instructional and independent level text is used • Students may represent a range of two or more reading levels • Lesson structure varies according to the teaching point and student need; always includes the components of explicit teaching: ∗ Tell Me—Teacher explains the skill/strategy ∗ Show Me–Teacher demonstrates skill/strategy ∗ Guide Me–Teacher and students engage in interactive practice ∗ Coach Me–Students apply the skill/strategy; teacher provides corrective feedback In addition to: ∗ Reading-Writing Connection—Students write in their Reading Response Journal ∗ Practice at the Literacy Center—Students practice the same skill/strategy at the center (Word Study, Fluency, or Comprehension)

To provide highly effective differentiated reading instruction, we vary the following:

1. **Content**
   skills and strategies
2. **Lesson structure**
   teaching sequence/format
3. **Reading material**
   level, genre, and text structure

In addition, we can vary the
- **Frequency of instruction**
  number of times we meet with each group
- **Intensity**
  number of students in the group
- **Pace of instruction**
  number of lessons in each skill or strategy

(GIBSON & HASBROUCK, 2007)

"*Guided reading* may not always be the appropriate lesson structure to implement with all small groups of students, especially struggling readers ... during a *guided reading* lesson it is difficult to build in the systematic review of critical knowledge and skills that struggling readers need."

(KOSANOVICH, LADINSKY, NELSON, & TORGESEN, P.3, 2006)

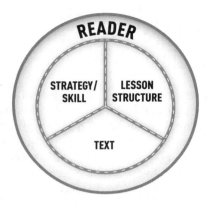

Figure 1.1 To meet the needs of all students, we differentiate the strategy or skill, lesson structure, and text.

The Students: Forming Differentiated Reading Groups

What information drives the grouping of our students?

At the heart of the problem in the guided reading scenario were the criteria for student grouping. Students were organized into groups based on the level of accuracy they achieved with our leveled series, rather than on a common instructional goal. In this approach to grouping, you have three to six students sitting in front of you who achieve similar accuracy scores on the same passage, yet each one operates with a differing set of skills, strategy use, and reading behaviors.

In comparison, a differentiated small-group reading program requires more than determining students' reading accuracy rate. This first level of analysis provides a narrow picture of the student as a reader. The teaching response is then guided only by decoding skills. Without integrating sources of information on students' fluency skills and comprehension strategy use, the instructional response is limited. Differentiated reading instruction requires that student grouping be guided by a deeper analysis of assessment data in which student performance in each reading area informs instructional goals (see Ongoing Informal Assessment in Chapter 2, page 15). In this way, we use our data to establish clear instructional goals and to plan supporting lessons that build understanding and mastery.

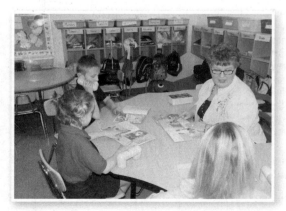

This group shares a common need in a specific fluency skill.

Teachers form a differentiated reading group when three to six students demonstrate the need for support in the same skill or strategy area, or share the same reading goal (see Student Reading Goals and Observations Form, Chapter 2, page 22). The lesson focus within these differentiated groups is strategically aligned with the current needs of its members. Membership in these differentiated reading groups will shift during the year because students move through stages of reading development at different rates, and their instructional goals therefore continue to change. It is not only the struggling readers who require such targeted instruction. Even on-grade and advanced students do not maintain a constant rate of growth; rather, they experience peaks and plateaus on their path to independence. The small-group reading lessons in this book are designed to support all students within a responsive reading program in which sets of leveled books are used as a vehicle to teaching skills and strategies.

The Lessons: Content, Structure, and Text

How can I make my small-group instruction more responsive to the differing needs/reading goals of my students?

Increasing the rate of student progress requires that we focus time and resources on specific areas of need. To achieve this, we will need to examine what (skills and strategies) and how (lesson format or sequence) we teach, along with the selection of materials (reading level, genre, text structure) that will support the instructional focus.

"Responding to student variance requires that two things change: what is taught and how it is presented."
(Gibson & Hasbrouck, p.3, 2007)

Lesson Content

How will I determine the teaching point for each group lesson?

What if we are at Lesson 13 in the core reading program on "identifying the main idea" and some students are still struggling with retelling? This is where the implementation of differentiated small-group reading lessons is critical. The skills and strategies in the *scope* and *sequence* of your core reading series or curriculum document provide a source of possible teaching points for different groups of students. By reviewing these guides and your students' assessment data you will be able to determine the next lesson focus or reading goal for groups of students. When there is more than one possible teaching point you will need to decide: Which teaching point is most important for these students now in their development as readers?

A common temptation is to try and teach too much in one lesson. Typically, the guidebooks that accompany any reading series present more than one teaching point in each lesson. Integrated strategy use during reading is an essential part of learning to read, but many of our younger readers have not yet developed sufficient understanding of each strategy to orchestrate multiple strategies simultaneously. These students require systematic instruction on a specific skill or strategy (their current reading goal) over a series of small-group lessons, cumulatively learning to integrate previously learned strategies in a step-by-step approach.

To assist you in this process of determining the appropriate teaching points, examine the When/Then charts on pages 20 to 21 in Chapter 2. These will provide you with a list of skills and strategies aligned with the lessons in Chapters 4 through 6.

Pacing Your Instruction

How many lessons will I need to teach on the same skill or strategy?

For instruction to be aligned with assessment data, it is essential that we monitor student progress carefully and adjust the pace of instruction accordingly. This attention helps us avoid moving students through a sequence of skills and strategies at a pace that is faster than their rate of learning. Two factors need to be taken into consideration: the students and the skill/strategy.

Firstly, when students are struggling with a concept or skill, they will require additional teaching time. This means scheduling more instructional minutes and allowing more time for students to apply the skill to the reading of connected text. They will also require varied modes of highly interactive instruction to consolidate their understanding and to ensure that we reach each and every student. To close the gap for low progress readers, we will need to implement explicit instruction that directly addresses their current deficits in skills and strategies over multiple small-group reading lessons.

Secondly, skills and strategies are not equally complex, and some require less or more instructional time. Unfortunately, not all reading programs vary the number of lessons or time spent on each one accordingly (Beck, 2006). The lessons in this book will enable you to provide supplementary lessons on more complex skills and to offer additional support when students experience difficulty.

A "touch and go" pace of instruction does not support the mastery and understanding that transfers to independent reading. Instruction remains responsive when teachers monitor and adjust lesson content continuously so that the *pace of teaching is correlated to the pace of student learning*. The result of too much, too fast is a slow rate of student progress. Suggestions for ongoing monitoring and responses to student progress are included in each lesson plan.

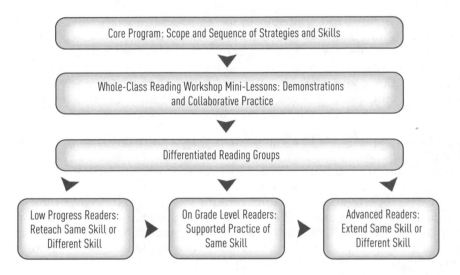

Figure 1.2 Linking differentiated reading group lessons to whole-class instruction

Lesson Structure

What is the teaching format or sequence?

To reach all students, we need flexibility in the design or structure of our lessons. This is especially true for low progress readers, who often require that we present the same skill in multiple ways to achieve mastery.

Kosanovich et al. (2006) identify the need for two types of small-group lesson structures in a differentiated reading program. The first type is guided reading, which is implemented with groups of students who have achieved grade-level expectations. The focus in these lessons is on integrated strategy use and the introduction of new genre and text structures. The second type is skill-focused lessons, which are designed for groups of students who are not achieving grade-level expectations, with the focus on specific skills in phonemic awareness, decoding, fluency, vocabulary, and comprehension (NICHD, 2000). Building on these two frameworks and my experience teaching strategy-based groups, where the focus is on neglected cues (visual, meaning, and self-monitoring strategies) identified in student running records (Morrison, 1994), I set about restructuring the design of my small-group lessons.

In common with guided reading, each lesson in Chapters 4 through 6 includes teacher-supported practice of a target skill/strategy while reading connected text. From my work with struggling readers, I know only too well the lack of transfer to independent reading if this component is not included and skills are left in isolation. In contrast to guided reading, and like the skill-focused lessons described above, these differentiated lessons include more flexibility in both the presentation and practice of the teaching point. For example, in a lesson with a decoding focus, students may engage in segmenting and blending words using tactile materials, and both fluency and comprehension lessons incorporate varied teaching techniques within shared and independent reading formats, as well as the use of a wide range of tactile learning aids (see Tools for Interactive Learning in Chapter 3).

It is important to note that the differentiated lessons in this book are not just for low progress readers. On-grade and advanced students also require challenging and extending lessons to continue to grow as readers (Walpole & McKenna, 2007). At times, the instructional goal with these students may be integrated strategy use, as in guided reading, but at other times during the year they will need a series of focused lessons on a specific teaching point, such as those provided in Chapters 4 through 6.

What will the lessons look and sound like?

In differentiated, responsive teaching, lessons will not look and sound the same for every group of students. Scan the lesson plans in Chapters 4 through 6 and you will see a range of teaching techniques and student responses designed to support specific areas of difficulty. Select the lesson that best supports your students' reading goals by examining the When/Then charts in Chapter 2, which align the lessons with common profiles of student need. Lessons are organized in an easy-to-follow, step-by-step lesson format based on the components of explicit instruction as cited in numerous studies on best practices. These lessons are characterized by a high level of interaction. If students are not engaged, they are not learning! Each step in the lesson plans is explained below, under Lesson Format/Sequence (page 12).

How are reading and writing integrated within the lesson structure?

If our goal is for struggling readers to see themselves as both readers and writers, then the reading response journal provides a powerful and integral part of our lessons. Students will write in their journals either during and/or after the lesson. Numerous research studies support the reciprocal relationship between reading and writing (Allington, 2005). By linking the focus skill to a writing application, we incorporate a critical step in long-term retention of taught skills. The type of writing incorporated in each lesson varies according to the instructional focus. In the word-solving lessons, there is a focus on using words representing the same phonics elements in shared or independent writing activities. In the comprehension lessons, scaffolds are provided so that students can write a personal response to the reading using strategy-based supports such as picture-cued sentence starters for generating questions and connections to support their opinions and insights. Further extensions may

"Skill-Focused Lessons are teacher-planned lessons that provide the opportunity for more systematic and focused practice on a relatively small number of critical elements at a time ...." (Kosanovich, Ladinsky, Nelson, & Torgesen, p. 3, 2006)

include using the same text structure to write a version of the story or informational text. For example, if the group is reading a descriptive text about an animal, students can follow the same text structure to write about an animal of their choice.

How do the lessons correlate with my literacy center program?

Each of the lesson plans includes suggested literacy center activities to practice the skill or strategy. These include activities for word study, fluency, and comprehension centers from my book *Differentiated Literacy Centers*.

Lesson Format/Sequence

The lesson format provides a cycle of support (Pearson & Gallagher, 1989). The cycle consists of four steps, plus practice at the literacy center and writing activities. Explain each of these steps and their purpose to students during the initial lessons.

Four-Step Cycle of Support

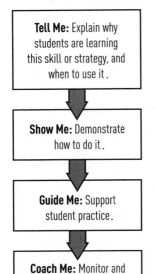

Tell Me Teacher introduces the strategy with a statement from the picture-cued strategy chart, explains the skill/strategy and how it will help the students grow as readers.

Show Me Teacher demonstrates how and when to use the skill/strategy, using consistent teaching language.

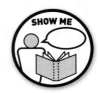

Guide Me Students practice the skill/strategy with teacher support in a highly interactive format.

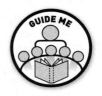

Coach Me Students apply the skill to the reading of connected text while the teacher provides corrective feedback, observing and documenting the students' level of understanding as a guide for future lessons. Students verbalize their strategy use with partners and with the group, using the sentence starters on the bookmark to support discussion. Teacher restates the teaching point and provides additional support for students who experience difficulty. The Monitoring and Responding to Student Difficulty chart outlines suggestions for responding with appropriate additional modeling, corrective feedback, and instruction. This four-step cycle is bolstered by the following.

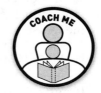

Reading-Writing Connection Students complete an independent writing activity that reinforces the skill/strategy in their reading response journal or on a graphic organizer.

Practice at the Literacy Center Students link the comprehension, fluency, or word-solving skill or strategy to independent and collaborative tasks at the literacy centers.

Lesson Text

What reading materials do I use to support differentiated small-group instruction?

Leveled texts are essential tools for differentiated instruction. The problem occurs when individual texts become the driving force for instruction and students are labeled by reading levels rather than their reading goals. Students in our differentiated reading program are described as reading text from a range of reading levels that varies depending on the demands that are placed upon the reader—whether the teaching point is word solving, fluency, or comprehension.

When selecting the text for the lesson consider the following:

1. The Teaching Point: The level of text students read during small-group instruction *will vary depending on the instructional focus.* For example, one of our students, Bella, is reading texts in her small-group lessons that range from levels J to H (Fountas & Pinnell, 2005). The passages, articles, and books the teacher selected for her small-group word-solving lessons are level J, which she can read with 90–94% accuracy. This provides her with the opportunity to practice applying word-solving strategies to 6–10% of the words in the text. In contrast, the text for comprehension lessons are selected so that she can read them with 95–100% accuracy (98%+ for more complex expository text structures). Easy level text enables Bella to focus on meaning-making strategies, and higher-level thinking text enables Bella to focus on meaning-making strategies and higher-level (metacognitive) thinking processes rather than decoding. When Bella (a speed demon) is working on her current fluency goal, adjusting the rate or pace at which she reads, her teacher selects a text she can read with 98–100% accuracy. Such a high degree of accuracy allows Bella to work on adjusting the rate of reading according to different sources of information in the text (e.g., dialogue, lists of facts) to ensure that she is also self-monitoring for comprehension. (See Figure 1.3, Selecting Text Based on the Teaching Point and Student Reading Levels.)

2. The Range of Student Reading Levels in the Group: When the focus is on word solving, you will be forming groups of students who decode text with a similar level of accuracy. The text selected for the lesson will need to be at the instructional level for every student in the group. This means that groups formed for word solving instruction are homogeneous in their level of decoding.

In contrast, groups that are formed for fluency and comprehension can be more heterogeneous; students do not all have to read the same text with the same accuracy rate in these groups. Their assessments reveal a range of reading levels and a common need in a fluency or comprehension skill. A fluency or comprehension focus requires that the text be at the independent level for every student in the group. This means that the guiding principle is to select text that is easy for the group member at the earliest stage in decoding. In this way every student will be able to decode at least 98% of the text with ease for fluency lessons, and 95% or more for comprehension lessons. This allows students to develop fluency and comprehension strategies without using precious mental energy and time figuring out the words. The fact that the text is easy is a good thing when you consider the difficulty so many students have reading with expression or engaging in

"Simply teaching students in smaller groups is not necessarily differentiating instruction. Grouping is a procedural change for how we teach. In order to differentiate, changes in what we teach are also needed. That means data-informed teaching using leveled materials that match text difficulty to student reading levels and leading skills-focused lessons that include more student engagement, and guided practice with constructive feedback from a teacher or peer."

(Gibson & Hasbrouck, p. 3, 2007)

higher-level thinking, such as making an inference. If the text is not easy, we are back to coaching students for word recognition during a comprehension lesson, or spending a disproportionate amount of time in a fluency lesson teaching words that cause hesitations.

Selecting Text Based on the Teaching Point and Student Reading Levels

Lesson Focus	Level of Accuracy	Guiding Principle for Selecting Group Text
Word Solving	90–94%	Instructional level for all students
Fluency	98–100%	Independent level text for all students
Comprehension	95–100% Narrative Text 98–100% Expository Text	Independent level for all students

Figure 1.3

Selecting Text to Support the Teaching of Specific Skills and Strategies

At the beginning of each chapter, I offer suggestions for selecting texts that specifically support the skills and strategies in the lessons. If you have difficulty locating an appropriately leveled text that directly supports a strategy, you can make a more challenging text accessible by adopting a shared reading format. When you have students who have a common comprehension strategy need, yet are reading at quite a range of levels, each student may practice with a different text and then share how they used the strategy with that title (see Chapter 6).

Whatever their functioning reading levels, all students benefit from reading authentic text that provides practice of the target skill or strategy. This is essential if they are to extend their understanding to new reading materials and internalize the thinking processes. By viewing leveled text as a means toward a goal and not the goal itself, our emphasis shifts from "doing the book" to closer examination of our students' development as readers.

In Chapter 2, you will be able to determine the appropriate teaching points for the demonstrated needs in your classroom. Together with the corresponding lessons from the following chapters, these points will enable you to successfully implement a differentiated small-group reading program where every student is both challenged and supported.

Summary of Key Principles:

- Students are organized in flexible small groups based upon current instructional goals, rather than placement along a continuum of text levels.

- Curriculum-based skills and strategies provide the scope and sequence for both whole class reading workshop mini-lessons and differentiated small-group reading instruction.

- Lesson content, teaching sequence, and learning materials are responsive to the needs of the learners.

QUESTIONS FOR PROFESSIONAL LEARNING DISCUSSIONS

1. How could you build upon your whole-class reading program and current lesson formats to provide more targeted practice in small-group lessons?

2. How will you provide independent practice for the rest of the class? What types of literacy centers would best support the learning?

Chapter 2

Planning Differentiated Small-Group Reading Instruction

Responsive instruction requires that we assess, teach, monitor progress, and reteach our students within small groups. This chapter describes how to determine the lessons that will be most effective for students at different points along the reading continuum. It is here we ask the crucial questions:

1. What information do I need to guide the formation of differentiated reading groups?
2. Which lessons support the reading goals identified in the assessment data?
3. How do I plan a sequence of reading instruction for groups of students with a common goal?

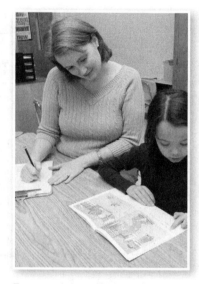

Frequent informal assessment during reading is essential to monitor transfer of skills and strategies to independent reading.

Ongoing Informal Assessment: The Information That Drives Differentiated Reading Instruction

What information do I need to guide the formation of differentiated reading groups?

Identifying the small-group reading lessons that will be most appropriate for our students requires ongoing assessment of their needs. Ongoing assessment ensures careful monitoring of student progress in the skills and strategies they require to continue to grow as readers. (See Figure 2.1.)

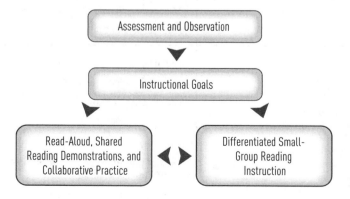

> "Knowing where they are and where they need to go and also knowing some strategies for getting them there on time is the real heart of a differentiated instructional plan."
>
> (WALPOLE & MCKENNA P. 7, 2007)

Figure 2.1 Assessment drives whole-class and small-group differentiated instruction.

Informal Assessment Tools

Walpole and McKenna (2006) recommend a set of informal assessments. These include a test of all levels of phonological awareness, including phoneme segmentation, a letter-name and letter-sound inventory, a phonics inventory, a pseudo-word decoding test, and a developmental spelling inventory, in addition to assessments of oral reading fluency and reading comprehension.

A "teaching toolkit" of informal assessment tools guides the selection of lessons for small-group instruction. These assessments are correlated with the areas of instruction addressed in Chapters 4 through 6 in the following chart.

Types of Informal Assessment

Differentiated Reading Lessons	Informal Assessments
Word Solving *Phonemic Awareness* *Phonics*	• All levels of phonological awareness, including phonemic blending and segmentation • Letter-name and letter-sound inventory • Phonics inventory • Pseudo-word decoding test • Graded word lists
Fluency *Oral Reading*	• Graded passages to assess accuracy and rate • Rubric for evaluating prosody • High-frequency word reading test
Comprehension *Strategy Use*	• Questions (literal, inferential, and evaluative) on narrative and expository text • Reading response journal (follow-up to small-group reading) • Collaborative discussion (what are students saying during whole-class and partner discussions that indicates strategy use?) • Teacher scripting of student dialogue

All Lessons
 	
Word Solving, Fluency, and Comprehension
 	
Self-Monitoring Strategies and Reading Behaviors
	• Running records
	• Informal reading inventories
	• Reading conferences
	• History as a reader
	Observation for evidence of:
	  ∗ Clarifying strategies (e.g., read on, reread, substitute a word, etc.)
	  ∗ Hesitations, persistence, passiveness, level of confidence, body language

Reading Strategy Conferences

Regularly scheduled reading strategy conferences provide another source of information to guide your instruction (Robb, 2008). During these conferences, we listen as students read for two to three minutes, ask questions to assess their understanding, record observational notes, and offer feedback on their progress as a reader (see Student Reading Goals and Observations Form, page 22). If you meet with two students each day, over a two-week period you will have provided all students with the constructive feedback they need to remain an engaged reader. During this time, the rest of the class participates in independent literacy centers (see Southall, 2007), partner reading, or independent reading or writing in their reading response journals. In a reading conference conversation, be sure to use consistent terminology for strategy use (making connections, summarizing, etc.), which empowers students to verbalize their reading goals.

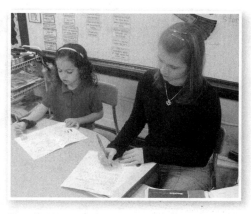

Step 2: While the student reads a short section of the text, the teacher uses an informal assessment tool to document her progress.

Steps in a Reading Conference

1. Prepare for the conference. Examine the assessment data on the student, including information you have recorded on the student observations form and their current goal set in the previous conference. This will help you to identify which skills and strategies will be the focus for this conference. Based on their progress with this goal, a new goal may be determined during the conference.

2. Review the current reading goal with the student and explain the purpose for the reading conference. Ask the student to read aloud a short excerpt from a familiar or an unfamiliar text (both are useful) to determine if the student can now apply previously taught skills independently and transfer their understanding of the concept to connected text. Note their progress on the current goal. Based on your observations, establish the next step in achieving the goal, or, if the student demonstrates readiness, identify a new goal.

3. Prompt students to verbalize how they applied the strategy in their current reading goal during reading (see prompt cards in Chapters 4 through 6). For example, ask them how they solved a tricky word or inferred the meaning of the passage. Refer to the classroom display of strategy statements (see Common Strategy Statements in Chapter 3, page 31), or the strategy charts or bookmarks in Chapters 4 through 6 to assist them to use the language of strategy use (see Interactive Tools for Responding to Text in Chapter 3, page 34).

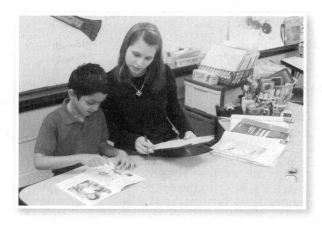

Step 3: The teacher prompts the student to explain how he applied the strategy during reading to determine his level of understanding.

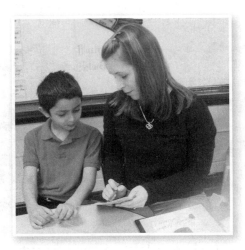

Step 4: Student motivation is enhanced by positive feedback on the current reading goal. Teachers may place "happy face" stickers alongside the strategy statement on student bookmarks (see Chapter 3) when this reading goal has been achieved.

"Well-timed and well-executed lessons from teaching professionals who are themselves thoughtful readers is often all it takes to begin the process of altering the fundamental view of reading that children hold. When we can match the reading profiles of our students with the instruction they need, we can put our children firmly on the road to effective, rewarding, and engaged reading throughout their entire lives."

(APPLEGATE, QUINN & APPLEGATE, P. 56, 2006)

4. Share your observations with students so they develop a greater self-awareness and ownership of their own progress as a reader. You may begin by asking them to reflect on their own progress by asking, "What did you learn about yourself as a reader today?" Share the strengths you noted, the strategies you observed the student apply successfully. Next, using your observations, explain an appropriate next step for the current reading goal, or set a new goal and discuss it. This becomes the teaching point for small-group instruction. Say something like, "This is what you need to work on next to continue to grow as a reader. It's your next reading goal, and this is how it will help you understand what you read."

5. Add new information to the student observation form to reflect current progress.

Assessment During the Small-Group Lesson: Making the Most of Your Time

I incorporate on-the-run, teacher-friendly informal assessment tools during each group lesson to maximize instructional time and to ensure I'm meeting students' current needs. These assessments include running records, skill/strategy use checklists or rubrics, and forms for observational note taking.

During each lesson I keep a copy of the Student Reading Goals and Observations Form (page 22) for one or two students on my clipboard. I listen to these students more than the others and document any signs of progress or difficulty. Often I add something to these notes right after the lesson. If I leave it longer than this, some of the details escape my memory.

Time for reflection on the assessment tools comes at the end of the literacy block or the day. Guidelines for setting up a planning notebook with sections for the different forms is described on page 31 in Chapter 3.

Planning Differentiated Reading Lessons

In this section, we will discuss how assessment data guides the selection of lessons in comprehension, fluency, and word solving. Students are placed together in a small group when they demonstrate need for instruction in the same skill or strategy. To decide upon an instructional focus and the corresponding lesson(s) for each group, we ask ourselves questions such as:

• What skills and strategies have these students mastered?

• What is the greatest area of need?

• What skill or strategy needs to be addressed?

• Which lesson will I use to address this need?

• How will I know if I need to reteach this skill/strategy or can I continue to the next reading goal?

The four steps outlined below address these questions so that the lessons meet the needs of our students. To plan and implement the lessons, review each of the four steps below. The fourth step is designed to ensure our instruction remains responsive to the rate of student learning. Keep in mind that some students will require more extensive teaching and practice in a skill or strategy than others. Assessment data and flexibility in our lesson planning can help to address the difference in the number of lessons on the same skill or strategy.

Four Steps to Differentiated Reading Lessons

1. Identify the appropriate lesson focus for your students. Use student assessment data to identify the skill or strategy that forms the appropriate reading goal for each student. Record on the Student Reading Goals and Observations Form, page 22.

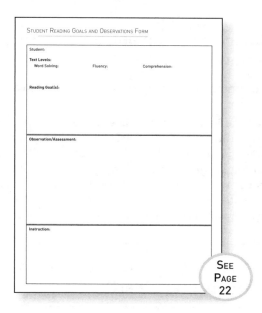

2. Form groups of students with a common reading goal. Review the Student Reading Goals and Observations Form from step 1 to identify groups of students who share a common reading goal. Record the goal and names of the students on the Planning for Group Instruction Form (page 23) and the Class Reading Goals Form (page 24).

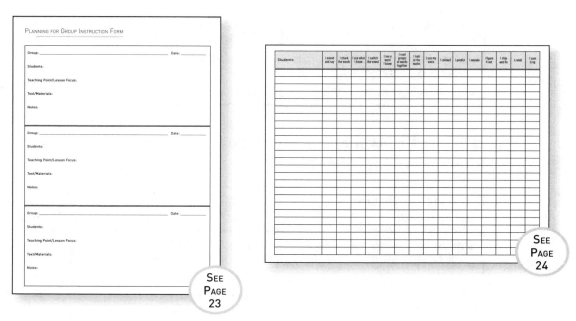

3. Plan lessons for groups of students. Refer to Aligning Student Need and Reading Lessons charts (pages 20–21) to select the lesson(s) that support(s) the goal on the Planning for Group Instruction Form.

4. Monitor student progress. Identify how you will monitor student progress (see Ongoing Informal Assessment on page 15 and Assessment During the Small-Group Lesson on page 18). Use this information to determine further lessons for reteaching or student readiness to move on to their next reading goal. Record further observations on the Student Reading Goals and Observations Form.

When/Then Charts for Planning Small-Group Reading Lessons

Which lessons support the reading goals identified in assessment data?

The following charts align student needs with relevant lessons in this book. The charts are organized into three key areas: word solving, fluency, and comprehension. I've also included some record-keeping and planning sheets that are helpful when forming groups and planning instruction—Student Reading Goals and Observations Form, Planning for Group Instruction Form, and Class Reading Goals Form—located on pages 22–24. Keep in mind that the lessons can be used with the same group more than once—simply vary the text.

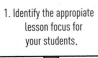
1. Identify the appropiate lesson focus for your students.

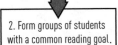
2. Form groups of students with a common reading goal.

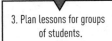
3. Plan lessons for groups of students.

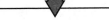
4. Monitor student progress.

Aligning Student Need and Reading Lessons: Word-Solving When/Then Chart

WHEN the student requires instruction in:	THEN provide these reading lessons:	Page Number
● Accurate and fluent blending	I Can Sound and Say:	43
	∗ Build and Blend	49
● Blending words in isolation and in context	∗ Blending Words in a List and Connected Text	51
● Recognition of common vowel patterns	I Can Chunk the Word:	54
	∗ Sound and Say the Chunk	60
● Using vowel patterns in familiar words to read new single and multisyllabic words	∗ I Can Use What I Know	63
● Flexibility with vowel pronunciations	∗ I Can Switch the Vowel	67

Aligning Student Need and Reading Lessons: Fluency When/Then Chart

WHEN the student requires instruction in:	THEN provide these reading lessons:	Page Number
● Increasing accuracy in reading irregular high-frequency words	I Can See Words I Know:	73
	∗ Train Your Reading Brain	79
	∗ X-Ray Eyes	81
● Increasing rate of reading irregular high-frequency words	∗ Countdown Game	83
● Reading with intonation and expression	I Can Use My Voice:	85
● Reading with meaningful phrasing	∗ I Can Read Groups of Words	87
● Attending to punctuation cues in the text	∗ I Can Look at the Marks	91

Aligning Student Need and Reading Lessons:
Comprehension When/Then Chart

WHEN the student requires instruction in:	THEN provide these reading lessons:	Page Number
• Making Connections	I Can Connect	103
• Predicting	I Can Predict	108
• Making Causal Inferences	I Can Figure It Out: Making Causal Inferences	116
• Making Relational Inferences	I Can Figure It Out: Making Relational Inferences	118
• Generating and answering literal questions	I Can Wonder: Literal Questions	126
• Generating and answering inferential and evaluative questions	I Can Wonder: Inferential and Evaluative Questions	129
• Self-monitoring using clarifying strategies	I Can Stop and Fix	134
• Using story structure and vocabulary to retell narrative text	I Can Retell	141
• Summarizing informational text; determining important information	I Can Sum It Up	145
• Integrating the use of multiple comprehension strategies	I Can Code My Thinking	149

QUESTIONS FOR PROFESSIONAL LEARNING DISCUSSIONS

1. What is the basis for student grouping in your classrooms? What information do you use? Do you need any additional information?

2. How could the scope and sequence of skills and strategies in your curriculum/standards be used as a guide for student grouping and teaching points for the lessons?

STUDENT READING GOALS AND OBSERVATIONS FORM

Student:

Text Levels:
    Word Solving: Fluency: Comprehension:

Reading Goal(s):

Observation/Assessment:

Instruction:

Planning for Group Instruction Form

Group: _____ Date: _____

Students:

Teaching Point/Lesson Focus:

Text/Materials:

Notes:

Group: _____ Date: _____

Students:

Teaching Point/Lesson Focus:

Text/Materials:

Notes:

Group: _____ Date: _____

Students:

Teaching Point/Lesson Focus:

Text/Materials:

Notes:

Tracking Class Reading Goals Form

Students	I sound and say	I chunk the words	I use what I know	I switch the vowel	I see a word I know	I read groups of words together	I look at the marks	I use my voice	I connect	I predict	I wonder	I figure it out	I stop and fix	I retell	I sum it up

Chapter 3

Organizing for Differentiated Reading Groups

The most common concerns about small-group teaching that I hear from colleagues have to do with the daily management of students, time, and materials. Let's take a close look at these factors so we can make differentiated small-group reading instruction a reality in your classroom.

Grouping Students

How many students should there be in a differentiated reading group?

Groups in a differentiated reading program range from three to seven students. For low progress readers, the groups should be between three and five students; for students performing at or above grade level, from five to seven students (Kosanovich, Ladinsky, Nelson, & Torgesen, 2006). Research supports that *intervention is unlikely to be effective when there are more than five students in the group* (Torgesen, 2005). The fewer students in the group, the more intensive the instruction becomes. To sum up, the number in a reading group depends upon:

1. The level of student need
2. The number of students requiring instruction in the skill or strategy

Should every student be in a small reading group?

Ideally, all students will have an opportunity to participate in differentiated small-group instruction on an ongoing basis to receive differentiated instruction and constructive, positive feedback. However, we know that low progress students will require more time and instruction. The number of low progress students in a class may result in a schedule where not all students participate in small-group instruction every day or continuously throughout the year. The learning needs of on-grade and advanced students may be served for periods of time with partner reading, independent reading, and responding to text (see Reading-Writing Connection: The Reading Response Journal on page 39), or participation in a book club. Participation in a small group is therefore flexible and determined by the level of student need in any one classroom.

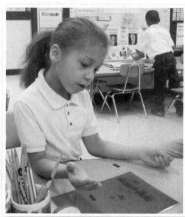

As a follow-up activity to a lesson on the I Can Chunk the Word strategy, students generate and build new words with the target vowel pattern. This supports recognition of these 'chunks' in new and more complex words.

Scheduling: Common Problems ... and Suggestions

Timeline

8:15	Entry Routines; Book Exchange
8:25	**Readers' Workshop: Whole-Class Mini-Lesson:** Read Aloud/Shared Reading; Demonstrations and Collaborative Practice
8:55	**Differentiated Small-Group Reading Lessons/Literacy Centers/Book Clubs**
9:45	Recess/Daily Fitness and Nutrition Break
10:00	**Differentiated Small-Group Reading Lessons/Literacy Centers/Book Clubs** (cont'd) **Reading Strategy Conferences**
10:25	**Word Study Workshop:** High Frequency Word Wall Practice; Group Rotation: Mini-Lesson/Word Sort Practice
10:45	**Writers' Workshop:** Mini-Lesson; Guided Writing Group/Independent Writing/Revision Stations
11:30	**Lunch Break**
12:00	**Reading Strategy Conferences**

Over the past two decades of small-group teaching, I have confronted each and every one of these challenges in my own classroom. Let's look at some problem-solving ideas to nip these issues in the bud.

I just can't seem to find enough time for small-group instruction

Perhaps you are trying to do it all—who isn't these days? But can you really keep doing everything you are now and fit more into the same time frame? Small-group reading instruction is not an add-on; it is essential if we are to provide the level of support each child deserves. *Maybe something you are doing now has to go* to make the time for it—and that something is whatever is giving you the least results for your teaching (and student learning) time. Here are some possible ways to crunch those teaching minutes in your schedule.

- Create a visual of your schedule to allow you to see the big picture. Draw a timeline of your literacy block (60 to 120 minutes) in five-minute increments vertically down the left of a sheet of chart paper. Alongside, list the instruction taking place, bracketing time intervals such as 10 or 25 minutes. Examine carefully each instructional activity you have listed. Take a highlighter and highlight the "must haves" in your schedule—the formats where you are seeing tangible student growth. What is left may need to go. Often what remains are activities and rituals we have always done. Prioritizing can be painful, but the effort is worth it—and you will see increased levels of student success.

- Student sharing during reading and writing workshop can be in partners or within small groups, with all groups meeting simultaneously. I trained my kindergarten and first-grade students to do this right from the beginning of school. One student in each circle of four was the group discussion leader and made sure every student got their "one minute" to share, passing the "talking stick" around the circle.

- Look for other time-eaters, such as transition time between short periods of instruction that require students to refocus and perhaps move or switch out their materials frequently. Note the time taken for transitions between different areas of instruction. Is there a more efficient order of activities or movement of students and their materials? Do the instructional formats flow into one another, e.g., shared reading into small-group reading?

- Integrate phonics and spelling into word study. We used to see spelling as a separate subject from phonics (letter-sound correspondences and vowel patterns), but research supports that students need to be learning to read and spell the same sets of words so they are learned in integration (see reading-writing connection activities in Chapter 4). For sight words that do not fit the phonics elements you are teaching, provide brief (five-minute) interactive activities three or four times a week alongside multisensory small-group and word study center activities.

- Teach grammar within writer's workshop mini-lessons using literature examples, and not as a separate subject.

- Integrate comprehension and vocabulary development with narrative and expository writing during content learning. Strategies for comprehending, summarizing, and writing informational text are appropriate across the curriculum, no matter what the grade level.

- In kindergarten and first grade, teach letter formation (handwriting) as you teach the letter-sound correspondences and monitor carefully for fine motor control and confusions. Handwriting should no longer be another subject on the list to fit into a day in second and third grade. I remember in my earlier teaching years how we used to spend as much as 20 minutes a day teaching cursive handwriting. Now there are scripts that are much more student friendly, that students learn right from kindergarten, and students don't use precious learning time mastering a second type of letter formation.

We are each trying very hard to maximize those minutes in our literacy block. I have come to the conclusion there will never be enough time to do everything I would like to do with my students. But I will always advocate for protected small-group teaching time: It is the heart of the reading program.

Our core reading program takes up so much time I don't have any left for small-group instruction.

Core reading programs or literature sets and small-group instruction are not mutually exclusive. They can both have their place in the program. Whole-class read-alouds, shared reading, and literature-driven discussions enable every student to have access to grade-level literature and the opportunity to grow from hearing the thinking of others. The proportion of time designated for these is the question. You must find the balance between whole-class and small-group instruction. Is it mandated in your school that you teach every lesson in the core program? Unless you are using a highly structured special education program, where following the sequence is critical to support cumulative skill-building, then you must be able to select from your program the lessons that correlate with student need. You may spend a longer or shorter time on different skills in response to student achievement levels. It is not a matter of "doing the book." You are a professional who is able to identify which skills and strategies from the core program and district standards require more intensive instruction within a small-group setting, and it is your responsibility to provide the responsive teaching that will make a difference for these children. It will be essential for you to document how you use student data to plan your lessons so that you have the necessary evidence to demonstrate how you are meeting both district literacy goals and student needs within your small-group instruction. The lesson planning forms in this chapter and the When/Then charts in Chapter 2 are designed to assist you with this. There is ample research supporting the efficacy of small-group instruction when it targets the data-based needs of students. (See the quotes throughout the book and references on page 159 that you can use to advocate for your students and provide the rationale for your program.)

What do I recommend as the proportion of time allocated to whole-class instruction, small-group lessons, and one-to-one conferences? If you think about a pyramid divided into three tiers, small group would be at the base of the pyramid, representing the most time, followed by whole-class instruction and then independent reading (in conjunction with a reading response journal, so that it is accountable time) alongside one-to-one teacher-student conferences.

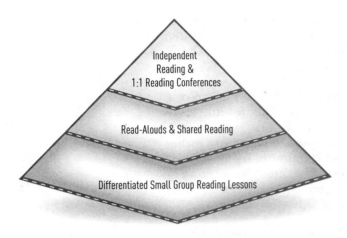

Figure 3.1 Allocating time for each component of a balanced reading program

I devote approximately 30 minutes to whole-class instruction using read-alouds and shared reading text and 45 to 60 minutes for small-group reading instruction. Some would argue that time conferring with individual students should represent the most time. I recognize the power of one-to-one tutoring and goal setting, and this could certainly be the second tier of the pyramid, where possible. I confer with and informally assess two students each day, which means over a two-week period every child has had individual feedback on his or her growth as a reader and current goals. I would like to see more time for individualized instruction, but in the majority of classrooms (and intervention programs), there are too many students for one teacher to tutor individual students with the frequency necessary to achieve learning goals. Practicality necessitates a small-group format.

How often should I meet with each group?

We vary not only the teaching point or content but also the frequency, duration, and intensity of group meetings (Gibson & Hasbrouck, 2007). For students who are not performing at grade level, daily small-group instruction is essential to bridge the gaps that have developed and achieve an increased rate of progress. Those performing at grade level should have the opportunity for small-group learning at least twice a week to extend their understanding of key concepts, and to take them higher in their critical thinking skills and deeper in their understanding of different genre and text structures. The peer discussion that takes place in small-group sessions is also an important growth opportunity for all students.

I find it difficult to watch the clock and end up running out of time for small-group instruction at the end of our literacy block.

If you find that whole-class instruction takes up a disproportionate amount of time and small-group instruction time suffers, begin the literacy block with small-group instruction and close with whole group or alternate periods of small-group and whole-class instruction.

I want to work with two groups a day, but my students can't remain independent for that long. Are there any scheduling options that would help me with this?

If you are meeting with multiple groups each day and this is not a realistic length of time for your students (developmentally and/or behaviorally) to work independently, schedule alternate periods of whole-class instruction and small-group lessons/literacy centers. For example, try small-group instruction for 20 to 30 minutes followed by a word study lesson or shared reading activity, then a second small-group session. This means students come together and refocus before going back to independent tasks at the centers.

How much time should I spend on each part of the lesson?

Create a visual time guide for yourself to represent the parts of your lesson. Draw a pie chart with three sections, the size of each section corresponding to the time you spend on teaching that part of the lesson, and write the time in your pie chart. How much time do you spend explaining and demonstrating the teaching point, guiding student practice, coaching students during reading, and restating the teaching point? In a 20-minute lesson, allow no more than five to six minutes for the first slice, seven to eight minutes for the second and eight to ten minutes for the last slice of your pie. If your lessons are 25 to 30 minutes, then adjust the guided practice time accordingly. Struggling readers require multiple demonstrations of a new skill, but be aware of the need to include student responses throughout your demonstration or you will lose their attention. Student practice should always be the largest part of the lesson; these are the activities under Guide Me and Coach Me in the lesson plans.

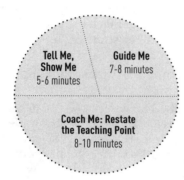

Plan your teaching time for each part of the lesson

I always run out of time before I finish the lesson.

Use a timer at the small-group table and set it for five minutes before the end of the lesson, so you will not run out of time to review the teaching point and have a group share of the roadblocks and successes students experienced during the reading (this is the Coach Me: Restate the Teaching Point part of the lesson; see Lesson Format/Sequence, Chapter 1).

Rotation Systems

In many classrooms, students rotate through literacy centers and the small-group teaching table using a rotation visual with icons representing each center (see Southall, 2007). You need to decide whether you want your small-group instruction to be part of the rotation system or separate from it. A rotation system where the teacher is part of the rotation means that the time for the lessons is the same amount of time students spend on a independent task at a literacy center, partner reading, etc. (see the first two rotation options). If you want flexibility in the lesson schedule, then do not include yourself in the rotation, but rather pull students to the teaching table from ongoing independent activities, based on common needs (see the bottom rotation option). You may also wish to have a follow-up task from the lesson as part of the rotation (see third rotation option).

Rotation Options

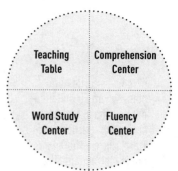

Small-Group Instruction
+ 3 Centers

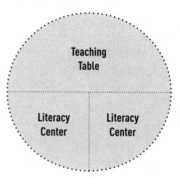

Small-Group Instruction
+ 2 Centers

Small-Group Instruction
+ Follow-Up Task + 2 Centers

Small-Group Follow-Up Task
+ 3 Centers

Working With Differentiated Reading Groups Within Response to Intervention (RTI) and Collaborative Teaching Models

How does this approach support the Response to Intervention model?

A growing number of districts across the country are implementing the Response to Intervention (RTI) model (Walpole & McKenna, 2007). If you are working with this three-tier model, the lessons in Chapters 4 through 6 will address the needs of Tier 1 students, who meet grade-level expectations but demonstrate varying instructional needs. The differentiated reading lessons are especially appropriate for Tier 2 students, who require more opportunities for small-group instruction to achieve grade-level goals. Low progress readers (Tier 2) can participate in the classroom teacher's group first, then work with a specialist in a second small-group session, and thus be supported by a double dose of targeted instruction on the same skill or strategy (Torgesen, 2005).

How would this work with a push-in model of classroom support?

A similar framework to the one described above is used for in-class support systems, where specialist teachers provide students with supplemental instruction on a regular basis. For example, the reading specialist, Title 1, or special education resource teacher works with a small group of students who have demonstrated need in a specific skill or strategy, while the classroom teacher also works with a small group. The benefit of having a second reading teacher is that low progress students are able to participate in small-group instruction on a daily basis.

Grouping Students From Multiple Classrooms

Some schools use their assessment data to form groups with common needs across classrooms, with students working with a second teacher during small-group reading instruction. The basis for distributing students among teachers is generally the students' functioning reading levels. For example, one teacher may work with low progress readers, while another works with students working at or near grade level and a third teacher works only with advanced readers.

The differentiated small-group reading framework can be readily implemented in a collaborative teaching model using skill-based grouping (with common instructional goals) instead of ability-based grouping. Individual teachers can then focus on a specific area of instruction, such as word solving, or have a dual-strategy focus, such as word solving and fluency. For example, one teacher can work with students requiring instruction in decoding skills and word-solving strategies; a second teacher on fluency aspects such as reading rate (correct words per minute), meaningful phrasing, and the use of expression; and a third teacher on comprehension strategies and vocabulary building. This would provide three reading "stations" at which students could participate depending on their current need. A fourth teacher may work with students engaged in partner reading or book clubs. In this way, students will spend time with different teachers based on their current reading goal(s). Of course, the numbers of students requiring instruction in each area will vary at different times of the year, and the instructional focus will not remain static for each teacher. Teachers will have the opportunity to teach two or more of the stations over the course of a year as they collaborate to meet the changing needs of students in their grade level(s).

Rotating Intervention Groups

Where there are two or more intervention teachers, each teacher can focus on a different aspect of reading. For example, during a 50- to 60-minute intervention schedule, students rotate between two "dual-strategy" reading stations (Torgesen, 2005). The first group begins with a 25- to 30-minute lesson on word solving and fluency, while a second intervention group works on vocabulary and comprehension strategies. After each lesson, the groups rotate to their next reading station for the remainder of the intervention schedule.

Materials to Support Instruction: Designing and Stocking Your Small-Group Teaching Space

What teaching and learning materials do I need during small-group lessons?

You need to have the necessary teaching materials at your fingertips to maintain student engagement and the pacing of the lesson. I have listed here the essential tools I use along with the interactive learning aids that are included in this book, such as strategy chart visuals, and student bookmarks. In each of the lessons in Chapters 4, 5, and 6 you will find suggestions for specific materials to support the skill or strategy.

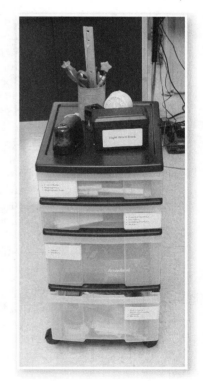

Small-Group Teaching Binder

I designed the lesson plans in this book in an at-a-glance format so that you will be able to refer to them during the lesson. In addition, I keep a binder at the table that contains the information that drives my small-group instruction. I divide my binder into the following sections:

1. District reading standards, strategy statements based on these (see below)

2. Tracking Class Reading Goals Form (page 24)

3. Planning for Group Instruction forms (page 23)

4. Student Reading Goals and Observation forms (page 22); I use dividers with tabs labeled in alphabetical order (available from office supply stores) to divide this section by students' last names

Labeled, stacked drawers store interactive tools designed to support each skill during the small-group lessons. What do you need in your teaching toolbox?'

Common Strategy Statements

The use of a set of common statements helps us achieve one of the criteria for explicit instruction—clear, consistent teacher wording (Hasbrouck & Denton, 2005). The importance of this cannot be underestimated.

Many of our low progress readers are confused by the conflicting terminology they hear from different teachers. I have followed students from classroom to intervention settings and heard different terminology being used for the same phonics element or comprehension strategy. These are the students who already struggle to grasp new concepts, and by neglecting to ensure consistency in our instruction, we slow the pace of student learning.

I've developed strategy statements to express the steps and thinking processes used for each reading strategy or skill. The strategy statements are based on my district standards, and I use them when discussing student reading goals, while making teaching points during small-group lessons, and during whole-class instruction. I've used these statements on the Strategy Charts, Student Bookmarks and Teacher Prompt Cards that are incorporated into each lesson sequence and referred to during group discussions, partner sharing, and independent reading.

Strategy statements are phrased in student-friendly language so young learners can verbalize and internalize their strategy use. The language used in our district standards is often too complex for young students and needs to be reworded for instructional purposes.

A number of schools and districts are making a concerted effort to build this school-wide consistency in their reading programs across classrooms and grade levels. A bulletin board display of grade-level strategy statements in each classroom can provide a central reference for teaching and learning goals. The strategy statements should be visible and accessible during whole-class and small-group instruction. The Classroom Bulletin Board of Reading Strategy Statements on page 33 shows how the strategies included in the lessons in this book could be displayed on a bulletin board or wall. You may add to or delete statements as appropriate for your grade level or range of grade levels your students represent. Each of the strategy statements is printed on a sentence strip and added to the display as it is taught, in the same way that words are added to a word wall. The three category headings on the bulletin board represent all five areas of instruction, where Word Solving includes both phonemic awareness and phonics, and Comprehension includes vocabulary development. I have used terms such as Word Workers (word solving), Smooth Talkers (fluency) and Meaning-Makers (comprehension) with young students, but whatever language you use it, needs to be consistent with the terminology they hear during instruction.

Assessment walls have become commonplace in schools, where student progress is monitored and student name cards organized according to level of need (benchmark, strategic, or intensive) or text levels. We know that linking assessment to instruction requires going beyond these categories to the identification of teaching points and instructional formats (see Chapter 2). During grade-level team and intervention meetings, the visual of common strategy statements is used to organize students into differentiated reading groups in the classroom and, where necessary, into intervention groups focusing on the same skill/strategy. During these meetings, each teacher refers to their copy of the skill/strategy statements to support the discussion process. You may decide to create a central bulletin board for your school or grade level, where student name cards (names on the back of the cards) or sticky notes are placed under the corresponding skill/strategy statements, that is their current instructional goal.

Classroom Bulletin Board

WORD SOLVING c ake	FLUENCY	COMPREHENSION
I can read the words.	**I can read smoothly.**	**I can understand what I read.**
I can sound and say. r-a-n ran	I can see words I know.	I can connect.
I can chunk the word. c ake = cake	I can read groups of words together.	I can predict.
I can use what I know. d(ay) pl(ay) ✓	I can look at the marks. ? ; !	I can figure it out.
I can switch the vowel.	I can use my voice.	I can wonder.
		I can stop and fix.
		I can retell.
		I can sum it up. 1 + 1 = 2

Differentiated Small Group Reading Lessons © 2009 by Margo Southall, Scholastic Teaching Resources page 33

Strategy Prompt Cards

The importance of responding to student need with consistent prompts for each skill area has been supported by numerous studies as essential for ensuring transfer from instructional to independent reading (Taylor, Pearson, Clark, & Walpole, 1999). I've included a teacher prompt card in each of Chapters 4 through 6 that uses the same terminology as the strategy charts. I recommend keeping a copy at the teaching table, so that when students have difficulty, you can quickly glance at the card for a prompt to use during coaching that corresponds to the strategy they are neglecting and need to apply to self-correct.

Anchor Strategy Charts

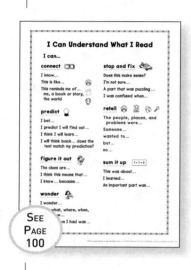

SEE PAGE 100

Using picture-cued strategy charts is another way to make the reading process more explicit for young learners. I use these charts at the teaching table during small-group instruction to ensure that every student can access the strategy statements. The lessons in this book integrate anchor strategy charts for word solving (Chapter 4, page 45), fluency (Chapter 5, page 76), and comprehension (Chapter 6, page 100). The strategies for each of these teaching areas are introduced cumulatively in each chapter, and together form the complete picture-cued Reading Strategy Chart on page 35 .

While lists of general good reader strategies and comprehension anchor charts are becoming more common, there are fewer word-solving and fluency-strategy charts available. I have been using a picture-cued word-solving strategy chart alongside similarly cued comprehension charts for nearly a decade. These picture-cued charts with their student-friendly language have made a real difference in the ease with which students have understood and applied the strategies.

I display the charts at the teaching table for each lesson. A tabletop whiteboard stand is useful for this purpose; simply clip the strategy chart onto the whiteboard. When I demonstrate and refer to specific strategies on the chart, I use a colored paper clip or clothespin and clip it alongside the icon for the strategy. To prepare for the lessons, copy the strategy charts on pages 45, 76, and 100 to make charts that you can use at the teaching table. To create wall-size copies of the strategy charts to display in your teaching area, enlarge on a photocopier and paste onto poster board. Students may have a copy of the Reading Strategy Chart pasted inside the cover of their reading response journal to refer to, in addition to the Reading Strategy Bookmark on page 38 in this chapter.

Interactive Tools for Responding to Text

The interactive tools described in this section, together with the routines for brief "turn and talk" formats, offer the solution to the dilemma of how to ensure every student in the group is accountable to respond in some way within a short timeframe. I have found each of these materials to be an invaluable aid in helping students to remain focused on the skill or strategy they are learning.

Reading Strategy Chart

I can read the words

I sound and say

I chunk the word = cake

I use what I know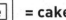

I switch the vowel

I can read smoothly

I see words I know

I read groups of words together

I look at the marks **? ; !**

I use my voice

I can understand what I read

I connect

I predict

I figure it out

I wonder

I stop and fix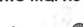

I retell

I sum it up | 1 + 1 = 2 |

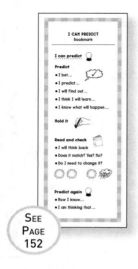

SEE
PAGE
152

Strategy Bookmarks

Reproducible student strategy bookmarks accompany each lesson and correspond to the Reading Strategy Chart on page 35. The bookmarks provide valuable tactile memory aids and support a high level of student engagement (Allen, 2007). Students can "think-pinch-share," using the strategy icon on their bookmark to help them verbalize their strategy use with a partner or the group (see page 38). The phrases on the bookmarks are meant as a support, but should be used flexibly so that students are not stifled in how they explain their strategy use. I do not confine responses to these phrases alone, but use them as a springboard to initiate and maintain discussion.

Preparation of the Bookmarks

Copy the bookmarks onto cardstock, making one for each student in the group. Use correction tape or a sticky note to conceal any strategy that is likely to pose a distraction or be a source of confusion to some students at this time.

Introducing the Bookmarks: Model Each Strategy Statement

Read a short section of text aloud and model how to use one of the phrases on the bookmark to think aloud about your strategy use during the reading. Invite students to practice by using the same statement or by selecting a statement and using it to compose a response to share with a partner or the group. Repeat for the other phrases in subsequent lessons until students understand and can use each of the statements with success.

Think-Pinch-Share Format

During the reading, pause at preplanned stopping points so students can respond to the text. When students may select from more than one statement and icon, ask them to hold up their bookmark and pinch the picture cue/ statement that represents their strategic thinking. For example, in the I Can Wonder: Inferential and Evaluative Questions lesson (page 129), students pinch different question starters and use these to share a question they have about the reading. One student might have a "What if" question, wondering what might have happened if the character had responded in a different way, while another student may have a "Should" question about something the character did.

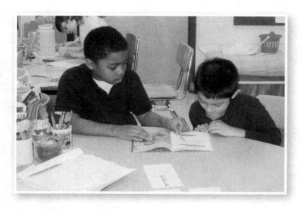

One partner reads, while the other partner coaches him to apply the word-solving strategies on the bookmark.

Designate partners before the lesson begins and have students sit next to their partner. I suggest varying the partners so that they benefit from exposure to multiple perspectives. These focused sharing formats will support writing in response to reading (see Reading-Writing Connection: The Reading Response Journal, page 39)—if they can't say it, they can't write it. Thinking aloud to an audience provides a valuable opportunity to clarify their thinking, piggyback on the thinking of others, and deepen their level of understanding, which leads to a more detailed written response.

Integrate Strategy Use

Provide cumulative practice by integrating the strategies on two bookmarks (copy two-sided or provide both copies) as you progress through the lessons. Once students have practiced all of the strategy bookmarks, then provide the Reading Strategy Bookmark on page 38 that integrates all strategies into a single bookmark. Allow students to choose the statement that best represents their thinking and use this to focus their response. For example, one student may make a connection while another generates a question about the reading.

Summary of Procedure:

- Review the statement(s) and icons on the bookmark
- Read to a key stopping point in the text
- Model strategic thinking by sharing your response to the reading using a cue from the bookmark
- Prompt students to use the same or a different statement to compose a response
- Provide a five-second wait time
- Ask students to hold up their bookmark and pinch their fingers next to the icon that best represents their thinking
- Invite sharing of these responses—in partners and with the group

We have read a few pages. Let's stop and talk about the story. Hold up your bookmark to let us know what you want to say. I see all kinds of questions. [For partner share:] Tell your partner what you are thinking. [For group share:] Let's hear what ___ has to say. [Or] __ , can I hear your thinking?

Other Tools: Sticky Notes, Flags, Page Markers, and Highlighter Tape

Many of the lessons suggest using consumable sticky notes for the interactive activities. These enable students to mark the text in places where they have a strategy-related response, such as an event they find confusing and need to "stop and fix" (clarify). By marking the text, students can then quickly locate their "thinking spots" to share with their "thinking partner" in the Think-Pinch-Share activity (see example on page 51).

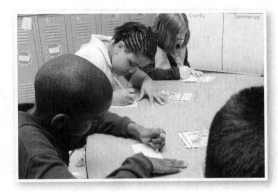

Students write their predictions on sticky notes to place on a group chart. This will provide a visual reference for confirming or adjusting predictions as they read.

An alternative material for this purpose that I include in my reading teacher's toolkit are sticky flags (one inch). I especially like these because they are reusable. I provide each student with a laminated strip of cardstock with a set number of these sticky flags. In the coding lesson on page 149, you will see an example of how to print codes on the flags with a permanent marker to represent specific types of responses. This provides a focus for student responses and develops application of integrated strategy use.

You can also provide sticky page markers that come in packs of four or five different colors. Several ways to use these include: marking the text with one color where students are to stop and make a prediction, then using a second color further in the text where they are to confirm or adjust their prediction; asking students to mark the clues that support their inference; and placing a marker where they generate a question and then another where they locate the answer. These page markers can also be kept on the strip of cardstock described above and reused in further lessons.

READING STRATEGY
Bookmark

I can read the words

I sound and say

I chunk the word

I use what I know dy ply ✓

I switch the vowel

I can read smoothly

I see words I know

I read groups of words together

I look at the marks **? ; !**

I use my voice

I can understand what I read

I connect

I predict

I figure it out

I wonder

I stop and fix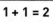

I retell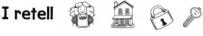

I sum it up | 1 + 1 = 2 |

READING STRATEGY
Bookmark

I can read the words

I sound and say

I chunk the word

I use what I know dy ply ✓

I switch the vowel

I can read smoothly

I see words I know

I read groups of words together

I look at the marks **? ; !**

I use my voice

I can understand what I read

I connect

I predict

I figure it out

I wonder

I stop and fix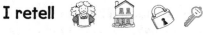

I retell

I sum it up | 1 + 1 = 2 |

Differentiated Small Group Reading Lessons © 2009 by Margo Southall, Scholastic Teaching Resources page 38

Other useful tools include highlighter tape that can be stored in strips on cardstock at the table. Students can highlight parts that were confusing or where a prediction was confirmed or disconfirmed, etc., and then place the tape back on the card when they have finished. Some teachers like to provide the student with special pointers, such as plastic fingers and popsicle sticks with "googly" eyes on the end to support tracking the text.

Together all of these tools support mastery of each strategy and also the goal of integrated strategy use during independent reading. Now let's look at what the students will need to record their responses.

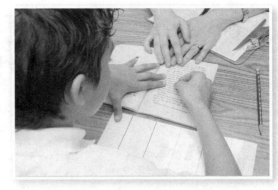

Students use highlighter tape to mark words and events that are puzzling or confusing during an I Can Stop and Fix (clarifying strategy) lesson (see Chapter 6). The group will practice using the "fix-up tools" on their strategy bookmark to solve problems and maintain comprehension during reading.

Reading-Writing Connection: The Reading Response Journal

As adults, we seldom remain silent about a novel we have just read. We look for others with whom to share our insights and reflections. Students are no different. Journals can be exchanged between reading partners and used as a springboard to more writing (a reply) or further discussion. Either way, students benefit from piggybacking their ideas off another student, extending their own understanding of the text. In each of the lessons in Chapters 4 through 6 there are suggestions for written responses that support the teaching point. See also, "How are reading and writing integrated within the lesson structure? in the Lesson Structure" section of Chapter 1, page 11, for an explanation of how the journal is used for different skills and strategies.

BUILDING CAPACITY IN YOUR SCHOOL—COMPILE AND SHARE A COLLECTION OF LESSONS

- As you plan and teach the lessons in this book, no doubt you will think of other ways to extend the skills and strategies in response to the needs of your students. Use the Planning for Group Instruction Form on page 23 to jot down an outline of your lesson. Reflect on the lesson, and what you might change next time. Place a copy in your small-group teaching notebook and share a second copy in a school or grade-level notebook of lessons organized by skills and strategies.

- As a literacy coach, I set out to share and compile a three-ring binder of lessons for specific skills and strategies that could be accessed by teachers across K–3 classrooms as an addition to our literacy resource room, or "teacher take-out" as I like to call it. Now other teachers have begun to contribute to this resource, the result of a professional learning focus on co-planning in grade-level teams.

Chapter 4

Word-Solving Lessons

....

The goal of word-solving instruction (phonemic awareness and phonics) is for students to be able to solve new words in running text while maintaining fluency. The lessons in this chapter address the most common difficulties students experience in acquiring word-solving strategies, including blending, recognizing vowel patterns, and using analogy. Students with word-solving difficulties can fall into the following categories.

- At-a-glance readers, who scan words ineffectively and do not attend to the successive elements in the word, such as final and medial sounds. They often use only initial letter cues.

- Huffers and puffers, who experience difficulty blending letter-sounds in words accurately and fluently. They may not yet be able to hold a sequence of sounds in their phonological memory to pronounce the word.

- Overly analytical readers, who often rely on smaller units of sound to decode (e.g., phonemes) rather than larger units, such as vowel patterns and affixes, and who over-analyze even familiar words.

- Word callers, who have not acquired the self-monitoring strategies required when problem-solving new single-syllable and multisyllabic words. They may substitute a nonsense word or omit words. These students do not use patterns in familiar words to decode new words (analogy).

- Isolationists, who do not transfer or apply their phonics knowledge in different contexts (e.g., from small-group lessons to independent reading) or to the reading of new text.

- Solo-strategy readers, who are unable to integrate strategy use to solve more complex words.

Word-Solving Lessons: An Overview

The word-solving lessons in this chapter progress in complexity, as organized below.

- Segmenting and blending successive phonemes
- Recognition of short and long vowel patterns
- Using familiar parts of words to decode new words
- Flexibility with vowel pronunciations

The first two lessons focus on accuracy and fluency in decoding words with phonetically regular spellings. Students segment and blend using a cumulative blending approach (see page 43) that has proven successful with students whose decoding is inaccurate, slow, and laborious (Beck, 2006). We teach segmenting and blending as we introduce letter-sound relationships. When we begin instruction with continuant consonant sounds (such as *m, f, s,* sounds that can be stretched) together with a vowel, students can form words even at the earliest stage of decoding, such as *am, sam, an, fan, man.*

Researchers from the Center for the Improvement of Early Reading Achievement (Taylor, Pearson, Clark, & Walpole, 1999) identified the qualities of effective word-solving instruction in the primary grades. "One major 'how' quality was that most teachers not only taught phonics in isolation but coached students or provided help to students as they attempted to use various phonics skills in real reading situations." (BLAIR, RUPLEY, & NICHOLS, P. 435, 2007)

Lesson	Skill/Strategy	Page
● I Can Sound and Say:	Accurate and fluent blending	43
＊Build and Blend		49
＊Blending Words in a List and Connected Text	Blending words in isolation and in context	51
● I Can Chunk the Word:	Recognition of common vowel patterns	54
＊Sound and Say the Chunk	Learning patterns in key words	60
＊I Can Use What I Know	Using vowel patterns in familiar words to problem-solve new and complex words (analogy)	63
＊I Can Switch the Vowel	Flexibility with vowel pronunciations	67

We teach students how to analyze words by phoneme and do not begin instruction with or rely solely on the teaching of rimes for two reasons. First, this ability to analyze words by phonemes is a precursor to storing and retrieving vowel patterns in both their phonological and visual (orthographic) memory. If students try to memorize the vowel pattern as a single unit without being able to segment and blend each phoneme, they may store an incomplete representation of the rime in their visual and phonological memory. This results in gaps in the recall of the rime and unsuccessful decoding during reading. Failure to retrieve all the letters in a vowel digraph or diphthong and silent consonants in a spelling pattern such as _ight, is a common outcome when students do not fully match, or when they mismatch, sounds to letters (see lessons under I Can Chunk the Word, page 54). Secondly, when students attempt to decode more complex words, where there is not always a rhyming word to help them figure it out, being able to analyze a sequence of phonemes and vowel units will be necessary for successful decoding. Word study center activities, such as word sorts and word building, are listed with the lessons to support independent practice of each skill.

The reproducible Word-Solving Prompt Card on page 44 provides suggested prompts for each strategy and can be used as a guide when responding to student difficulty. When a student comes to an unfamiliar word and begins to struggle, select a prompt that directs the student's attention to the neglected strategy. This prompting scaffolds the student's application of skills during reading to ensure transfer of taught skills to the reading process.

Clark (2004) describes the steps for prompting a student during reading: "Mrs. Green began the interaction by identifying a possible strategy and cueing a relevant sound, and then she become more specific by guiding the student through the strategy." (p. 445)

Monitoring and Responding to Student Progress in Word Solving

Reading accuracy depends upon a number of skills, including blending sounds in sequence and discriminating sound-spellings of common vowel patterns. Each of these also depends upon several phonological awareness skills (see suggestions in the chart under Monitoring and Responding to Student Difficulty, page 48). When a student's accuracy is a concern, assessment of these underlying skills will identify which requires more intensive small-group teaching.

In addition to the lessons in this chapter, you will also find detailed suggestions on how to address specific difficulties students may encounter while acquiring each of these skills. Just like the When/Then charts in Chapter 2, these charts list the type of difficulty paired with ways in which the teacher can support the particular area of need.

Tools for Interactive Learning

In the following section we examine picture-cued visuals and materials specifically designed to scaffold the application of word-solving strategies during reading, so that students internalize the process. When used in conjunction with supportive text, and practice in reading and writing the same words, we provide our students with a systematic, integrated approach to the learning of word-solving strategies.

Anchor Strategy Chart

Each strategy is represented on the picture-cued I Can Read the Words anchor chart on page 45. Photocopy and laminate the chart so you can display it and refer to it during the lessons. The student-friendly key words and phrases allow struggling readers access to the language of word solving so that they can successfully internalize the process of problem-solving new and complex words. My word-solving chart has evolved over the years, and I have revised and extended it after observing how other teachers used visuals to demonstrate a strategy (Lynch, 2002).

Strategy Bookmark

The reproducible, picture-cued Word-Solving Bookmark (page 46) helps students verbalize word-solving strategies. The bookmarks also encourage a high level of student engagement during lessons as students "think-pinch-share," using the statements on their bookmark to apply the strategy. Together, these activities support long-lasting understanding and application of each strategy. By cumulatively practicing each one, students become independent, flexible word-solvers who are able to integrate multiple strategies to solve new words they encounter in text.

The Text: How to Select

Students benefit from reading words in running text that contain the same decodable elements they are learning (Blevins, 2006), which raises the question of whether to use decodable text or uncontrolled text in the lessons. Low progress readers who are struggling at the earliest level of decoding may benefit from more controlled text that incorporates a significant proportion of the phonics elements they are learning within instructional contexts. However, a diet of controlled texts alone would likely pose a barrier to these students successfully reading the books they self-select or other classroom materials.

Fortunately, some of the newer series of books that are designed to support word solving have addressed the problems of being overly contrived, which impedes comprehension. I have included examples from several of these texts in the lessons. First, select the appropriate level of text for word-solving lessons (90–94%) and scan the text for words with decodable elements students know and are currently learning. Next, choose words for analysis (Show Me) and support transfer by reading them both in isolation and within connected text (Guide Me, Coach Me). Some publishers list them at the back of the book or in an accompanying teacher guide.

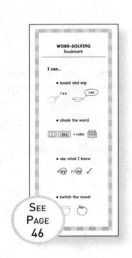

SEE PAGE 45

SEE PAGE 46

Other Materials

Other materials that support the word-solving lessons include:

- Blank index cards for masking words and parts of words (they close in on the word/part like automated sliding doors)
- Translucent highlighters, such as counters found in math catalogs, for locating parts in words
- Small whiteboard for illustrating how words work
- Lowercase magnetic letters and magnetic boards
- Picture-cued alphabet chart to use when prompting for recognition

Reading-Writing Connection

As a follow-up to a lesson, students compose sentences containing words with the same spelling elements in shared or independent writing. You may dictate a sentence or compose a language experience story that incorporates the target phonics elements and/or high-frequency words. I try to use children's names in the stories we compose.

Generate charts of words with the same patterns and display for students to use as a source of possible words they can incorporate in their writing. Poems are often the easiest for students to write when you are working on rimes.

Reading and spelling words with the same features helps students consolidate their understanding of how words work and accelerates the transfer of skills to independent reading.

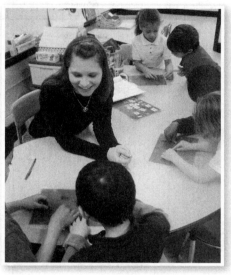

When the students' reading goal is increased accuracy and fluency with high frequency words, teachers provide practice with developmentally appropriate tactile materials, and support recognition of these same words during reading.

I Can Sound and Say: Accurate and Fluent Blending

The successive blending technique used in this series of lessons, in which students cumulatively blend the sounds together as they decode a word, has proven to be more effective with struggling readers than the final blending approach, which requires the student to segment each phoneme and then recall a string of individual phonemes to pronounce a whole word, e.g., /c/ /a/ /t/, *cat* (O'Connor, 2007). Beck (2006) notes that "the strong advantage of successive blending is that it is less taxing for short-term memory because blending occurs immediately after each new phoneme is pronounced ... at no time must more than two sounds be held in memory, and at no time must more than two sound units be blended" (page 50). This instructional technique is especially supportive for children with phonological memory difficulties.

The National Reading Panel (NICHD, 2000) noted that while phonics programs address letter-sound relationships, not enough attention is placed on teaching children *how* to blend efficiently to decode new words. Even fewer programs provide information on how teachers can avoid the most common problems children experience as they learn to blend letter sounds. The following lessons address this common gap in our teaching materials.

"Blending can be an area of great difficulty for many youngsters with reading difficulties. ... It is recommended that teachers teach letter-by-letter decoding as students' first reading strategy, followed by other strategies to augment this approach as children gain skills and confidence."

(O'Connor, 2007, p. 61, on results of the National Reading Panel, 2000)

WORD-SOLVING PROMPT CARD

Strategy	Prompt
Sound and Say	• Get your mouth ready ... say the first sound(s) • Does that fit with your first sound? • Say it slow. Touch and say each sound. • Use your eyes, finger and mouth to check it. • Run your finger under it to check the sounds. • Blend the sounds together to say the word. • Say it fast ... Bulldoze it ... Keep your motor running. • Look across the word. What are the other letters in the word? • Did you look to see what letters the word began and ended with? • You said _____. What letter would you expect to see at the beginning/end of _____? Does it match? • Check that it makes sense and matches the letters.
Chunk the Word	• Look inside the word. Is there a chunk (part) you know? • Use your fingers to find the parts you know. • Cover up part of the word so you can see the chunk. • Karate-chop this word into parts you can say. • Find a part of the word you can say. • Blend the parts together/crash the parts together (if student pauses between onset and rime).
Use What I Know	• Is this like a word you know? • What is the same about this word and the new word? (show familiar word on whiteboard). • Where would you break this word to see a part that's the same as the word you know? (underline chunks or use slashes to demonstrate) • You can use the part you know to help you read the new word. • Cover the beginning/prefix ... and ending/suffix. What word/root word is that? Now, uncover the beginning/prefix and ending/suffix ... the word is _____.
Switch the Vowel	• What sound does the vowel stand for in this word? • What do you think that (vowel) sounds like? • What other sound can you try? • Is that a word you know? Is it a real word? Does it make sense? • Try changing the vowel to the [short/long] sound. • Flip the sound.

I Can Read the Words

Sound and Say (r-a-n) (ran)

Sound out the letters   r a n   (r-a-n)

Blend the sounds together   r + a + n = ran

Say the word   (ran)

Chunk the Word   [c] [ake] = cake

Karate-chop the word   c ake   h ab it at

Say the parts I know   (c) (ake)   (ab) (it) (at)

Blend the parts together   c + ake = cake

Use What I Know   d(ay) pl(ay) ✓

Think of other words that look like this one   (day)

Think about what is the same about this word   d(ay) pl(ay)

I know _____, and the chunk is _____, so this
is _____.

Switch the Vowel   ⧄

Does it make sense?   ¢

Does it sound like a real word?   yes/no

Try the other sound—switch it

Differentiated Small Group Reading Lessons © 2009 by Margo Southall, Scholastic Teaching Resources page 45

WORD-SOLVING
Bookmark

I can...

- **sound and say**

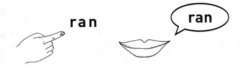

- **chunk the word**

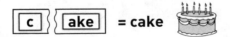

- **use what I know**

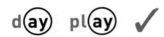

- **switch the vowel**

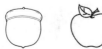

WORD-SOLVING
Bookmark

I can...

- **sound and say**

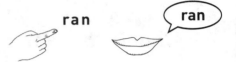

- **chunk the word**

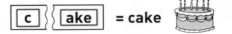

- **use what I know**

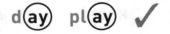

- **switch the vowel**

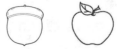

Teaching Tips

Review letter names and sounds before beginning to ensure the focus is on blending rather than letter-sound correspondences. Monitor student letter-sound recognition during guided practice and independent applications. Reteach any that cause hesitations. Provide repeated practice cumulatively blending letter sounds to decode words with common syllable patterns. During reading, prompt for:

• Saying successive sounds quickly

• Using context and sentence structure to self-monitor and self-correct nonsense errors

Student Profiles

We all have students who "huff and puff" and "hiss and spit" their way through words, laboriously sounding out each phoneme in a word: /ka/ – /a/ – /tuh/." By the time they get to the second or third phoneme they have forgotten what the first one was. Not only does this leave no mental energy for comprehension, but it is an inefficient way to decode words. I have found that the successive, or cumulative, approach to blending prevents this common problem.

The following lessons provide practice in cumulatively blending letter sounds to decode words with CVC, CCVC, and CVCC syllable patterns and applying the strategy to reading new words within connected text. They are designed to meet the needs of students who:

• Over-rely on initial consonants to predict a word in running text (accuracy)

• Recognize sounds and letters in isolation, but have difficulty blending a sequence of sounds to pronounce a word (fluency)

• Laboriously sound their way through words and continue to overanalyze familiar words

After sufficient practice, students internalize this process. They can scan a sequence of phonemes and pronounce a word without having to segment and blend each time. You will observe students in the transitional phase stretching and blending the first two or three phonemes and then pronouncing the word. At this stage, they no longer need to go through cumulatively blending every phoneme in the word.

The next section describes ways to support students who may experience initial difficulty in blending letter sounds.

Monitoring and Responding to Student Difficulty with Accurate and Fluent Blending

Teacher observation of students during guided practice and independent reading provides an insight into the specific letter-sound relationships that may be causing them difficulty. The teacher can then provide the appropriate additional modeling, corrective feedback, and instruction, and can monitor student understanding during reading by having students point to a word and blend it. The chart below describes common difficulties students may experience in blending letter sounds to decode and the corresponding instructional response.

In a study of struggling readers that compared student outcomes from three approaches to teaching blending—1. initial bigrams with a final consonant (*mo-p*) 2. onset-rime (*m-op*) and 3. three letter sounds (*m-o-p*) ... "Children who learned to blend the initial bigrams (*fi-x*) read significantly more of the transfer words correctly than any other group." (O'CONNOR, P. 59, 2007)

"Blending is one of the few strategies that children can transfer to words they have never seen before." (O'CONNOR, P. 64, 2007)

Student Difficulty With Accurate and Fluent Blending	Teaching Response/Next Steps
Student Fails to recognize a sound-symbol correspondence/confuses letters	**Teacher** ● Reviews letter names and sounds. Points to a letter and cues the student: 　* Letter?　* Sound? ● Reteaches the sound-symbol correspondence using memory aids such as a picture-cued alphabet card and corresponding action or song ● Reviews letter names and sounds before beginning to ensure focus is on blending rather than recognizing letter-sound correspondences ● Monitors student letter-sound recognition during guided practice and independent applications, and reteaches any that cause hesitations ● Places tactile letters (e.g., magnetic letters) above the letters causing hesitation in the word to support recognition ● Has student discriminate the problem letters from an array of letter cards or magnetic letters and remove them from the array, e.g., *b's* or *d's* (see Dufresne, 2002)
Pauses between phonemes when stretching the sounds (blending is not continuous)	● Assesses phonemic awareness skills: oral blending and segmentation ● Stops the student and models the process. Has them slide their finger under the word and cues them to hold the sounds as if singing the word (two seconds for continuant sounds, one second for stop sounds): 　* Pull the sounds together so it sounds like talking 　* Say the sounds fast. Say the word 　* Bulldoze the word ... keep your motor running ● Provides practice in cued, timed blending (see lessons page 50 and 53)
Omits or substitutes a phoneme	● Points to the letter and asks the student to say the phoneme. If student is unable to, the teacher silently mouths the sound ● Prompts the student to "touch and say" the sounds in the word ● Prompts for meaning cues when the student pronounces a nonsense word or one that does not fit the context
Adds schwa sound after the consonant (when it is a stop sound—*b, c, d, g, h, j, k, p, q, t, x*—that cannot be stretched). This distorts the pronunciation of the medial vowel and prevents accurate decoding of the word	● Begins by having student locate and identify the medial vowel (which can be stretched), then blend this with initial consonant, followed by identifying the last consonant and blending all three phonemes, e.g., [student points at letter *a*; teachers asks] *What sound does this letter stand for?* [/a/] [Teacher points to first letter] *And this letter?* [/c/] *Blend these sounds together.* [/ca/] [Points to last letter] *What sound does this letter stand for?* [/t/] *Now blend the sounds: /cat/. What's the word?* cat (O'Connor, 2007)
Inaccurately decodes medial sounds	● Reteaches the vowel sounds ● Has students build and sort words that differ by medial vowel (minimal pairs such as *cat, cot, cut*) ● Presents sentences that require the student to distinguish the correct word to complete a sentence
Inaccurately decodes final sounds	● Prompts for visual scanning across the word: Say __. What letter would you expect to see at the end of the word? ● See further prompts for the strategy on the Word-Solving Prompt Card, page 44 ● Isolates and highlights the final letter(s) ● Teaches common rimes and affixes (-*ed*, -*ing*)

Reading Materials to Support Accurate and Fluent Blending

Select words from the text that contain previously taught letter-sound correspondences and that are in students' listening vocabulary. Decodable words in order of difficulty are:

- VC and CVC words that begin with continuous sounds (vowels, the consonants *m, n, f, l, r,* and *s*), e.g., *am, sit*
- VCC and CVCC words that begin with a continuous sound (e.g., *ask, rest*)
- CVC words that begin with a stop sound that cannot be stretched (*b, c, d, g, h, j, k, p, q, t, x*), e.g., *jam, pen*
- CVCC words that begin with a stop sound and end with a consonant *blend*, e.g., *past, desk, hand, gift*
- CCVC words that begin with a consonant blend, e.g., *plan, spin*
- CCVCC, CCCVC, and CCCVCC words that begin and end with a consonant blend, e.g., *spend, trust, scrap, sprint*

The following letter positions represent the highest error rate for struggling readers in order of increasing frequency: 1. final consonants; 2. medial vowels; 3. second consonant in a blend or digraph; 4. first consonant in a final consonant blend (McCandliss et al., 2003). Procedures for blending CVC, CVVC, and CVCC words are provided in lessons to address these common miscues. Select words from your text appropriate for your students.

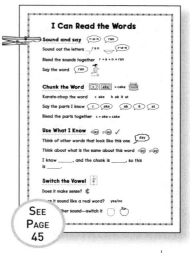

SEE
PAGE
45

LESSON: BUILD AND BLEND

Preparation

- Copy the reproducible Word-Solving Strategy Chart (page 45) onto cardstock.
- Copy the reproducible Sound and Say Bookmark (page 55) onto cardstock. Make one for every student.
- Copy the Word-Solving Prompt Card (page 44).
- Gather a large colored paper clip or clothespin and magnetic whiteboards and letters for each student.
- Select practice words.
- Select a text or create sentences containing the practice words.

Tell Me

Point to the icon for the Sound and Say strategy on the Word-Solving Strategy Chart. You may place a paper clip or clothespin alongside the icon.

> *When readers see a new word they quickly sound the letters and say the word. Today we will use the Sound and Say strategy on our Word-Solving Chart to build and read words from our story. We will sound out the letters and quickly blend them together to say the word.*

Show Me

Point to the icons and statements you use on the chart or bookmark.

> *I will build an important word from our story today. I will say each sound and then blend the sounds together to say the word.*

Place your letters across the top of your magnetic board in alphabetical order. Leave a two-finger space between each letter. Slide each letter down in sequence to form the word as you touch and say the sound. In this example, I use the word *Sam.*

Tip

Procedures for blending CVC words are provided in this lesson. The easiest words to decode are VC and CVC words beginning with a continuant sound—which can be stretched and held.

s a m

←

sa m

←

sam

Touch the first letter (C) and say the phoneme, /s/.
Touch the second letter (V) and say the phoneme, /a/.
Slide the second letter alongside the first letter.
Run your finger under the two letters and blend, /sa/.
Slide the third letter (C) alongside the second letter.
Touch the third letter and say the phoneme, /m/.
Blend the first two (CV) and last (C) sounds without pausing: /sa/ /m/.
Slide your finger under the three letters and say the word: /sam/.
Say, "This is the word *Sam.*"

Guide Me

Distribute the magnetic boards and letters. Have students place the letters across the top of their boards. Model and practice sliding down the letters they need for each word before you begin the build-and-blend procedure.

> *Pull down the letters* M A T *like this. Leave a two-finger space between each letter like mine. Now we are ready to build and blend.*

Prompt and support students to build and blend each word. Provide verbal and physical cues to guide them. Touch the letters and say the sounds together. Then guide students through the following steps, repeating three to four times with different words.

○ **Sound /Say It Slow**

> *Let's stretch and blend an important word from our story today. Touch and say each sound in the word with me.*

m a t

←

ma t

←

mat

Touch the letter *m*. Say the sound /m/.
Touch the letter *a*. Say the sound /a/.
Slide *a* over to *m*. Run your finger under *m-a*. Blend /ma/.
Touch the letter *t*. Say the sound /t/.
Slide the *t* over to *a*. Run your finger under m-a-t. Blend /mat/.
What word is this?

○ **Say/Say It Fast: Cued, Timed Blending**
Print or build the words you have practiced on your whiteboard. Point to the words one at a time. Signal students to say the sounds in their head, then pronounce the word.

Provide a silent, timed cue. Hold up one finger at a time with your other hand to the count of three, then ask students to say the word. Reduce this time in further lessons from three to two seconds, and finally, allow only one second, which is the goal for fluency. Cued, timed blending develops the necessary processing speed for fluency in decoding. With sufficient practice, students will no longer continue to overanalyze each word they meet in running text.

> *Say the sounds in your head.*

Finger-cue the wait time: 1-2-3. Students may mouth the sounds only.

> *What word is this? Yes, the word is _____.*

Coach Me

Introduce the text. Ask students to read these same words in sentences to ensure the transfer of skills to connected text. You may provide a teacher-created sentence on a chart or a short story to read.

> *We know these words. Now let's read them in the story to find out* [*something about your particular text*].

Students now begin to read the story independently and at their own pace using a whisper voice. Cue individual students to read a sentence or two aloud to you so that you can monitor their understanding, and prompt as necessary. The rest of the group continues to read as you listen in to each student in turn (see Prompts on Word-Solving Prompt Card page 44).

○ **Partner Think-Pinch-Share**

Invite students to share a word they sounded out and blended with a partner by repeating the process they used by sounding and saying the word aloud. Ask them to use the bookmark, "pinching" the correct strategy icon/phrase, to help them verbalize their strategy use.

○ **Group Share**

Invite partners to share a word they discussed with the rest of the group. Write the word they share on the whiteboard and demonstrate again how to apply the strategy.

○ **Restate the Teaching Point**

When we sound out the letters and quickly blend them to say the word, we can solve new words in the story.

Reading-Writing Connection

After reading, compose a sentence together to summarize the story. Have students repeat the sentence, counting each word on their fingers to aid in recalling the sentence and to support self-checking. Invite individual students to write a word from the sentence on the chart in an interactive writing format. The rest of the group provides feedback and/or writes the word on their whiteboards at the same time. Read the sentence to and with the students several times to check it. Students may copy this sentence in their reading journal.

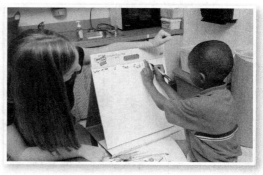

The group composes and records a sentence using the words they have segmented and blended. Students copy the sentence in their reading response journal.

Practice at the Word-Study Center

○ **Sentence Puzzle**

＊ Copy the shared writing sentence you created in the Reading-Writing Connection onto a sentence strip.

＊ Cut the sentence into individual words and store in an envelope or baggie along with a complete copy of the sentence on a 3″ x 9″ flash card or index card.

＊ Place this at the word study center. Label the activity with the reading group logo so they will know to complete this task at the center.

＊ Students will reconstruct and read the sentence, first with the model as a guide. Next they will turn over the model sentence, mix up the words, and rebuild it (without looking at the model).

The following supporting center activities can be found in *Differentiated Literacy Centers* (Southall, 2007):

● Word Sorts: Initial, Final, and Medial Letter Cues; Initial Blends; Final Blends
● ABC Pick Up: Initial Blends and Digraphs

LESSON: BLENDING WORDS IN A LIST AND CONNECTED TEXT

Preparation

● Copy the reproducible Word-Solving Strategy Chart (page 45) onto cardstock.
● Copy the reproducible Sound and Say Bookmark (page 55) onto cardstock. Make one for every student.
● Copy the Word-Solving Prompt Card (page 44).
● Have on hand a colored paper clip or clothespin.
● Select text containing words with the target syllable patterns (CVC, CCVC, CVCC). This may be a book, a poem, or a teacher-created sentence or story.
● Print the selected words in large letters on a chart or whiteboard.

Lesson Text Example:

Meg and Jim's Sled Trip by Laura Appleton-Smith (1998)

Tell Me

Point to the icon for the Sound and Say strategy on the Word-Solving Strategy Chart. You may place a paper clip or clothespin alongside the icon.

When readers see new words in stories, I they sound the letters in their head and quickly blend them together to say the whole word. We need to be able to do this quickly while we read so we can think about what is happening in the story.

Show Me

Demonstrate the strategy with the words you have printed on the chart.

I will sound and say a word from our story today. I will say the sounds and blend them together as I go across the word.

Words are in order of increasing difficulty:

SEE PAGE 45

CVC Words

Point to the *s* and say /s/.
Point to the *u* and say /u/.
Slide your finger under the *su* and say /su/.
Point to the *n* and say /n/.
Slowly slide your finger under *sun* and say /sun/ (stretch the sounds).
Quickly slide your finger under the word and say /sun/ at a natural speed, so it sounds like talking.
Circle the word with your finger say, "The word is *sun*."

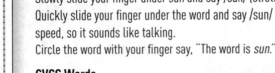

CVCC Words

Point to the *s* and say /s/.
Point to the *o* and say /o/.
Slide your finger under the *so* and say /so/.
Point to the *f* and say /f/.
Slide your finger under *sof* and say /sof/.
Point to the *t* and say /t/.
Slowly slide your finger under *soft* and say /soft/ (stretch the sounds).
Quickly slide your finger under the word and say /soft/ at a natural speed, so it sounds like talking.
Circle the word with your finger say, "The word is *soft*."

CCVC Words

Point to the *t* and say /t/.
Point to the *r* and say /r/.
Slide your finger under the *tr* and say /tr/.
Point to the *i* and say /i/.
Slide your finger under *tri* and say /tri/.
Point to the *p* and say /p/.
Slowly slide your finger under *trip* and say /trip/ (stretch the sounds).
Quickly slide your finger under the word and say /trip/ at a natural speed, so it sounds like talking.
Circle the word with your finger say, "The word is *trip*."

Repeat the same procedure with two more words from the text.

CVC Words

Meg	sun
Jim	wet
den	mugs
sit	

CVCC Words

fast	rest
soft	gust

CCVC Words

sled	drag
trip	spin
snug	

Guide Me

Prompt and support students to apply the same strategy that you demonstrated to further words on the chart.

○ **Sound /Say It Slow**

Let's stretch and blend another word we will read in our story. Say each sound with me, and blend them together as we go.

Repeat the procedure with three or four other words from the story. Gradually remove the cues as you progress to further words or in subsequent teaching sessions for this strategy:

1. Provide sounds and cues, and use finger pointing.

2. Cue the students verbally for each step, but do not say the sounds; continue to use finger pointing.

3. Use finger pointing only, with no verbal cues or sounds.

When all the words have been stretched and blended, have the students choral read through the list of words on the chart without analyzing each word.

Coach Me

Point to each word on the chart one by one. Cue students to say the sounds in their head and then pronounce the word, following the guidelines below.

○ **Say/Say It Fast**

Say the sounds in your head. What word is this? *Yes, the word is _____ .*

Ask students to choral read these same words in sentences located in the story to ensure transfer of word analysis skills to connected text.

> *We know these words. Now let's read them in the story to see how the author used them to tell us what happens in* Meg and Jim's Sled Trip.

You may have students find and frame these words in the text on one or two pages, then read the sentence to see how the word is used in context. This supports transfer to independent reading of the text. Prompt them to identify the initial, medial, and final sounds to guide the process of locating them in the text. Emphasize initial sounds by stretching them out or repeating the sound.

> *What letter would you expect to see at the beginning of the word* w-w-w-wet*? What is the second letter in* w–eee-t*? What is the last letter in* wet*? Find it and frame it with your fingers* [or framing tool, such as translucent counter or strip of highlighter tape].

> Repeat with two or three more words.

Have students read the story (from the beginning) independently at their own pace using a whisper voice. Listen in to each student as they read a sentence or two, and prompt as necessary (see Word-Solving Prompt Card, page 44)

> ∗ *Touch and say each sound. Run your finger under it to check the sounds.*
> ∗ *Use your eyes, mouth, and finger to check it.*
> ∗ *Look across the word. What are the other letters in the word?*
> ∗ *Blend the sounds together to say the word.*
> ∗ *Bulldoze the word ... keep your motor running.*

○ **Partner Think-Pinch-Share**

Have students share how they sounded out and blended a word during the reading with a partner. Ask them to use the bookmark, "pinching" the correct strategy, to help them verbalize their strategy use.

○ **Group Share**

Invite partners to share an example with the rest of the group. Write the word they share on the whiteboard and demonstrate again how to apply the strategy.

○ **Restate the Teaching Point**

When we sound out the letters and quickly blend them we can keep on reading the rest of the story [*focus on the meaning*].

Reading-Writing Connection

Have students use the words on the list to compose a sentence or retelling of the story.

Practice at the Word-Study Center

Build and Blend Dominoes

● Students pronounce the first consonant(s) and vowel together and then connect this to a final consonant(s), blending them together to pronounce the word, e.g., /do/, /g/ - /dog/.

● Cut index cards in half. Print Beginning and Final Sounds on cards. Students match the cards to build, blend and read words.

Example:

Beginning Sound Cards   Final Sound Cards

| mi | ha | | x | s |

I Can Chunk the Word: Vowel Patterns and Onset-Rime Analogy

To be fluent readers at the third-grade level, students need to be able to recognize 80,000 words (Juel & Minden-Cupp, 2000). That is far too many words for students to memorize. All students will need strategies for problem-solving new words they meet in print every day. For reading efficiency, they must recognize larger units in words, such as the vowel pattern in a syllable or chunk. I also use the term chunks to refer to diphthongs like *oi, oy, ou, ow,* and other syllable patterns like *–ion,* because they all begin with a vowel.

Teaching Tips

To help students decode successfully, I teach them to scan words by first attending to the initial consonant(s) and then identifying the first vowel and the letters that follow in the syllable (the chunk). I want them to learn how to visually scan words and look for familiar patterns that begin with a vowel and use these to decode.

Guiding principles for teaching vowel patterns include the following.

1. Introduce rimes cumulatively as you teach the letter-sound correspondences. For example, teaching the letters *s, a, t, c, m, e, p, n* enables students to read words with the rimes *–at, –an, –am, –ap,* and *–ee,* such as *sat, pan, map,* etc.

2. Teach the analogy phrase so that students internalize it as a strategy for decoding unfamiliar words: "I know *cat* (familiar word) and the chunk is *at,* this is *bat* (new word)." Have students practice problem-solving words aloud using this dialogue during reading (Gaskins et al., 1997).

"Teaching procedures like phonics instruction, use of context cues for word recognition, and solving words by analogy to know words are designed to foster searching strategies." (SCHWARTZ, P. 176, 1997)

SOUND AND SAY
Bookmark

I can...

- sound out the letters

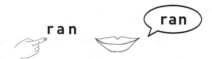

- blend the sounds together

$$r + a + n = ran$$

- say the word

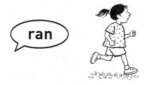

- check it makes sense

SOUND AND SAY
Bookmark

I can...

- sound out the letters

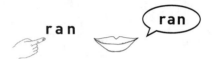

- blend the sounds together

$$r + a + n = ran$$

- say the word

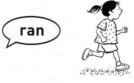

- check it makes sense

3. Display a key word for each rime on a bulletin board or chunking word wall for reference during reading and writing (Wagstaff, 1999).

4. Plan multiple practice opportunities for students to recognize and apply the key words in a variety of reading and writing contexts.

Students should cumulatively practice words with more than one syllable as they learn different vowel patterns. Use simple words like *napkin* and *catnap* for students at the earliest stages of reading. This prepares them for reading authentic text, which contains words with more than one syllable in all but the first few text levels.

Word Wall

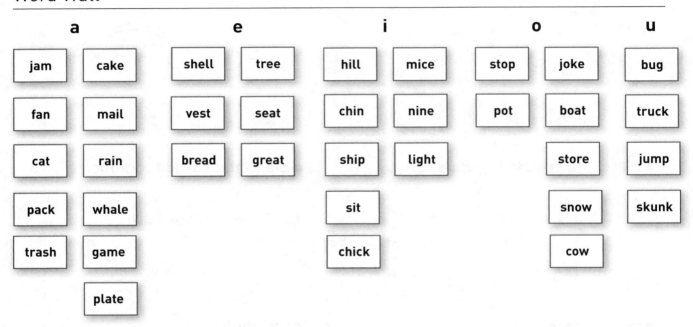

a		e		i		o		u
jam	cake	shell	tree	hill	mice	stop	joke	bug
fan	mail	vest	seat	chin	nine	pot	boat	truck
cat	rain	bread	great	ship	light		store	jump
pack	whale			sit			snow	skunk
trash	game			chick			cow	
	plate							

"Because some poor readers have difficulty with rimes, rimes are broken down into their individual sounds after being presented as wholes."

(JUEL & MINDEN-CUPP, 2000, IN GUNNING, P. 247, 2002)

I use a chunking word wall with a category heading for each vowel and one key word for each vowel pattern (not multiple words) on cards organized by their first vowel (Wagstaff, 1999). The rime is printed in a different color or underlined. I also include the letter *y*, with key words such as *baby* and *fly* to represent both pronunciations. As we progress to vowel digraphs, I display one word for each pronunciation, such as *seat*, *bread*, and *great* for *–ea*, *snow* and *cow* for *–ow* (see I Can Switch the Vowel lesson, page 67).

To foster the transfer of this skill to reading, when we come to a new word in the text, I ask students to touch the first vowel and look at the word wall words displayed under that vowel. Then I ask, "Is there a word we know that can help us (that contains the same chunk)?" We use the analogy dialogue to verbalize how we use a word wall word to solve a new word: "We know *seat* (familiar key), [and] the chunk is *eat*, so this word is *wheat* (new word)."

When teaching intervention groups, I use a project display board and have a different set of key words on each side, as groups are at different developmental stages. Continual reinforcement of this strategy in whole- and small-group instruction increases the rate at which students transfer these patterns to their independent reading.

Student Profiles

Vowels are not friendly, and their sounds vary depending upon the letters that surround them. The advantage to teaching rimes is that the vowel is part of a stable unit that students can rely on to decode—rimes are pronounced in the same way 95% of the time. Beyond common rimes, though, students will require flexibility with vowel sounds. We teach the most common pronunciations for each vowel pattern first, and then introduce the other pronunciations for the same spelling.

There are three profiles of need I see in this area again and again, and the following lessons are designed to address them. The first profile describes students who have difficulty storing and retrieving vowel patterns in their phonological and visual memory. They simply do not recognize these parts in words, whether they are presented in isolation, in words, or in running text.

In the second profile, students may perform satisfactorily on assessments that require them to recognize words in isolation, yet something happens when they open up the page of a book. They don't transfer their phonics knowledge to problem-solving new words in running text or use analogy from words they know.

A third profile describes students who rely on one pronunciation for the vowel or vowel pattern. When their miscue is a nonsense word or does not make sense in the context of the story, they are unable to self-correct their miscues by trying other possible sounds for the vowel or pattern.

Monitoring and Responding to Student Difficulty With Vowel Patterns and Onset-Rime Analogy

Struggling readers often try to memorize words one by one and soon reach a plateau in the number of words they can recall. They need strategies for solving words in running text like the Chunk the Word, Use What I Know, and Switch the Vowel strategies. Many phonics programs do a good job of teaching letter-sound relationships and vowel patterns but neglect to show students how to use these to read new words. It is critical to teach this skill explicitly, or it will not transfer to reading. What makes the difference for struggling readers is the metacognitive dialogue or self-talk that is part of the I Can Sound and Say the Chunk lesson:

> Whenever you come to a word you don't know, think of a word you know that looks like this one (contains the same chunk) and say: I know _____, and the chunk is __, so the word/this is _____.

The steps in this process are based on the Word Analysis Chart developed by Gaskins et al. (1997). Students learn the step-by-step approach to using their phonics knowledge rather than remaining passive (and inaccurate) readers. If this dialogue is too challenging for some students to remember and say, simply ask them to find a part of the word they can say, say that part, and blend the parts together through the word (Gunning, 2002).

Strategy Prompts

↑ **Most Support**

- Make the word with magnetic letters and help the student break the word apart.

- Write a known word on an index card and place beneath the new word. Say: *This word has a chunk you know that can help you. What's the chunk? Use that chunk to help you say the new word.* Scaffold segmenting and blending the parts.

- Cover the beginning consonant(s) with a finger and prompt: *You know this chunk. Say this chunk.*

- *Where could you break that word? Put your finger there and break the word apart.* Direct student to cover part of the word.

- *Do you see something that might help you? Do you see a chunk you know?* Use a masking card or finger to cover the initial letter and isolate a familiar word part; or use a translucent counter to highlight the chunk.

- *Is there a part of the word you can say?*

↓ **Least Support**

Student Difficulty With Vowel Patterns and Onset-Rime Analogy	Teaching Response/Next Steps
Student Has difficulty with auditory discrimination (discriminating parts of words that sound the same)	**Teacher** ● Assesses phonological awareness and provides instruction in areas not yet developed: 　* rhyme discrimination tasks: *Do these words have a part at the end of the word that sounds the same?* cat, cap 　* rhyme production tasks: *I'm going to tell you a word and I want you to tell me a word that rhymes with it. Tell me a word that rhymes with* cat. 　* onset-rime blending: *I'll say the sounds of a word. You guess what word it is:* /m/ /ap/ [*map*] 　* onset-rime segmentation: *Say the* [*two*] *parts you hear in* map. [/m/ /ap/] 　* phoneme deletion: *Say* map. *Now say it again, but don't say* /m/. [/ap/]
Is not able to retrieve the spelling of the vowel pattern to decode	● Demonstrates how to listen to and record the sounds of a word in sequence using sound boxes or a series of lines to represent the position of each letter (see Reading-Writing Connection in I Can Sound and Say the Chunk lesson); guides student to do the same ● Dictates words with the pattern ● Incorporates word building ("making words") and word sorting
Has difficulty (visually) locating chunks or familiar parts in words	● Covers up the onset, as described in the list of scaffolds prior to this chart, so they can focus on the rime; asks child to do the same, copying their model: *Can you show me that part?* ● Provides lists of the words with the pattern in a different color; helps students blend the word parts ● Presents lists of words and has student circle or highlight the vowel pattern ● Has student build the word with magnetic letters, then break it apart at the chunk(s), reading the chunk and then blending with the letters in the rest of the word ● Incorporates word sorting into daily instruction, where the student is required to discriminate between two or three patterns ● Provides concrete models, such as environmental print (see Reading Materials to Support using Vowel Patterns and Onset-Rime Analogy, page 59)
Does not use familiar word parts to read new words; struggles to apply the analogy strategy to single-syllable and multisyllabic words.	● Builds a word bank of known words (regular high-frequency words such as *see*, *that*) on which to base analogies (like the key words on the word wall); extends on the parts in these words to build new words (known word: *cake*; new word: *take*) ● Shows the student how a known part of a word can be used to build and read a new one; uses magnetic letters to pull a rime from the word and add a different onset to form a new word (see I Can Use What I Know lesson, page 63; Dufresne, 2002, for more examples) ● Pulls two known words from text containing two different chunks and prints on cards, then presents a new word with the same pattern as one of the words and has child match it up to the known word that will help him or her read it: *Which one of our two words will help us to solve this tricky word?*; asks student to verbalize strategy, using part of a known word to read a new word ● Coaches during reading by modeling the analogy dialogue ● Prints a known word containing the rime on an index card and places this directly below the tricky word in the text (or syllable in a multisyllabic word); models and has student use the analogy phrase: "*I know* cake, *and the chunk is* ake (points to rime in *cake*), *so the word is* rake" ● Provides daily chunking word wall practice to read and write new words ● Incorporates challenge words and writing sorts activities where students write dictated words, chunk by chunk (see Reading-Writing Connection in I Can Use What I Know: Problem-Solving New and Complex Words lesson, page 63)

Student Difficulty With Vowel Patterns and Onset–Rime Analogy	Teaching Response/Next Steps
Student Is unable to break apart a complex word at the syllable boundaries to decode	**Teacher** ● Has student say the word with him/her, tap/clap the syllables, and identify the number of syllables: *How many vowels are there? Are they together or apart? Is there a silent* e*?* ● Has student build the word, then break it into that number of syllables by sliding their letters to the right (this may take trial and error, as first attempts may not always sound right); students move letters from one syllable to another until it matches what they say and looks right: *What is the first syllable? Where will you break your word? Say the word again. What is the second syllable? Where will you break your word?* ● Writes the new word with familiar words directly underneath that contain the same syllable patterns, and demonstrates how to use these to decode (see I Can Use What I Know lesson, page 63) ● Dictates the word; has students build the word, then rewrite it and examine the difference in the two spellings to demonstrate the need to analyze each syllable
Mispronounces word using incorrect vowel sound; does not attempt to self-correct by trying other pronunciations for this vowel	● Teaches the multiple pronunciations for vowels in isolation, and teaches vowel digraphs (e.g., *ea, ie*) cumulatively in the program ● Uses a picture-cued visual to support student attempts (Bear et al., 2004; Vogt & Nagano, 2003; see I Can Switch the Vowel lesson, page 67) ● Displays key words on the word wall to represent each sound ● Incorporates sound-based word-sorting activities, e.g., for *ea*, short *e* sound (*bread*) and long *e* sound (*seat*), and long *a* (*great*) ● Provides practice reading words in connected text that have more than one possible sound and use meaning cues to adjust pronunciation of the vowel ● Coaches the student during reading to apply the strategy with a hand signal to "flip" the sound, or uses a concrete visual, such as a light switch, to model the procedure of being flexible with our vowel pronunciations

Reading Materials to Support Using Vowel Patterns and Onset-Rime Analogy

There are a number of reading series for beginning readers that include sets of books that focus on word families. I often use poetry to support the transfer of strategies because it can provide a short, humorous text for rereading. Two of the books I have used include *Phonics Poetry* by Timothy Rasinski and Belinda Zimmerman (2001) and *Phonics Through Poetry* by Babs Bell Hajdusiewicz (1999). I copy these onto chart paper.

Create your own decodable text with ideas and topics generated by your students, using a list of possible words that contain the elements you are teaching for reference. This can be completed in a shared or interactive writing format. I include students' names in the stories we compose together. We also write about nonfiction topics we are studying. I type them up for the students to take home in their I Can Read folders, so they can show off their newly acquired skills and gain increased motivation for reading from positive feedback.

I also include environmental print, such as food wrappers, on the word wall because they provide a concrete example of the usefulness of chunks.

Before it goes on the wall, I highlight the pattern on the wrapper, and attach it to the top of the chart. We use this as a reference to generate more words with the pattern.

Homographs are examples of words to use to practice the I Can Switch the Vowel strategy and my students enjoy books such as *The Dove Dove: Funny Homograph Riddles* by Marvin Terban (1998), in which there is a play on words that requires flexibility in vowel pronunciations.

LESSON: SOUND AND SAY THE CHUNK

Preparation

- Copy the reproducible Word-Solving Strategy Chart (page 45) onto cardstock.
- Copy the reproducible Chunk the Word Bookmark (page 66) onto cardstock. Make one for every student.
- Copy the Word-Solving Prompt Card (page 44).
- Copy the I Can Sound and Say the Chunk steps on a chart and laminate for use with a wipe-off pen, or write the chart on a whiteboard (see lesson).
- Have available a large colored paper clip or clothespin.
- Select text containing words with the target vowel patterns.
- Print selected words in large letters on chart or whiteboard where the vowel in the pattern is printed in red, consonants in green or black.
- Unwrap a chocolate bar (optional).

Tell Me

Point to the icon for the I Can Chunk the Word strategy on the Word-Solving Strategy Chart. You may place a paper clip or clothespin alongside the icon.

You may break apart a chocolate bar into chunks to demonstrate the concept.

> *Words are like chocolate bars; they are made up of chunks. Today we will practice the I Can Chunk the Word strategy on our chart and look for chunks we know in the words we read.*

Present a word on a chart or whiteboard (with color-coded vowels and consonants). Point to the vowel and the letters that follow in the syllable to form the chunk.

> *When we read, we look for the biggest chunk of the word we can say. This helps us read words without having to sound out every letter, and we have more time to think about what we are reading. We can find chunks in words because they always start with a vowel, like the -at in* cat *or the -ug in* bug *on our chunking word wall.*

Show Me

Review the steps on the chart and bookmark with the demonstration below. Show a word with a familiar chunk (rime or vowel pattern). Point to the statement "[I can] karate-chop the word" on the Word-Solving Strategy Chart. Tell students that you will karate-chop (segment) a word at the chunk. Demonstrate how to find the chunk in the word by scanning the word from the first vowel. Run your finger under the initial consonant(s) and then touch the first vowel in the chunk. Pretend to karate-chop the word at the chunk. I use *trap* in the example below.

> *We can karate-chop a word into chunks. Here is a new word I need to read. I know the first letters,* t *and* r, *stand for /tr/. Now I will look for a chunk I know. I will touch the vowel and look at the next letter(s) to see if it is part of a chunk I know.*

Run your finger across the chunk in the word. Use the statements on the Word-Solving Strategy Chart to demonstrate the strategy.

This chunk begins with the letter a, *and the next letter is* p. *I know this chunk; it is /ap/. Now I will say the parts and blend the parts together to say the word: /tr/, /ap/, trap. Cat trap. That makes sense, so I can read on.*

Guide Me

We need to know lots of chunks so we can read any book we choose. Let's learn a new chunk today that is found in many words in our books. First we stretch the word and listen for the sounds. Then we use the sounds to figure out the letters. We hook the sounds to the letters so our brain will remember the chunk and use it to read new words.

Follow the steps on the Sound and Say the Chunk chart. Here is an example of the process, using the word *lake*.

- Say the key word containing the chunk (*lake*). Ask students to repeat it.
- Model how to stretch the word: "*llllaaak.*"
- Support students by stretching the word slowly together. Ask students to count the sounds they hear and hold up one finger for each sound (begin with thumb, raise fingers of left hand one at a time).
- Say, *I hear three sounds in the word.*
- Display the key word. Count the number of letters with the students. Record the number on the chart.
- Examine whether the number of sounds matches the number of letters. Note that the silent *e* at the end gives the vowel a long sound, but does not make any sound of its own. In short-vowel (closed-syllable) words, there will be a one-to-one correspondence between sounds and letters. For example, in the word *fun* the teacher would record on the chart: *It has three letters because each sound is spelled with one letter.*

In addition to words with the silent *e* pattern (such as *lake*), words with vowel digraphs and r-controlled vowels also have a mismatch of sounds to letters because two letters stand for one sound. This is important for students to note. Discuss the reason why there is a match or mismatch of sounds and letters. Note: Consonant blends (*bl, tr*) have one sound for each letter, while in consonant digraphs (*th, wh, ch, sh, qu*) one sound is spelled with two letters. You can explain it by saying:

I hear _____ sounds, and/but I see _____ letters because _____.

To review, identify the vowel pattern or chunk and have students state it.

The chunk is _ake.

You can make the match or mismatch more evident by writing the number of sounds under each letter or drawing a Y-shape line from the two letters that form a sound to the number of sounds.

```
l a k e          s a i l
| | |            | Y |
1 2 3            1 2 3
```

Repeat the steps with another word from the story that shares the same syllable pattern or represents the same phonics principle, for example, closed syllable (short vowel, *dog*), silent *e* (*lake*), open syllable (*me, tiger*), vowel digraph (*keep*), r-controlled (*car*).

Sound and Say the Chunk

1. The word is
_____.

2. S-t-r-e-t-c-h the word.
It has _____ sounds.

3. It has _____ letters because _____.

4. The chunk is _____.

○ **Review the Spelling and Sound of the Chunk**

Example:
What letters stand for the _ake sound? a-k-e
What sound does a-k-e *stand for?* /ake/

Coach Me

Review how to find the chunk in a word by scanning the word from the first vowel, using a further example on the whiteboard.

Put your finger on the word. Say all the letters.

Touch the vowel. Look for a chunk you know. Say the chunk, then blend the parts together.

Introduce the text. Next, distribute the bookmarks, reviewing the strategy of recognizing familiar parts in words to read new ones. As students read the text independently, prompt them to identify familiar parts of words and blend the parts together to pronounce the word (see Word-Solving Prompt Card, page 44 and Monitoring and Responding to Student Difficulty, page 58, for levels of support in coaching).

Examples:
- *Do you see something that might help you? Do you see a chunk you know?* Use a masking card or finger to cover initial letter and isolate a familiar word part; or a translucent counter to highlight the chunk.
- Cover the beginning consonant(s) with a finger and prompt: *You know this chunk. Say this chunk.*
- *Look for chunks you know. Use your fingers to find the parts you know.*
- *Where could you break [karate-chop] that word? Put your finger there and break the word apart.* Direct student to cover part of the word.
- *Break the word apart and put it back together. Chunk and crash the parts together.*
- *Is there a part of the word you can say?*
- *What could you try?*

○ **Partner Think-Pinch-Share**

After reading, have students share how they figured out a tricky word during the reading. You may have students share with partners before sharing with the group to make sure everyone verbalizes their strategy use. Ask them to use the bookmark (by "pinching" it) to help them verbalize their strategy use.

○ **Group Share**

Have partners share an example with the group. Write the word on the whiteboard and underline the chunk. Invite students to demonstrate how they used the chunk to say the word.

○ **Restate the Teaching Point**

Reaffirm strategy use with positive feedback. Tell them what they did so they will use it again:

You used a part of the word that you knew to help you say the whole word.

Reading-Writing Connection

- Generate more words with each pattern and record them on a chart labelled Our Chunk Chart. Use these words in a shared writing activity. Copy the story for student reading folders and partner reading. We call these our I Can Read folders, and they go home regularly for repeated readings.

- Invite students to write a poem using the Chunk Chart word list.

- Practice with sound boxes. These are a series of connecting boxes also known as Elkonin boxes (Clay, 1997). The number of the boxes corresponds to the number of sounds in the word. Have students say and stretch the sounds in the word, and then indicate how many sounds they hear with their fingers. Then have them draw that many boxes (or provide a form with the required number of interconnected sound boxes). Stretch and say each sound in the word and have students record the letter(s) they would expect to see to represent that sound: *What is the first sound you hear in* lake? *What letter would you expect to see?* Stretch the sound again. *What is the second sound you hear?* Chant and check the letter sequence and have students draw a dot under each letter in sequence as they say it to ensure self-checking (Wagstaff, 1999; Gaskins et al., 1997).

- Practice with word or sentence dictation. Dictate three to five words and have students stretch and spell each one. Alternatively, dictate a sentence for students to write: Say the sentence, then say each word one by one, then repeat the sentence. Students check their own writing for spelling errors, writing the correct spelling underneath, where necessary.

Practice at the Word-Study Center

Provide independent practice with the following activities from *Differentiated Literacy Centers* (Southall, 2007)

- Magic Mat
- Cut and Sort
- House of Rimes
- Wrapper Rimes
- Find a Rime
- Flap Book
- Story Rimes
- Word Games
- Tic Tac Rime

LESSON: I CAN USE WHAT I KNOW: PROBLEM-SOLVING NEW AND COMPLEX WORDS

Preparation

- Copy the reproducible Word-Solving Strategy Chart (page 45) onto cardstock.
- Copy the reproducible Chunking Bookmark (page 66) onto cardstock. Make one for every student.
- Copy the Word-Solving Prompt Card (page 44).
- Have large paper clip or clothespin on hand.
- Select a text containing words with the target vowel patterns.
- Print practice words that contain familiar chunks or vowel patterns on a whiteboard.

Tell Me

Point to the icon for the I Can Use What I Know strategy on the Word-Solving Strategy Chart. You may place a paper clip or clothespin alongside the icon.

> *Good readers think about what they know to help them solve new words. Today we will use chunks in words that we already know to read a new word. Remember a chunk always begins with a vowel—a, e, i, o, u. We can break apart (karate-chop) a word at the vowel to find the chunk.*

Show Me

Take a word from the story and write on your whiteboard. Examine the letters in the word and think aloud about words you know that contain the same parts (rimes, vowel patterns, consonant clusters).

Model the analogy strategy of using a familiar word to decode a new word with the steps:

> *If I don't know a word, I can think of another word I know that looks like it.*
> *I know a word that looks like this one. This is like our key word _____. I will it use it to help me.*
> *I am thinking, what is the same about this word and the new word? They both have the same chunk.*
> *The chunk is _____.*

Write the supporting known word directly underneath the new word. Begin with words that contain the same rime and progress to words that contain the same digraph or diphthong and are not part of a rime. Say and sound the consonant blends and then identify the vowel pattern using the dialogue structure.

New Word:	str<u>ay</u>	bl<u>eat</u>ed	st<u>ee</u>d
Familiar 'Key' Word:	d**ay**	**eat**	f**eed**

Use the structured dialogue below to verbalize how you used words (parts) you knew to assign a pronunciation to each part/syllable in the new word:

I know [day], *and the chunk is* _ay, *so this is* [stray].

Guide Me

Write a sentence from the story on your whiteboard. Underline a word in the sentence that contains a familiar chunk or syllable pattern. Direct students to look for a word on the Chunking Word Wall or Chunk Chart with the same chunk or think of another word they know that looks like this one (see Teaching Tips).

Select another sentence containing a word with a familiar chunk. Repeat the procedure that you have modeled, which is summarized below.

○ **Summary of Steps**
  * Present the new word on the whiteboard.
  * Invite students to suggest words they know that will help them problem-solve this tricky word.
  * Write these directly underneath the corresponding syllable (see example above).
  * Have students verbalize how they figured it out using known words.

Multisyllabic Words

If the word is a multisyllabic word, students repeat the process for each chunk. Challenge students to figure out these big "college" words.

● Count the number of vowels and note that there is more than one pattern in the multisyllabic word.

● Blend each pronounceable part as you go through the word, then say the whole word (see dialogue below). Sight words from the group's word bank can also be used in analogy lessons (see example below).

<u>umbrella</u>	e s t i m a t e	d <u>if</u> f <u>er</u> ent	<u>adventure</u>
gum well	**best him**	**if her went**	**dad ten sure**

I know if, *so this is* dif. *I know* her, *so this is* fer. *Blend together:* differ. *I know* went, *so this is* ent. *Blend together:* different

If students have difficulty dividing into syllables, have the students first build the word with magnetic letters and then divide the word by syllables (see Monitoring and Responding to Student Difficulty chart, page 58).

Next Steps

When students demonstrate understanding of the steps, model the strategy without using familiar words. Simply say the chunks (vowel patterns or syllables) and blend to say the word.

Coach Me

Introduce the text. Distribute the bookmarks and review the strategy icons. As students read, prompt them to verbalize how they used the strategy to solve a word (see Word- Solving Prompt Card, page 44).

Examples:

- *Is this word like another word you know?*
- *You know a word that looks like this one.*
- *Where would you break this word to see a part that's the same as the word you know?*
- *What do you know in this word?*
- *You can use the chunk you know to help you read the new word.*

○ **Partner Think-Pinch-Share**

Invite students to use their bookmarks, "pinching" the strategy, to help them share how they figured out a tricky word using the analogy strategy with a partner.

○ **Group Share**

Take up examples that students have shared with the whole group.

○ **Restate the Teaching Point**

Provide positive feedback on how students applied the strategy during reading and review the steps they used to successfully solve new words.

We used chunks in words we know to solve new words.

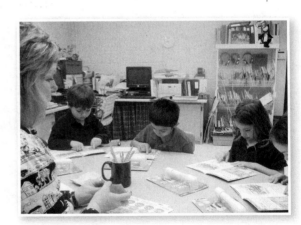

Present new words for students to locate and solve, and provide an opportunity for them to verbalize their strategy use

Reading-Writing Connection

- Invite students to use the words on the Chunk Chart they have generated with the target vowel patterns to write stories and poems.

- Dictate words containing familiar chunks, including multisyllabic words.

- Have students tap out the syllables and draw the same number of lines on the page as there are syllables.

- Say the word syllable by syllable and have students listen for the chunks they know and use those chunks to spell new words. Say, *When we write, we say the word and listen for a chunk we know. Then we think about how that part is spelled, the letters that stand for the chunk.*

Practice at the Word-Study Center

Provide independent practice with the following activities from *Differentiated Literacy Centers* (Southall, 2007):

- Wrapper Rimes
- Cut and Sort
- Story Rimes
- Word Games
- Find a Rime

CHUNK THE WORD
Bookmark

I can...

- karate-chop the word

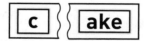

- say the parts

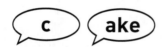

- blend the parts together

c + ake = cake

- use what I know

day play ✓

- check it makes sense

CHUNK THE WORD
Bookmark

I can...

- karate-chop the word

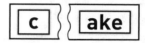

- say the parts

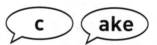

- blend the parts together

c + ake = cake

- use what I know

day play ✓

- check it makes sense

I CAN SWITCH THE VOWEL: FLEXIBILITY WITH SINGLE VOWELS, VOWEL DIGRAPHS, AND DIPHTHONGS

Preparation

- Copy the reproducible Word-Solving Strategy Chart (page 45) onto cardstock.
- Copy the reproducible Chunk the Word Bookmark (page 66) onto cardstock. Make one for every student.
- Copy the Vowel Switch card (page 70) onto cardstock.
- Copy of the Word-Solving Prompt Card (page 44).
- Have available a large colored paper clip or clothespin.
- Select words from a text that contain vowels with more than one pronunciation.

Tell Me

Point to the icon for the I Can Switch the Vowel strategy on the Word-Solving Strategy Chart. Display the Vowel Switch picture card. Say:

We know that vowels can have more than one sound. Sometimes we need to switch the sound so the word makes sense and sounds right in the story. There is a word from our story today that has a vowel with more than one sound. We will use the pictures on our Vowel Switch card to try both sounds and check which one makes sense.

Show Me

Let's practice using some words from our book.

Proceed through the lesson using words in which a single vowel sound must be switched, or in which a vowel digraph or diphthong must be switched. I provide examples of each below.

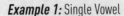

Example 1: Single Vowel

Present the word from the book on the whiteboard. In this example, the target word is *wiped*. Underline the first vowel. Guide students in attempting all pronunciations by referring to key words on the I Can Switch the Vowel card that represent each sound.

This word has the vowel i. *First we will try* /ĭ/ *as in* igloo, *because that is the most common sound for* i. *If that does not sound like a real word we will try* /ī/ *as in* ice cream. Point to the picture cues on the vowel switch card as you say each sound and picture name. *What are you going to try?*

Have students repeat the vowel sound and key word—/ĭ/ like *igloo*, or /ī/ like *ice cream*. Demonstrate application to independent reading.

I will use the vowel switch card to help me figure out this tricky word. First I will try /ĭ/ *as in* igloo [pronounce the word]. *Now I will read the sentence to check that it makes sense in the story.* Henry's mother wiped Henry's nose. *Does it make sense in the story? No.*

Now I will try /ī/ *as in* ice cream *and see if that makes sense. Let's read the sentence together and check.* Henry's mother wiped Henry's nose. *Yes, that makes sense and sounds right.*

wi ped

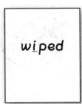

Vowel Switch

Short Vowels	Long Vowels
a	a
e	e
i	i
o	o
u	u

SEE PAGE 70

Guide Me

After briefly introducing the text:

● Have students locate another sentence in the story and find and frame the target word. Practice trying two different vowel sounds in several words from the text, using the same dialogue structure that you modeled.

● Ask students to read the word in context to check that it is a real word, makes sense, and sounds right grammatically.

● Remind students to check the I Can Switch the Vowel card using the self-monitoring dialogue structure you used in the Show Me part of the lesson.

● Remodel the self-monitoring statements, then say them together as necessary to support student understanding.

Coach Me

Prompt students to apply the strategy as they read the text independently, using the Word-Solving Prompt Card.

What sound does the vowel stand for in this word?
What other sound can you try?
Try changing the vowel to the short/long sound.
Is that a word you know? Is it a real word? Does it make sense?

○ **Restate the Teaching Point**
Restate the word-solving strategy of trying different pronunciations and checking that it makes sense in the story:

We switched the vowel when it did not sound right or make sense.

> **Example 2:** Vowel Digraph *ea*

Show Me

There is a word from our article today that has the vowel team ea. We will use the pictures on our Vowel Switch card to try both sounds and check which one makes sense.

Present the word on the whiteboard. Underline the vowel digraph *ea* in *ready*.

When I see the vowel team ea, what sounds can I try? Let's check our vowel switch card. First, I will try /ē/ as in eagle, because that is the most common sound for ea. If that does not sound like a real word, I will try /ĕ/ as in egg. [Point to the picture cues on the card as you say the sound and picture name: /reedy/.] I am thinking, Is this a word I have heard before? Is it a real word? No. I need to switch the sound. I will try /ĕ/ as in egg and see if that makes a word that sounds right and makes sense: /reddy/. Yes, sounds right, and it makes sense. [Discuss meaning in context of the story.] I used the vowel switch strategy and what was happening in the story to figure out the word with a vowel team. When I came to the vowel team ea I tried e /ē/ as in eagle, then /ĕ/ as in egg and checked what made sense in the story.

You may demonstrate the multiple sounds of the digraph by mapping the letters in the word to the sounds to show two or three possible pronunciations for the two vowels (see below).

Provide guided practice with further examples from the text.

meat	**bread**	**great**
Y	Y	Y
/Ē/	/Ĕ/	/Ā/

○ **Restate the Teaching Point**

Review how students applied the Switch the Vowel strategy.

When we came to the vowel team ea *we tried /ē/ as in* eagle *and when it did not sound right we tried /e/ as in* egg, *and it made sense.*

Example 3: Vowel Diphthong *ow*

When teaching flexibility with vowel diphthongs *ow*, *ou*, and variant vowels such as *oo*, use a familiar word with the same pronunciation, such as *look* for *crooked* and *zoo* for *scoop*, to guide students to attempt all pronunciations.

Show Me

When I see o-w, *what sound will I try? First I will try /ow/ as in* snow, *because that is the most common sound for* ow. *If that does not sound like a real word, I will try /ow/ as in* cow. Point to the key words printed on cards as you say each one.

Present the word from the story on a card and place above the two key words. Model how to apply previously introduced word-solving strategies, such as I Can Sound and Say and I Can Chunk the Word to decode the spelling elements before and after the vowel pattern. For example, the *ow* in *chow*:

I will try the word with ow *as in* snow

Pronounce the word *chow* with /ow/ as in *snow*.

Does that sound like a word you know? Does it make sense in the story? No. Now I will try the other sound, /ow/ as in cow *and see if that makes a word we know.*

Pronounce the word with /ow/ as in *cow*.

Yes, that's a word we know. Let's read the sentence to check that it makes sense in the story.

Provide guided practice with further examples from the text.

| sn**ow** | c**ow** |

| ch**ow** |

○ **Restate the Teaching Point**

Restate the word-solving strategy and how students applied it in combination with meaning-making strategies to successfully problem-solve this word. Extend upon the meaning of the word where appropriate to ensure transfer to different contexts:

When we came to the vowel team ow, *we tried* ow *as in* snow *then* ow *as in* cow *and checked what made sense in the story.*

This strategy can also be used for hard and soft consonant sounds, each using a picture cue. For example *c* as in *cat*, and *c* as in *centipede*, *g* as in *goat* and *g* as in *giraffe*, as well as *b* and *d* confusions—with a key word for each consonant, e.g., *b* as in *bear*, *d* as in *dog*.

Reading-Writing Connection

● Have students write their own homograph riddles using riddle books as a model (see Reading Materials to Support the Strategy, page 59).

Practice at the Word-Study Center

● Word sorts with words that contain more than one possible vowel sound.

Guidelines for the most common pronunciations in order include:

When a vowel is in isolation—try short sound first

ea—long *e* as in *eagle*, short *e* as in *bread*, then long *a* as in *great*

ow as in *snow*, *ow* as in *cow*

oo as in *zoo*, *oo* as in *book*

Vowel Switch

Short Vowels	Long Vowels
a	a
e	e
i	i
o	o
u	u

Chapter 5

Fluency Lessons

As students learn how to decode words accurately, we encourage them to read with the same rate and expression they use when they talk—that is, with fluency—so they can focus on comprehension. Profiles of students who will benefit from the lessons in this chapter include the following.

- Word stumblers or bumper car drivers (stop and go, stop and go), who lack automaticity with irregular sight words (such as *eight*, *would*) due to difficulties in storing and retrieving the sequences of letters in words in their visual or orthographic memory

- Robot readers, who read in a monotone voice, without expression

- Impersonators or false positives, who attend to punctuation cues and use appropriate expression, but do not make inferences about the character's intent or use this information to determine cause-and-effect relationships

- Stoplight runners, who take no notice of the signals on the highway, such as punctuation marks and text features (lists, questions, and so on) or other "yellow lights" in the text that tell them they need to adjust their reading speed

- Speed demons or stopwatch readers, who see reading as a race to get to the end as soon as possible, with a negative impact on comprehension

Fluency Lessons: An Overview

Fluency includes reading accurately, at a pace like talking, with phrasing and expression appropriate to the content of the message. Word-solving lessons provide a foundation on which fluency skills develop. The lessons in this chapter move students along the reading continuum so they read accurately at a fluent rate, recognize phrase boundaries, and attend to intonation cues in the text. The Fluency Prompt Card on page 74 has statements and questions to encourage students to apply these fluency skills.

Lesson	Skill/Strategy	Page
● I Can See Words I Know:		73
∗ Train Your Reading Brain	Increasing accuracy in reading irregular high-frequency words	79
∗ X-Ray Eyes		81
∗ Countdown Game	Increasing rate of reading irregular high frequency words	83
● I Can Use My Voice:	Attending to punctuation cues in the text	85
∗ I Can Read Groups of Words	Reading with meaningful phrasing	88
∗ I Can Look at the Marks	Reading with intonation and expression	91

Monitoring and Responding to Student Progress in Fluency

We know that students need to build reading stamina and read at a rate that supports their thinking, or they will struggle as text becomes more lengthy and complex. We also know there is a danger in focusing our fluency training solely on how many correct words they read per minute. There is not a direct one-to-one causal relationship between reading rate and comprehension. We will need to monitor growth in *both* areas and determine how much time we devote to each in small-group instruction. A dual-strategy approach fosters the integrated strategy use characteristic of effective readers.

Reading fluency incorporates a number of foundational skills, and a gap in any one of these presents a stumbling block requiring instructional support. Assessment data and teacher observation will identify whether the roadblock is decoding, sight word recognition (accuracy and rate), vocabulary development, recognition of phrases and punctuation, or text-based aspects such as the students' experience with the topic, vocabulary, language structures, writing style, genre, or text structure. We observe students during reading for information such as the following.

- Where and why are students hesitating? Which parts did they read slower? Which parts more quickly?

- Which words require corrective feedback? Which words represent unfamiliar concepts?

- Do they understand what they are reading?

- Are they repeatedly rereading and then self-correcting/not self-correcting? Rereading is usually seen as a constructive reading behavior, but it can also be a sign that the words or text is too challenging, or that the student has come to over-rely on rereading as a clarifying strategy and needs to develop others. They may also lack confidence as a reader.

- What is their reading experience? Are they familiar with this topic, vocabulary, or text structure?

- Is the text too challenging?

Self-monitoring is an important part of fluency. In *Differentiated Literacy Centers* (2007), I provide a Fluency Feedback Form for partner reading and a Tell-a-Tape form on which students self-evaluate their own recorded reading.

Fluency Feedback Form

Name: _____ Date: _____

I read: _____.

Reading # 2: Here's how my reading got better:

Circle the face that best fits the reading

- Knew more words ✓✓✓   ☺ ☺ ☹
- Read more smoothly 〜〜   ☺ ☺ ☹
- Sounded like talking ⬯   ☺ ☺ ☹
- Used the punctuation ! ? .   ☺ ☺ ☹

Reading # 3: Here's how my reading got better:

Circle the face that best fits the reading

- Knew more words ✓✓✓   ☺ ☺ ☹
- Read more smoothly 〜   ☺ ☺ ☹
- Sounded like talking ⬯   ☺ ☺ ☹
- Used the punctuation ! ? .   ☺ ☺ ☹

My goal is to: _____

_____

A picture-cued form enables students to evaluate each aspect of their reading fluency and set goals for improvement

---

Tools for Interactive Learning

I have several tools in my reading toolbox that I use to support fluency, and to which I refer to in the Monitoring and Responding to Student Difficulty Charts (pages 78 and 87) and in the lessons in this chapter. For example, I use tracking aids such as soft, translucent pocket-chart highlighters, which are available from teacher resource stores. Students place these directly under the line of text they are reading to help maintain their focus. Another advantage of pocket-chart highlighters is that they do not block the return sweep, so students can sustain a fluent pace and do not hesitate in the middle of a phrase, which in some cases can alter the meaning.

To provide auditory feedback, I recommend providing reading phones so students can monitor their own rate of reading and use of expression. Reading phones also help students focus while reading aloud in a whisper voice in a small group. There are two types of reading phones available, the type made with PVC pipe elbows and the hands-free Whisper Phones® that allow students to use both hands (available from www.whisperphones.com).

The fluency strategy chart (page 76) and bookmark (page 77) provide a visual reminder of the skills students can apply to maintain fluency. These are incorporated into each lesson as students share their strategy use with a partner and the group.

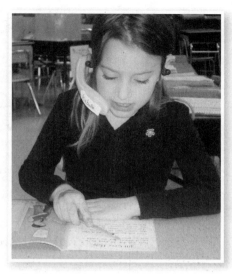

Reading phones provide auditory feedback and keep voice-levels to a whisper, so that each student can read at their own pace without interrupting those seated beside them.

Reading Materials to Support Fluency Instruction

Different types of texts support different types of fluency training: word level for reading rate, phrase level and connected text for expression and intonation. Fluency training at the word level requires materials containing words students know, but not always automatically (i.e., words they can decode within one second). This means the accuracy rate must be at least 98% if the student is to read the text *independently*. To achieve this accuracy rate, the materials used in fluency training are often familiar readings, texts that have been used several times in a shared reading format, in which the teacher reads with students to model and support a fluent rate of reading.

To help students recognize phrase boundaries, we look for text that contains clear phrases, sometimes identified by commas, but most often phrases that represent the subject of the sentence, the action, or are prepositional phrases. To help students read with expression, I use poetry, Readers Theater scripts, stories with lots of dialogue, and nonfiction text with questions and opinions that require adjusting both reading speed and intonation. (See the introductions to the following sections for more details on materials for each type of fluency training.)

I Can See Words I Know: Fluency Training With High-Frequency Words

High-frequency words are often referred to as "glue words" because they hold the meaningful parts of a sentence together. Knowing how to read these words fluently greatly improves accuracy and reading rate and sets the reader up for success with the content nouns in the sentence that tend to be more challenging. Although approximately 87% of our words follow regular orthographic patterns, the remaining words have irregular sound-spelling relationships, and their spelling gives little

"Once a word can be read fluently, the reader no longer has any need to rely on context. Fluency does not describe a stage in which the reader is able to decode all words instantly; rather we become fluent word by word." (Shaywitz, p. 105, 2003)

Fluency Prompt Card

Strategy	Prompt
See words I know	• Do you see a little word you know? Look and say the word. • You know that word. Show me that word. • Do you spy words you know? (Play "I spy with my little eye" on the page.) • Can you see the word in your mind's eye? (Look up and to the right.)
Read groups of words	• Look for words that belong together. • Where could you take a quick breath? • What does that phrase tell you? (Isolate phrase with masking cards.) • Where would it make sense to break the sentence?
Look at the marks	• Stop at the periods. • Take a quick breath at the commas. • Watch for signs along the way … exclamation marks … question marks.
Use my voice	• How would the character say that? • How is the character feeling when they say this? • Can you read it like you're talking? • Speed up at the exciting parts. • Slow down when there is lots of new information. • Try reading it without your finger.

clue to their pronunciation (think of *one*, *of*). Even high-frequency words with regular spellings often include advanced phonics elements, such as which, each, and how (Gunning, 2002). Students do not learn irregularly spelled high-frequency words as easily or quickly as regular ones. These words lack a distinctive appearance and are easily confused. For example, the words *of*, *for*, and *from*; the reversible words *on/no* and *was/saw*; and words with *th*, *wh*, and *w* such as *there*, *their*, *where*, *were* (Blevins, 2006) are frequent sources of confusion.

Teaching Tips

The lessons on irregular high-frequency words focus on developing visual memory for letter sequences that are not decodable. Students typically require more practice recognizing these irregularly spelled words, and repeated practice with them in isolation and in text is necessary. Analyzing the letter sequences in the words to determine the regular and irregular parts helps build orthographic (visual) memory for these words. Useful strategies for teaching irregular high-frequency words include the following.

"Because words with irregular spellings still offer clues to their identities, it is helpful to students when teachers require them to examine all letters in these words and to determine how each letter functions to contribute towards the pronunciation of the word."

(O'Connor, p. 81, 2007)

- Pointing out the supporting letter-sound correspondences, usually initial and final consonants, for example, *said*, *find*
- Highlighting the patterns or repeated letter sequences that can be found in some irregular words, such as *-ould* in *would*, *should*, and *could*, *-ere* in *here*, *there*, *where*

- Providing visual memory training for parts that are not pronounceable: Students visualize the word on a large screen, such as they see at the ball-park, or a digital sign where the letters come up one by one (according to brain research, we look up and to the right when we try to recall a visual image, so you can ask students to try this when they are visualizing a letter sequence)
- Using a time delay technique, where you cue students to say the word after three, then two, then one second; providing a visual or kinesthetic cue increases attention and engages the brain
- Displaying on a word wall and providing brief, interactive practice throughout the week (regular sight words such as *can* and *did* should not be on a Words We Know word wall as they are decodable and can be displayed under the first vowel on the Chunking Word Wall (see Teaching Tips for the I Can Chunk the Word strategy on page 54–56)
- Including repeated reading of irregular words in text
- Asking students to locate the word and read it within context; you can play the I Spy game during this word-find activity using the terminology of the strategy statement: *I see (spy) a word I know, the word is _____*

Create word banks of target words you have pulled from text by writing them on index cards. Store the word cards in an index card holder, using dividers labeled for each group of students. To quickly locate the words that require additional practice, mark new words with a green sticky dot and words causing difficulty with an orange sticky dot.

Student Profiles

In this section we address the needs of our "word-stumblers" or "bumper car drivers," who continue to hesitate at these tricky little words that cannot be completely decoded. These students often demonstrate the following reading behaviors.

- Have difficulty recalling irregular words because they have not stored (and retrieved) a complete sequence of letters from their visual memory
- Often over-rely on phonics; they try and sound out irregularly spelled words that are not fully decodable
- Spell what they hear and so use phonetic spellings for irregular words such as *because*
- Frequently confuse words where there is a minimal difference, such as *where* and *were*
- Have difficulty recognizing the spellings of words that share the same pronunciation, such as *write* and *right*
- Try to memorize a "picture image" of each word, which is futile as learning words by sight (logographic) is limited to about 40 words because there are not sufficient distinctive features to remember each word in this way (Gunning, 2002)

"Students who lack orthographic awareness [awareness of letters and letter sequences in words] over rely on phonics and are slower in their reading... they may continue to sound out words that they have encountered many times ... they tend to confuse words such as what and want that are orthographically similar and may continue to reverse and transpose letters."
(Badian, N.A. (2000) in Gunning, p. 44-45, 2002)

I Can Read Smoothly

I can...

see words I know

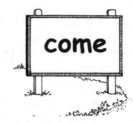

I see a word I know   said

I see 2 little words I know   some thing

I see words I know inside big words   re read ing

read groups of words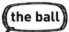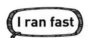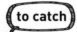

Look for groups of words

Read the words in one breath

look at the marks ? ; !

Use the signs on the way

use my voice

Make it sound like talking

I CAN READ SMOOTHLY
Bookmark

I can...

- **see words I know**

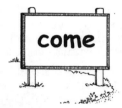

- **read groups of words**

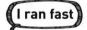 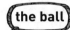

- **look at the marks**

- **use my voice**

I CAN READ SMOOTHLY
Bookmark

I can...

- **see words I know**

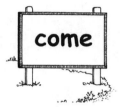

- **read groups of words**

  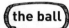

- **look at the marks**

- **use my voice**

Monitoring and Responding to Student Difficulty with High Frequency Words

Struggling readers who over-rely on context clues will find a problem when trying to predict irregular high-frequency words because they often have little meaning of their own. The following chart lists teaching techniques designed to support our word-stumblers who must develop the ability to recognize these words on sight, within a second, to reach their fluency goals.

Student Difficulty With High Frequency Words	Teaching Response/Next Steps
Student Unable to immediately recognize irregular sight words in isolation and in running text	**Teacher** • Has student build the word with magnetic letters. Says the word, touches and says each letter in sequence, and reads the word again. Mixes up the order of the letters and has the student rebuild it • Places two or three target words written on sticky notes across the front of the student's desk. Provides two-minute daily one-to-one coaching sessions by pointing to the word and signaling the student to read the word using a countdown format—a show of fingers for 3-2-1 (see Countdown Game lesson, page 83) • Provides personal word banks with word cards written on index cards held with O-rings. Writes the word on one side and the word in a phrase or sentence on the other to check for meaning • Includes kinesthetic movement to learn the letter sequence where this is helpful, such as *where* vs. *were*. Students spell the word by stretching tall for the tall letters, touching hips for letters that sit on the midline, and touching their toes for letters below the midline • Uses music and rhymes with high-frequency words • Plays "guess the missing letters" in a game show format. Omits the tricky medial vowels and silent consonants in the word and replaces with a line for each mystery letter • Incorporates word sorting using word cards that require attending to letters in confusable words (see lesson Train Your Reading Brain on page 79) • Cumulatively teaches the words in sight word phrases, adding a new word to previously taught words • Provides meaning cues, such as highlighting the word in a sentence, using the word within a student-dictated sentence to add to their personal word bank, having student build and read rebus sentences with picture and word cards • Incorporates word games like "flip up" (concentration), go fish, lotto, bingo

Reading Materials to Support Accuracy with High Frequency Words

Any text contains high-frequency words. Examine the text and identify opportunities for repeated practice of target words. Reading materials with predictable sentence structures and familiar vocabulary, along with texts specifically designed to support instruction, such as reading series that introduce the words cumulatively, are suitable resources for fluency training with high-frequency words.

Preparation

- Copy the reproducible I Can Read Smoothly Strategy Chart (page 76) onto cardstock.
- Copy the reproducible I Can Read Smoothly Bookmark (page 77) onto cardstock. Make one for every student.
- Copy the Fluency Prompt Card (page 74).
- Have large paper clip or clothespin on hand.
- Select target high-frequency words and make word cards for sorting for each pair, or make individual sets (see categories in the lesson).
- Select reading material that contains target high-frequency words.

Tell Me

Point to the icon for the I Can See Words I Know strategy on the I Can Read Smoothly Strategy Chart. You may place a paper clip or clothespin alongside the icon.

Today we will use the I Can See Words I Know strategy on our chart. To read smoothly we need to know all the words. But there are tricky little words in every book that can trip up our reading brain. Our word-solving strategies alone will not work with these words. We need to train our brain to remember them as soon as we see them—to see the word and know it instantly, so we can keep on reading and thinking about the story. To help our reading brain know these words the second we see them, we will look carefully at each letter in the word so our brain remembers it.

Show Me

Show the first word card to students and model how to analyze the order of letters in the word, pointing out the regular and irregular parts of the word. Demonstrate how students need to look carefully at the medial letter(s), because the vowel sound may be an exception to the usual pronunciation. Illustrate the mismatch with other words containing the same pattern, such as *rain* and *said* in the example below.

Here is a word from our story that is on nearly every page. [Read a sentence with the target word to illustrate its usefulness.] *There are parts of this word that we can sound out and parts that we cannot. In the word* said, *we hear /s/ at the beginning of the word and /d/ at the end of the word. The tricky part is in the middle, where we see the letters* ai. *In many words, like* rain *and* mail [use examples they know], *the* ai *stands for the /ā/ sound, but in the word* said, *it has a different sound. The* ai *stands for /e/. We will need to remember that when we read this word in our book today.*

Guide Me

Introduce another irregular sight word from the text and have students analyze it:

As I show you each of the tricky words in our book today, look carefully for the easy parts and the tricky parts. The first word is _____. What's the word? What are the easy parts that we can sound out in _____? What are the tricky parts? [Saying parts encourages risk-taking because it implies there is no single correct answer but several possibilities.] *Now let's read the word together again and say each letter so they will stick like glue in our brain. What's the word? Spell it!*

The next word is _____. [Repeat the process for one or two more words.]

○ **Sort the Words From the Story**

Word sorts support student learning of high-frequency words when one or more words are exceptions to phonics rules or are "out of sorts." You can label a category heading with a question mark to designate these or call them "oddballs" (Ganske, 2000).

Model the procedure of sorting the word cards into categories. You may provide partners or individual students with a set of the cards for independently sorting the words you have been reading. Introduce the process by saying something like the following.

When we compare words, we find they have letters that are the same and letters that are different. Watch me sort these words. We will look closely at the letters in each word to see what is the same and what is different. Now let's sort these words together.

Explain each category for the guided word sort. Provide partners or individual students with a set of cards for sorting. Read and review the words together before supporting students as they sort them.

Categories for word sorts include:
* **Initial Consonant or Consonant Clusters (blend, digraph)** Example: words that begin with *t* and *th*, *w* and *wh*
* **Pattern** Example: *-ould* words, *-ere* words
* **Sound** Example: homophones, where students need to distinguish the different spellings, such as *their* and *there*, *where* and *wear*

Provide sight-word sorts according to appropriate level of difficulty.

Level 1
* Beginning Letters: Same/Different, e.g., *me, my* vs. *can, will*
* Final Letters: Same/Different, e.g., *was, his* vs. *was, saw*
* Word Shape (where this varies), e.g. *the, and, you, for*
* How Many Letters? e.g., two-, three-, and four-letter sight words

Level 2
* Single Initial Consonant vs. Blend or Digraph, e.g., *t* vs *th*, *w* vs. *wh*
* Same/Different Final Letters, e.g., *went, want; the, them, then, there, their, they*
* Same/Different Medial Vowels, e.g., *went, want; come, came; __a__, __e__, __o__*
* Pattern, e.g., *_ould, _ere, _en*

Level 3
* Silent Consonants: Yes/No, e.g., *could, laugh* vs. *sleep, best*
* Silent Vowels: Yes/No, e.g., *does* vs. *well*
* Same Sound, Two Spellings (homophones), e.g., *to, two*

Yes	No
was	saw
his	him

Level 1: Final Letters

w	wh
were	where
work	what

Level 2: Single Initial Consonant vs. Blend or Digraph

Yes	No
you	me
read	with

Level 3: Silent Vowels

Coach Me

Introduce the reading material. Play I Spy by having students locate the practiced words on several pages. Help students read the words in context fluently. Students continue to read the rest of the text independently at their own pace. Have each student read a sentence or two to you aloud, in turn, and prompt as necessary (see Fluency Prompt Card).

You know that word. Tell me that word. Read that word in the sentence. Read the words smoothly.

○ **Partner Think-Pinch-Share**
Students share a part in the story where they saw a word they know, and could read instantly.

○ **Group Share**
Ask partners to share one of the words they found with the group. Have students locate the word in the text, and read in context of the sentence together. Discuss the meaning of the sentence.

Show us where you can see a word you know (like the I Spy game).

○ **Restate the Teaching Point**

Provide positive feedback on how students looked for words they knew. Review the strategy and how it helped them as readers (link to statements you used in Tell Me).

Today you looked for words you know in the story. You used your reading brain to see and say the word quickly, without having to stop. This helped you to stay focused on the meaning of the story.

Reading-Writing Connection

- Students use the words they sorted to write a sentence or short story. This can be a shared or independent activity.
- Word sorts may be recorded in word study journals. Have students record the words in columns with category headings.

Practice at the Fluency Center

Select independent practice activities from the following center tasks found in *Differentiated Literacy Centers* (Southall, 2007):

- Mix and Fix
- Partner Tic Tac Read
- Word Windows
- Sight Word Sort
- Flip Up Sight Words
- Sight Word Hunt
- Rebus Sentence
- Homophone Flip Up

LESSON: X-RAY EYES

Preparation

- Copy the reproducible I Can Read Smoothly Strategy Chart (page 76) onto cardstock.
- Copy the reproducible I Can Read Smoothly Bookmark (page 77) onto cardstock. Make one for every student.
- Copy the Fluency Prompt Card (page 74).
- Have large paper clip or clothespin on hand.
- Stock table with whiteboard and erasable pen.
- Select reading material that contains target high-frequency words.
- Select high-frequency words for practice. Print on index cards.

Tell Me

Point to the icon for the I Can See Words I Know strategy on the strategy chart. You may place a paper clip or clothespin alongside the icon.

Today we will use the I Can See Words I Know strategy on our chart. We are going to play the X-Ray Eyes game to help our brain remember the tricky little words we see in our books. This game helps you see the letters for a word in your head, just like on a big screen or digital sign. When you have a complete picture of a word in your head, you will know that word each time you see it in a book, and you won't have to stop and try to remember it.

Show Me

Let me show you how we play the X-Ray Eyes game.

Print the high-frequency word from the book on a whiteboard. Point to the word and read it.

Here is our new word: would.

Touch and say each letter in sequence, then read the whole word again as you sweep a finger under it in a single, quick movement.

I am going to erase one of the letters in the word and see if my brain can remember it.

Erase a letter from the word. (The easiest letters to recall are usually in the initial and final position; the hardest are the medial vowels and silent consonants.) You may draw a short line to represent the missing letter (as in "guess the missing letter" games) or simply leave a blank space. With longer words, such as *because*, students may require this visual support when naming letters that have been erased.

_ould

I will use my x-ray eyes to see and say the missing letter.

Touch and say each letter, including the letter that has been erased, touching the blank space as you say this "invisible" letter.

w-o-u-l-d

Guide Me

Ask a student to choose a second letter they would like you to erase from the word. The letter can be in any position in the word. The group reads the word, chants all the letters along with you (including those that have been erased) as you point to each letter or space, then reads the word again.

_ o u l_

Let's use our x-ray eyes to see and say the missing letters.
What's the word?
Everybody, spell it.
What was that word?

If you wish to role-play the act of using your x-ray eyes, ask students to form circles with their thumb and finger around their eyes, to represent the special glasses that enable them to see invisible letters (like a superhero!).

Continue by asking another student to choose a third letter to erase, until all the letters have been erased and students have successfully retrieved the complete letter sequence for the word from their visual memory. Ask students to visualize the letters in the word coming up on a big screen, letter by letter (like a digital sign or big screen at a football/baseball stadium) as they spell it aloud.

Print the word a second time on the whiteboard and say, *Let me quickly write the word again. Now you know how to play the X-Ray Eyes game. It's your turn to play the game together without my help.*

Repeat the process of erasing a student-selected letter and chanting the spelling, but this time, do not say the letters with them. The group reads the word, chants the letters in sequence as you point to each letter or space, and reads the word again. Repeat the process you modeled and practiced together above, removing one more student-selected letter each time until none are left and students have to recall the entire word. Check that the students say each letter in the word in the correct sequence. If students have difficulty recalling the correct letter, display the word on a card or write on the whiteboard as a visual reference, ask them to locate the correct letter, and highlight this in the word.

Coach Me

Introduce the reading material containing the target word. Ask students to locate the target word they have practiced by framing with their fingers or highlighting with a transparent counter.

Find the tricky word we practiced today on this page. What's the word? Now that you know it you can each read the story on your own.

Students read independently, at their own pace, all at the same time. Coach individual students to apply fluency strategies during reading (see Fluency Prompt Card page 74).

○ **Partner Think-Pinch-Share**

Students share with their partner a page in the story where they saw a high-frequency word they know.

○ **Group Share**

Have partners share an example of a high-frequency word they found with the group and read the word in the sentence.

○ **Restate the Teaching Point**

Provide positive feedback on how students read high-frequency words without hesitating, and trying to remember them.

Today you looked for words you know in the story. Your reading brain remembered the words and you said them quickly so you could keep on reading the story.

Reading-Writing Connection

● Have students build and write/draw rebus sentences using word cards and pictures.

Practice at the Fluency Center

● Make a set of word cards omitting one or more letters, replacing the missing letter with a line. Students are to copy and complete the word. Laminated cards can be used with an erasable pen.
● Partners or small groups can play the X-Ray Eyes game, with one student being the recorder.

Provide these activities from *Differentiated Literacy Centers* (Southall, 2007):
● Word Pyramids
● Tic Tac Look and Say
● Homophone Flip Up

LESSON: COUNTDOWN GAME

Preparation

● Copy the reproducible I Can Read Smoothly Strategy Chart (page 76) onto cardstock.
● Copy the reproducible I Can Read Smoothly Bookmark (page 77) onto cardstock. Make one for every student.
● Copy the Fluency Prompt Card (page 74).
● Have large paper clip or clothespin on hand.
● Create high-frequency word cards. Make four to six word cards from the group word bank (words students have been introduced to and have read in context in previous lessons, but do not recognize within the one-second fluency rule). The number of words you present in the lesson depends on the developmental level of the students.
● Select reading material that contains the target high-frequency words.

Tell Me

Point to the icon for I Can See Words I Know on the strategy chart. You may place a paper clip or clothespin alongside the icon.

Today we will play the Countdown Game with our words. When we read, we need to know our word bank words fast. If we have to stop each time we see these words, we may forget what the story is about.

Show Me

Sometimes when I see a tricky word, I have to stop and think about where I have seen it before. Then I often forget what I was just reading. Today we will play a countdown game that will help us to read these words fast, without having to stop and try to remember them.

Point to the target word in the text and read it aloud.

Here is the word ___.

Show the same word on a card.

I am going to practice reading this word fast using the word card. First, I will give myself three seconds, then two, then only one second to read it. Let's see how I do.

Hold up the word card and use the fingers on your other hand to count to three, holding up one finger at a time, until you show three fingers. Read the word. Repeat the process of finger-counting to two, then, finally, only counting to one before reading the word.

Guide Me

Now it's your turn.

Present the set of word cards to the students one by one. Each time you read through the set of cards, reduce the time by one second just as you demonstrated, using the time-delay countdown format. Remind the students to read the word aloud together (choral-read) on your cue. Brain research tells us that a physical cue increases student
engagement and attention.

As I show you each word from our word bank, look carefully, wait, and watch my fingers count down from three, then read the word out loud together. Three, two, one (finger-count). What's the word?

Repeat for each word card in the set. For the next round, reduce the time by one second.

This time, when I count down from two, read the word. Two, one. What's the word?

In later sessions, repeat the process until students are able to say the words within one second.

Now that you have a picture of this word in your brain, when I hold it up and ask you, "What's the word?" you will all say it together.

When students meet the one-second goal over three consecutive sessions, the words retire from the bank.

Next step: The following activity provides practice in discriminating between the high-frequency words. As students progress, present common confusions, such as *where* and *were*, and have students practice reading these words in context with your support.

○ 3-2-1, Pick-Up Cards
Provide each student with a set of two to four word cards to place face up in a row in front of them

Say one of the words and ask students to select the correct word card and hold it up upon hearing your cue: *Three, two, one! Cards up!* Students now hold up their word cards all at the same time.

When the students have held up their cards, acknowledge with a "Yes!" Next, give the cue, *Cards down!* Students place their card back in the array in front of them, face up.

Provide corrective feedback as necessary. If a student holds up the incorrect card, support him or her in analyzing the letter sequence, touching and saying each letter in sequence, and reading the word.

With confusable words, ask them to discriminate between the two possible words, pointing to the differences in their spellings (e.g., *there/ their*).

Coach Me

Introduce the reading material containing the target words. Have students locate the words on specific pages in the text, framing with their fingers or using a highlighting tool. Students will read independently (whisper or silent reading) while you coach individuals.

- ○ **Think-Pinch-Share**
  Students share with their partner a page in the story where they saw a high-frequency word they know.

- ○ **Group Share**
  Partners share an example of a high-frequency word they found with the group. The group locates the word and choral reads the word in the sentence.

- ○ **Restate the Teaching Point**
  Provide positive feedback on how students recognized high-frequency words in the story without pausing to try and recall them, and read smoothly.

  You used your reading brain to quickly say the words you know in the story.

Reading-Writing Connection

- Students copy and illustrate the sentence from the book containing a high-frequency word they know. The high-frequency word is printed in color.
- Have students write a retelling using one or more of the target high-frequency words.

Practice at the Fluency Center

Activities from *Differentiated Literacy Centers* (Southall, 2007):
- Word Reading Relay
- Flip-Up Sight Words

I Can Use My Voice: Phrasing and Expression

We have all heard students who read in a robotic manner, without emotion, neglecting to attend to punctuation and context cues. This can interfere with understanding and even alter the meaning of the text. In the following lessons we focus on recognizing meaningful phrases in the text and adjusting the use of expression and emphasis to reflect the author's intent.

Teaching Tips

Phrasing requires a great deal of practice with supportive text. By practicing with the same text, students grow from reading the words to understanding what they read to presenting it orally in a meaningful, well-phrased way.

As I teach each high-frequency word, I integrate it cumulatively with previously taught high-frequency words to form phrases. In this way, students have repeated practice and review of these glue words in a sentence. The Frog and Toad series by Arnold Lobel abounds with high-frequency word phrases. We teach high-frequency phrases in isolation, but we always practice reading them within context in the same lesson to ensure transfer to independent reading. When you examine the reading materials for the group, you will notice that many of our prepositional phrases are almost entirely high-frequency words.

Reading in phrases supports comprehension, and the same phrases can be used to support the retelling. Authors of both narrative and informational text locate important facts within phrases. I integrate phrasing with comprehension by sorting the phrases under story structure elements or topic subheadings. This is equally useful in both fiction and nonfiction text. We are all familiar with the "who, what, where, when" categories that lend themselves well to sorting phrases, e.g., "The bear is eating honey in the woods today."

I extend this with sentence-building activities, in which I pull phrases from familiar literature—characters we have read about, the settings where the story occurred, the character's actions—and print these on 9" x 3" flash cards. I color code these: green for the first phrase in a sentence, yellow for the second, and red for the last phrase, like a traffic light sequence. Students use these to construct "silly sentences." They mix them up to create innovations on familiar stories, placing Arthur in a setting where Junie B's story took place and so on. We build upon this in our writing by using story structure phrases as springboards for writing a complete story.

Example:

Arthur	is writing a postcard	at the beach

When students demonstrate poor use of expression, we focus their attention on the intent of the character, what he or she might be thinking and feeling at that moment, what is happening in this part of the story, and the punctuation marks on the page that the author provides as signposts that tell us how this passage should be read to convey the meaning.

Provide a reason and motivation for rereading for fluency by varying the focus each time you read the same passage. The first reading is for meaning and enjoyment of the text (comprehension), the second for locating high-frequency words (accuracy and rate), the third for reading in phrases, and the fourth reading for practicing expression and intonation, including attention to punctuation.

Student Profiles

Students who require fluency training demonstrate a range of reading behaviors. Many students continue to read word by word and benefit from small-group instruction in recognizing phrases in the text, which are meaningful groups of words. When students are able to read phrases, their reading becomes smoother and their comprehension is enhanced. In oral reading, phrasing impacts the understanding of the listener. Word-by-word readers also benefit from learning when to adjust the pace of reading, such as increasing the rate with independent level text that is being read for enjoyment. Prior experience with timed fluency tests can lead some students to view successful reading as a matter of accuracy and speed—and they become "stopwatch readers," whose aim is to get to the end of the text as soon as possible.

Monitoring and Responding to Student Difficulty with Phrasing and Expression

In this section you will find techniques that have proven to be successful when working with the student profiles described above.

Student Difficulty With Phrasing and Expression	Teaching Response/Next Steps
Student Reads word by word; does not use phrasing and reading is choppy	**Teacher** ● Makes concept concrete: ＊ Uses the "phrase steps" activity: writes phrases from stories and poems on cards and places on the floor so students can step from one to the other as they read to tell a complete sentence or short story (see Step to the Beat activity in Southall, 2007) ＊ Displays a vertical sentence: cuts apart familiar sentences into phrases; places phrases vertically on the table, and reads to and with the students, supporting appropriate pauses (see I Can Read Groups of Words lesson) ＊ Scaffolds during reading: frames a two- or three-word phrase with two masking cards, helps student read the phrase, and prompts: *Read across these words* *Now read these two/three words together* ＊ Constructs phrase pyramids (see I Can Read Groups of Words lesson) ＊ Marks slashes in the text with pencil or marker if using a photocopy so students can practice reading attending to the phrase marks; then erases the marks or provides an unmarked copy and monitors for transfer (Blevins, 2006) ＊ Draws arcs under phrases in chart sentences for student to read ＊ Provides phrase sorts (see Teaching Tips and I Can Read Groups of Words lesson)
Does not attend to punctuation	● Has student use a colored pencil to mark the punctuation on a photocopy of the text; the same as we use to edit our writing, and then provide repeated oral reading opportunities with the marked text: ＊ underline capitals in green ＊ circle end marks with red ＊ mark commas in yellow or brown ＊ mark dialogue with purple
Does not adjust their reading speed	● Has students choral read a short part of the text, holds up a color-cued card in places where the students need to slow down (yellow) and speed up (green) to play the "flag game," as if students are driving a racing car ● Marks the text with color-coded sticky flags to indicate change in reading speed is required
Reads without expression and intonation	● Provides short text, such as comic strips, for repeated reading, where getting the joke depends upon the use and understanding of expression ● Displays picture-cued emotion cards (see I Can Look at the Marks, I Can Use My Voice lesson). Substitutes a different emotion cue and has the student reread, adjusting their use of expression according to the character's motives, feelings, actions and to reflect the student's personal responses to the story ● Incorporates performance oral reading, where each student reads the part of a character or a specific part of the text for the purpose of presenting the information in a way that is enjoyable for the audience (class or group)
Reads with frequent repetitions; stops and rereads one to three words	● Slides a masking card over the words, covering them as they are read, to train the student to look beyond the word they are saying (students need to be able to scan three to five words ahead as they read to maintain fluency)

These speed demons and stoplight runners ignore the traffic signals on the road, such as punctuation cues and text structure. They neglect to adjust reading speed, slowing down for important information, such as dates and names, and they may lose the gist of what they are reading.

The use of expression in reading requires that students make inferences about a character's emotions and also use intonation that demonstrates their personal response to the reading. Some students use expression, but can be described as impersonators or false-positives. They are adept at using punctuation cues to mimic the appropriate intonation, but are not processing the meaning of what they read. By including comprehension checks within our fluency instruction we can monitor student understanding and adjust our teaching to include shorter text, with frequent student interaction.

Reading Materials to Support Phrasing and Expression

Short, motivating text, such as comic strips, are ideal resources because getting the joke depends upon the use of intonation and expression. Readers Theater scripts and books that rely heavily on dialogue can be found at different reading levels with many reading series. Rhythmical text, such as poetry, also supports phrasing. For beginning readers, look for books that include poems for phonics and sight words to address both accuracy and fluency. Web sites that provide downloadable copies of the Dolch sight words in phrases at no cost include www.createdbyteachers.com and www.schoolbell.com. A list of Edward Fry's sight words in phrases can be found at www.flashcardexchange.com and in Timothy Rasinski's book *The Fluent Reader* (2003).

LESSON: I CAN READ GROUPS OF WORDS

Preparation

- Copy the reproducible I Can Read Smoothly Strategy Chart (page 76) onto cardstock.
- Copy the reproducible I Can Read Smoothly Bookmark (page 77) onto cardstock. Make one for every student.
- Copy of the Fluency Prompt Card (page 74).
- Have large paper clip or clothespin on hand.
- Provide one sticky note for each student.
- Select reading material.
- Print a sentence from the text onto sentence strips and cut apart into phrases; print a second sentence and cut apart to form a cumulative sequence of phrases (see example on next page).
- Print labels Who, What, Where, When, How on index cards.
- 4–6 blank index cards.

Tell Me

Point to the icon for the I Can Read Groups of Words on the strategy chart. You may place a paper clip or clothespin alongside the icon.

To read smoothly, we read groups of words together. When authors write, they put important information into groups of words called phrases. A phrase might be two or more words. As readers, we look for these groups of words to help us understand the story. When we talk, we say words that belong together; we talk in phrases. When we take a quick breath after each phrase, it gives the other person a chance to think about each phrase as we say it.

Show Me

Read the sentence (that you cut apart) word by word (choppy), then read it again and pause at the phrases. Do not show the text to the students. Ask students what they noticed about your reading. Which reading was easier to understand? Why?

Display the sentence you cut into phrases, placing phrases vertically on the table. Read it to and with the students, pointing to each phrase as you read. Use the phrases to generate predictions about and connections to the story or topic.

Here is a sentence from our book today. In your book, the phrases are written across the page, but I am showing them to you like this so you can see how the author put important information in phrases. What have we already found out about this book from reading the phrases (the characters, what they like to do)? Notice James Howe didn't just write "Dolores," he wrote "mostly Dolores." What information does that tell us? What do you predict? What might happen in a story about three mice who love adventure? Turn to your partner and share your prediction. Begin your sentence with "I predict," "I think," or "I bet"

Example: *Horace and Morris but Mostly Dolores* by James Howe (1999)

Horace and Morris	but mostly Dolores	loved adventure

Guide Me

Display the second sentence you cut apart to form a cumulative sequence. Read the pyramid sentence to the students. Discuss the phrase breaks. Read the sentence together, attending to the phrases. You can mark the phrase boundaries with a sticky dot or slash mark.

Here is another sentence from the book today. What do you notice about the way these strips look? (They get longer as you progress to the bottom.) That is because I have added on one more phrase to each line until we have the whole sentence at the bottom.

I'll read it to you. Listen for groups of words that belong together—the phrases. You will need to know where the phrases are so you take a quick breath there. Where is the first phrase? Now look at the next strip. Can you spot the phrases? It's getting tougher. Now look at the third strip. Take a breath; now let's read together.

I'll bet•

I'll bet• Horace and Morris•

I'll bet• Horace and Morris• couldn't do that,•

I'll bet• Horace and Morris• couldn't do that,• she thought.•

Have students read to the first stopping point in the story. They use their sticky notes to mark a place where they find a group of words that belong together and can be read in one breath.

We will read the first part of our story and look for groups of words that tell us about the characters and what happens to them. Use your sticky note to mark a group of words you read together, a phrase.

After students read, have students retell the story, and then use the following activities.

○ **Partner Think-Pinch-Share**
Ask them to share with a partner the spot in the book where they placed their sticky note, and to read their phrase.

○ **Group Share**
Ask partners to share one of their phrases with the group. Record the phrases on index cards. Display to the group. Have students locate each phrase within the text, if possible, and read it together. Discuss the information it gives the reader. Keep the cards for later.

Let's hear a group of words you found that you read with one breath.

Coach Me

Students read the next part (or the rest of the story, if short) and move their sticky notes to a new phrase. Coach individual students to read with appropriate phrasing.

Support individual students by framing two to three words in the text with a masking card, and reading the phrases to and with the student.

Read across these words.

Now read these two words together.

Next step: Students will collaboratively sort the phrases they located according to meaningful categories and use these to retell the story.

○ **Group Phrase Sort**
Ask students to share the phrases they found and record these on index cards. Add these to the ones you recorded earlier together and display all on the table. Read them together. Pause after each card and ask students if they notice something the same about two phrases; do they tell us who, what, where, etc.? Sort the phrase cards by meaning under the index cards you labeled. Ask students to identify additional categories by which they could be sorted.

Example:

When	What	Where
One day	They sailed	the seven sewers
Now-and-forever	They climbed	Mount Ever-Rust
Next day	go exploring	clubhouse
	build a fort	

○ **Restate the Teaching Point**
We read groups of words together, smoothly, so our reading of the story made sense.

Reading-Writing Connection

Students can:
● Use the phrases to write a retelling or an innovation to the story.
● Find more phrases and identify possible categories for a phrase sort.
● Illustrate phrases from the book.
● Copy sentences and cut into phrases.

Practice at the Fluency Center:

Provide independent practice with center tasks from *Differentiated Literacy Centers* (Southall, 2007):

- ● Fast Phrases
- ● Froggy Phrase Slide
- ● Phrase Sort
- ● Step to the Beat

LESSON: I CAN LOOK AT THE MARKS

Preparation

- ● Copy the reproducible I Can Read Smoothly Strategy Chart (page 76) onto cardstock.
- ● Copy the reproducible I Can Read Smoothly Bookmark (page 77) onto cardstock. Make one for every student.
- ● Copy the Fluency Prompt Card (page 74).
- ● Have large paper clip or clothespin on hand.
- ● Make picture-cued emotion cards; see image at right.
- ● Write punctuation marks on sticky notes or flags (see lesson example) for each student or distribute one blank sticky note and pencil to each student. Store sticky flags on a bookmark made of cardstock.
- ● Select a text with dialogue and/or varied punctuation.
- ● Write a sentence from the text with an exclamation mark on whiteboard or chart.

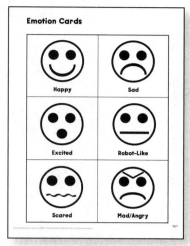

Picture-cued emotion cards are used as a visual prompt to indicate when students need to adjust their use of intonation and expression, so they will gain increased understanding of the author's intent

Tell Me

Point to the icons for the I Can Look at the Marks, I Can Use My Voice on the strategy chart. You may place a paper clip or clothespin alongside the icons.

Today we will look for punctuation marks in the text and use our voice to help us read smoothly and understand what we are reading.

How we use our voice when we are talking tells the listener many different things. Are we serious or joking? Are we happy or upset? The author of this book knew he/she would not be here to read it to us, so we wouldn't hear his/her voice, but he/she gave us clues so we know how to read it! We can use clues like the punctuation marks on the page. If we see a question mark like this [point to ? in text], then we know our voice will go up at the end of the sentence. If we see an exclamation point, then we say it like we really mean it, or maybe as if we are surprised. When we see quotation marks, we know someone is talking, and we need to know something about just how they might say the words. Authors also give clues to help us with the dialogue. They tell us about the characters and how they might be thinking and feeling, and they describe what is happening when they say it. Then we know what emotion to use when we read it so we get the meaning. Emotion and thinking are both part of reading. Today we will look for clues or signposts in the book/poem that tell us what kind of emotion we should use when we read it.

Show Me

Read a poem or dialogue from a story without emotion. Then read it again with expression and have students brainstorm what they noticed, prompting them to note the different types of inflection, emphasis, intonation, and expression, including the type of body movement you used. List these on a chart as students share them and discuss how these are all part of fluency.

Display the sentence you wrote on a whiteboard to the group. Read it to and with the students. Introduce the emotion cards and choose and display the one that matches your sample text.

Here is a sentence from our book. I will show you how I use my voice to help me, and you, understand the meaning of what I am reading. The author gave me two clues so I know how to read it. The clues are an exclamation point and the word cheered. *I can also use what I know, my schema; I know how excited we get on the last day of school!*

Example: *Arthur's Family Vacation* by Marc Brown (Scholastic, 1993)

Excited

"...school's out!" Everyone cheered.

Now I will switch out the punctuation and put a period there instead. [Erase and replace on whiteboard or put a sticky note with a period over the exclamation mark on chart.] *How will that sound?* [Read sentence without excitement.] *Does that change the meaning? I don't sound excited about it anymore.*

What if I switch the emotion card for mad/angry? [Read with angry voice.] *Now that would mean the character was feeling very differently about this, and that could change what happens in the story.*

Here is another sentence where Arthur is talking to Buster. I don't see any punctuation clues. I will have to think about how Arthur is feeling when he says this. What emotion would he use to say this? How do you think he is feeling? What emotion should I use? [Display emotion card.] *What would that sound like?* [Choral read using appropriate expression. Repeat the process, switching out the emotion card and rereading.] *I wonder why Arthur doesn't want to go on vacation. Turn to you partner and share why you think Arthur isn't happy about going.* [Students share their thinking—what they predict is the answer to this question.] *We will have to read and find out.*

"I wish I didn't have to go on vacation with my family," said Arthur.

Guide Me

Review the emotion cards and punctuation sticky notes. Then read two to four more sentences or phrases from the text together. Switch the punctuation and/or emotion icons to reread the same sentence in two or three ways. Read it first as a statement, then switch the emotion icon and read again using different intonation and expression. Discuss how this affects the meaning and possible storyline.

Examples:
"I can't wait for baseball practice to start," said Francine.
"I'm taking a computer course," the Brain announced.
"I'll really miss you at Camp Meadowcroak this year, Arthur," Buster said.

Introduce the next section of the text. After working with the sample sentences, students read to the first stopping point in the text. Provide each student with the bookmark and sticky flags with punctuation marks (or have students print a question or exclamation mark on a blank sticky note). Have students match the punctuation sticky note to a sentence with the same punctuation in the text. Display the punctuation cards on the table as a visual reference for students.

As you read page ___ to ___, look for sentences with each of these punctuation marks. Place a sticky with that punctuation mark in the margin next to the sentence. Read it to yourself and think about how the author uses these marks so you know how it will sound, which emotion to use.

Next step: During the following small-group session(s), have students substitute different punctuation marks in the text and read with a different emotion. Display the emotion cards as a visual reference.

Choose one sentence. Switch the punctuation mark and read again. How does that change the story? Try reading one thing the character says with a different emotion. Use the emotion cards to help you. How would it sound? Would it change the story? Think about the clues the author gives you so you know how this would sound. Be ready to read something the character said to your partner, to show how they are feeling.

Coach Me

Ask students to show you a part they marked with their punctuation sticky note. Prompt them to read the sentence with the appropriate expression and intonation. Probe to monitor student understanding of the author's intent or the meaning associated with the punctuation and emotion clues in the text.

○ **Partner Think-Pinch-Share**

Have students read to their partner the sentence where they matched [or switched] the punctuation mark and used a different emotion to guide their expression.

○ **Group Share**

Ask partners to share their sentences with the group. You may have the group locate and read two or three sentences together and use the same emotion, expression, and intonation.

○ **Restate the Teaching Point**

We looked at the punctuation marks and used our voice to help us read smoothly and understand the story.

Reading-Writing Connection

Students can write an innovation on the story using different punctuation marks and altering the emotion so that the storyline is changed. They could show how a character reacted in a different way, using dialogue and description to illustrate the emotion.

Practice at the Fluency Center

Provide independent practice with these activities from *Differentiated Literacy Centers* (Southall, 2007):
● Say That Again
● Say It With Feeling
● Comics and Riddles
● Get the Beat
● Read-a-Round

Chapter 6

Comprehension Lessons

The lessons in this chapter address challenges students often experience in developing effective comprehension strategies. Students with these difficulties can fall into the following categories.

- Storytellers, who over-rely on background knowledge. They make up their minds about what is going to happen before they read the text and do not integrate new information.

- Under-predictive readers (no map, no GPS), who read without anticipating events or information, do not revise predictions when they do not match the text, and fail to monitor for meaning during reading.

- Literalists, who depend solely on what is written in the text and have difficulty responding to questions that require inferring or integrating multiple sources of information.

- Left fielders, who are unable to answer questions, or who offer responses that are unrelated to the events, information, or topic.

- Unequipped readers, who lack fix-up strategies to solve problems in comprehension.

- Solo strategists, who apply strategies in isolation rather than integrating them, resulting in a superficial level of comprehension.

Comprehension Lessons: An Overview

Many intervention programs focus primarily on developing decoding skills. We know that word analysis is a barrier to comprehension for many students. However, even when working with appropriate leveled text, we need to use a dual-strategy approach in our small-group instruction, teaching a balance of word recognition and fluency alongside comprehension; otherwise, a gap in comprehension will develop (Walpole & McKenna, 2007).

I have worked with many second-, third-, and fourth-grade students who have gaps between their word-solving skills and their comprehension. They look blankly at me when I ask for responses to the text; they can decode the words but don't understand what they have read. The assessments currently being implemented across the country reflect a greater emphasis on higher-order thinking. We can't wait until our students are fluent decoders before we begin to work on comprehension. When the teaching point is word solving, we do integrate dual strategy use through sharing our connections, questions, and retellings in brief partner and group discussions. But this is not the primary focus of the time allocated to direct instruction in the lesson. Each comprehension strategy needs to be taught more explicitly and over a period of time. The scaffolds incorporated into the following lessons are designed to make these higher-order thinking processes accessible to *every* student.

In each of the following lessons you will notice that the key emphasis is on interacting with the text *during* reading as opposed to the traditional emphasis on often lengthy book introductions before reading and answering teacher questions *after* reading. The teacher prompts on the Comprehension Prompt Card on page 98 are organized by strategy and enable teachers to question and probe student understanding during reading. These are part of the Coach Me step in the lesson sequence.

Lesson	Skill/Strategy	Page
• I Can Connect	Making connections	103
• I Can Predict	Predicting	108
• I Can Figure It Out	Making Causal Inferences	116
• I Can Figure It Out	Making Relational Inferences	118
• I Can Wonder	Generating and answering literal questions	126
• I Can Wonder	Generating and answering inferential and evaluative questions	129
• I Can Stop and Fix	Self-monitoring using clarifying strategies	134
• I Can Retell	Using story structure and vocabulary to retell fictional text	141
• I Can Sum It Up	Summarizing informational text; determining important information	145
• I Can Code My Thinking	Integrating strategy use by coding the text with multiple strategic responses during reading	149

Monitoring and Responding to Student Progress in Comprehension

As you know, children can experience a wide range of challenges in comprehension and we need more than one teaching technique at our fingertips. The same approach may not work for each child, so look at the charts accompanying the lessons as menus *from which you can select additional levels of support* to meet the varied needs of your students.

Tools for Interactive Learning

Using the interactive learning tools listed below ensures every student is continuously interacting with the text. These memory aids are incorporated into the reading, talking, and writing applications so that every student is accountable for his or her strategy use during the lessons. The strategy chart and bookmark use the same language for each strategy as the classroom bulletin board display described in Chapter 3 (See Common Strategy Statements page 31) to support students in verbalizing and internalizing their strategy use. Further interactive props and materials are described in the introduction to each strategy and preparation section of the lessons.

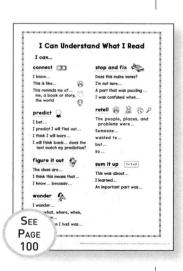

SEE PAGE 100

Anchor Strategy Chart

The strategies are introduced cumulatively to correspond to the *picture-cued comprehension anchor chart* found on page 100.

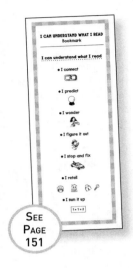

SEE PAGE 151

Strategy Bookmarks

Each lesson has a bookmark with visual cues for each step in applying the strategy. These are copied onto cardstock for each student in the group. Use white-out before copying to erase any icon that is not being taught at that time (see Chapter 3).

Strategy Hats and Masks

To help students develop self-talk skills and the ability to think aloud, props such as masks and hats labeled with strategy icons can be incorporated into the lessons. Teachers explain and model their purpose during the Show Me part of the lessons. As part of the think-aloud, point to the page in the text you are reading and then to the prop as you share your thinking, demonstrating the process of responding to the text during reading. During the Guide Me and Coach Me parts of the lesson, students hold/wear the mask or hat as they share their thinking in group and partner discussions.

Some teachers use specific types of hats to establish the purpose for reading, the genre, and the type of thinking it requires (Marcell, 2007). For example, students don a construction hat when reading expository text (challenging text) for the purpose of learning important facts about a topic; baseball caps for narrative text, where the purpose is recreational reading; and a visor when "skimming and scanning" text to locate information or examining text for research purposes. I also use the visor when reading magazines, which we seldom read in sequence cover to cover, as well as catalogues, comics, the newspaper, and other text that we tend to flip through.

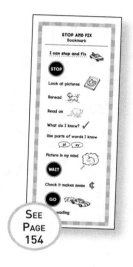

SEE PAGE 154

To make the mask, draw a large thinking bubble on poster board and cut out a circle in the center large enough for the students to see through. Cut a rectangle of poster board for the handle or use a craft stick. Draw a series of connected bubbles on the handle. Copy the icons from the strategy charts on pages 45, 76 and 100 and attach the appropriate label at the top of the mask using Velcro so you can quickly switch it out for different lessons. If you are using the genre hats described above, attach strategy labels in the same way.

Selecting Text for the Lesson

In each lesson in this chapter there are recommendations for reading materials that support the strategy. As you browse your reading materials you may wish to code them by the strategies they lend themselves to with a sticky dot or marker on the back of the book. For example, I use I for inference, C for connecting, CL for clarifying, and so on. I devote separate pages for listing books and other reading materials by level and comprehension strategy in my planning notebook. I add to this throughout the year to save time later when I am looking for a book at that reading level to support a specific strategy.

Reading-Writing Connection: The Reading Response

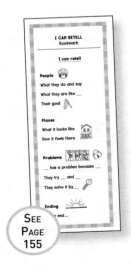

SEE PAGE 155

Some students who provide minimal responses in oral discussions may provide a more expanded answer in writing (with appropriate scaffolds). Other students participate enthusiastically within group discussions, yet use an economy of words in their written responses. It can be frustrating as a teacher to know a student has valuable points to share, yet is not able to convey them either orally or in writing.

As students learn to respond to the text, they often begin with a simple retelling or summary, even in a list format. We move students beyond this rote retell by providing frameworks in which students can share what the story or information means to them. These tasks include making connections to familiar experiences, people, or other readings, and generating questions. Such responses require students to analyze what they have read on a deeper level, reflecting on the information and the author's purpose. Journals can be shared with a partner or the group so students can gain ideas from each other and expand upon their thinking. As you read through student journals, look for patterns in their responses and evidence of their thinking. Do they go beyond the text?

Writing Prompts

You may provide prompts like the following to support students' writing about their thinking on the text:

- Write about what you know.
- Write an "I wonder" question.
- Think about the book and write about the ideas/facts the author shared with you.

Alternatively, select a powerful sentence from the text you are reading and use it as a focus for discussion and writing a personal response or as a model of sentence structure for writing an innovation.

Mentor authors and texts provide a valuable springboard for student writing. Students gain a model for their own writing style, and practice a variety of writing techniques. For example, Joy Cowley's narratives often use animal characters, humor, and a twist at the end. Once we identify what is characteristic about each author's works, we can then challenge students to write an innovation or extension on the text by integrating these same techniques.

Likewise, the text structure can provide a model for student writing. This approach can be used with students at even the earliest level of literacy development. For example, a nonfiction book that describes the life cycle and habits of an animal provides a model for students to use as they organize the facts about an animal they know and write a descriptive text. A text that invites students to express their opinions, such as *Should We Have Pets?* by Sylvia Lollis (2002) can form the model for students to write a persuasive piece. Connecting your reading and writing program by focusing on the same text structure will enhance both comprehension and writing skills.

Graphic Organizers

A blank page can be daunting to many young readers and writers. Incorporate simple graphic organizers that are designed to support students in synthesizing the information in the text.

Charts

Students can use the two- or three-column format in their notebooks outlined in Chapter 3 (page 39) to provide a supportive format for writing in response to reading. See example at right.

It says	I think

Comprehension Prompt Card

Strategy	Key Phrase
Making Connections	• What do you already know about _____? • What does this remind you of/make you think about? • How are you connecting this to your life? Did something like this happen to you or someone you know? What experiences have you had like _____'s? • Does this remind you of a book you read, something you saw on the Internet or TV, or something that has happened in the real world?
Predicting	• Skim and scan. Run your fingers down the sides of the page and look for clues. • What do you think might happen/you will find out? • What makes you say that? (evidence) • Now you know _____. Does that match your prediction?
Generating and Answering Literal Questions	• Ask a who, what, where, or when question about what you read. • What might a teacher ask about what happened/this information? • Show me the part that supports your answer. • Show me where it says that.
Generating and Answering Inferential Questions	• What makes you say that? How do you know _____? • What are you thinking about the character or information? • What might the character be thinking? • Why do you think the character did/said that? • How do you think the character feels now? • What was the effect of _____? What do you think caused that to happen?
Inferring	• Use the clues the author has given you in the book and what you already know to figure it out. • On page ___ the author says _____. What does that tell you? How does that help you figure it out? • What did you notice that helped you figure it out?
Clarifying (fix-up tools), Self-Monitoring	• Is there a part/word that is puzzling or confusing, that is not clear? • Show me that part/word. • Which fix-up tool could you use?
Retelling	• Where does the story happen? Who has the problem? What was the problem? Why was it a problem? • What was their goal? What did they want? What stands in the way of _____ achieving their goal? How do they solve the problem? What happens that explains how they solve the problem? • What can you tell me about [topic]? What more do you know? What have you read?
Summarizing/ Determining Importance	• What does the author most want us to remember? • What is the most important idea or event? • Can you summarize what you read in one sentence? • Think about your reason for reading this. What are you trying to find out? Look for words that will help you to sum it up.

Text Structure-Based Organizers

Graphic organizers that allow the information to be organized according to the text structure support a variety of comprehension strategies, such as summarizing and writing skills, and organization of ideas and facts. For example, a book comparing seals and sea lions lends itself to a Venn diagram, whereas an article on the life cycle of the butterfly is a sequential text structure that can best be represented by a flow chart with a series of connected boxes. The facts in a descriptive text on a specific animal can be organized into categories of information in a web. Problem and solution in both fiction and nonfiction text such as environmental issues can be represented in a two-column chart. Bring students' attention to the signal words and phrases that indicate each text structure at stopping points during the reading.

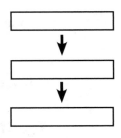

Flow chart

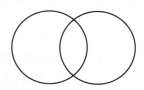

Venn diagram

Making Connections

When readers connect to prior knowledge, they build a bridge in their minds from the known to the new. The experience the reader brings to the reading is also referred to as our schema (Miller, 2002) or the compilation of all our life experiences, ideas, and opinions. As each of our schemas differ, because of varied experiences, student connections will also differ.

Teaching Tips

A teaching sequence progresses from helping students make connections to their own lives to making connections with other sources of information acquired in reading, listening, and viewing experiences, to making connections with larger themes found across literature, such as friendship, and world issues or events, such as protecting endangered animals. These three levels of connection are described below and are incorporated into the following lesson. Begin by focusing on text to self, then introduce the other two types of connections one at a time, responding to the readiness of your students.

"The background knowledge we bring to reading colors every aspect of our learning and understanding. If readers have nothing to hook new information to, it's pretty hard to construct meaning ... when we know little about a topic or are unfamiliar with the format, we often find ourselves mired in confusion."
(Harvey & Goudvis, p. 92, 2007).

Text to Self

Help students make text-to-self connections by focusing on events, ideas, or facts that convey key information or the author's purpose. They are, in order of difficulty:

● Personal experiences, feelings, opinions
● Other people I know and places I have seen

Text to Text

These include connections to other books, television programs, movies, or Internet content. Display a cumulative chart listing different types of texts that you have read together as a class and the types of text-to-text connections students made (Harvey & Goudvis, 2007), which may include:

● Comparing characters: what they do, say, and think
● Comparing the events in a story or facts in a book on the same topic
● Identifying the different themes or author's messages in stories
● Identifying the style of an author
● Comparing how different authors write about the same theme or topic
● Identifying what is the same and what is different in two versions of the same story

I Can Understand What I Read

I can...

connect

I know...

This is like...

This reminds me of...
   me, a book or story,
   the world

predict

I bet...

I predict I will find out...

I think I will learn...

I will think back... does the
   text match my prediction?

figure it out

The clues are...

I think this means that...

I know... because...

wonder

I wonder...

Who, what, where, when,
   why, how...

One question I had was...

stop and fix

Does this make sense?

I'm not sure...

A part that was puzzling...

I was confused when...

retell

The people, places, and
   problems were...

Someone...

wanted to...

but...

so...

sum it up $1 + 1 = 2$

This was about...

I learned...

An important part was...

Differentiated Small Group Reading Lessons © 2009 by Margo Southall, Scholastic Teaching Resources page 100

Text to World

Text-to-world connections require students to notice new information as they read and link it to what they already know. Students can make connections to:

- New information: family, community, state, country, world
- Global theme: friendship, courage, bullying, honesty, kindness, prejudice, tolerance, survival, responsibility

Student Profiles

Many struggling readers do not connect with what they read. They do not see something or someone in the text that is relevant to their life and remain disengaged readers. To avoid this, making connections is typically where we begin when introducing a new text to students; we try to hook them to the book in some way to engage them both personally and intellectually with the theme or topic.

Two profiles of need we often encounter when teaching this strategy are the following.

1. Disconnected students, who lack the background knowledge necessary to build a bridge between known and new concepts.

2. Off-track connectors, who become distracted by other ideas that come to mind that are unrelated to the events or facts in the text. These students would happily talk about everything from their dog's favorite toy to what they had for breakfast this morning, if given the opportunity. This requires we tread a delicate balance of protecting the learning opportunities of the rest of the students while also respecting individuals within the group.

I describe techniques that I have found to be successful with these two profiles in the chart on page 102.

Reading Materials to Support Making Connections

We have all taught a reading lesson when students express a lack of connection to the title you have selected, often saying "I just don't get it." It doesn't engage them because the concepts are not within their range of experience, interest, or imagination. If you can't make an on-the-spot switch, it's best to carry on, admit to yourself this wasn't a good choice for this group, and find a text that they can relate to for the next session.

It is often easier to narrow down nonfiction topics, where a few questions can quickly determine whether or not students have any background knowledge. Determining fictional themes that will support connections can require more probing as they are less finite, but this will save precious teaching time later.

To support text-to-self connections, incorporate books with characters and experiences that students can identify with, such as a boy or girl in their own age range and/or from sociocultural contexts they can relate to.

Series books that revolve around consistent characters make excellent resources for learning text-to-text connections. Students build upon their connections by reading and comparing several books in a series, each time learning more about how and why a familiar character responds to different events and issues in a characteristic way. Reading a nonfiction and a fiction title on the same topic or theme also supports making text-to-text connections, as students are able to build upon prior knowledge on a topic they might otherwise have little experience with.

Student Difficulty With Making Connections	Teaching Response/Next Steps

Student
 	
Has difficulty making connections to the character, event, or information; may lack supporting background knowledge or experience
	Teacher
	
	● Provides text with picture supports for new vocabulary and concepts in a familiar text structure
	
	  ✻ Models making a connection with a think-aloud
	
	  ✻ Provides an example based on a shared classroom experience: *What is happening in the story is like what happened …*
	
	● Reads text/section with students before beginning strategy instruction, so that the content is familiar and a higher level of analysis is possible
	
	● Provides background information on the topic
	
	● Rereads a sentence or two, points to the illustrations, prompts for possible school-based or personal experiences that could connect to this: *How is this like* [a familiar experience, book or concept]?
	
	● Incorporates concrete props, such as interconnecting plastic math links (students each have a link that they place on the book page as they describe the link or connection they have made)

Shares connections that are *not related to the text*, or fails to make the connection clear; these connections may be personal and superficial in nature, such as having a cat the same color	● Demonstrates how off-track connections get in the way of understanding what you are reading:
	
	  ✻ Thinks aloud how to refocus back on the text by stopping and self-monitoring their understanding: *Does what I am thinking have anything to do with this story? If it doesn't, I need to be thinking about what is happening in the story to get back on track with my understanding*
	
	● Brings students' attention to how their thinking does or does not help them understand the text:
	
	  ✻ Asks them to explain the link they are making between their experience (schema) to an event or fact; rephrases what the student said, asking *How are you connecting to this?*
	
	● Rereads the same part from the text and prompts:
	
	  ✻ *What in the book/what I have just read reminds you of* [student example]?
	
	● Records student connections during the lesson on large sticky notes; after reading, the group collaboratively sorts these into two columns: connections that are "important to me" (unrelated) and connections that "helped us understand" (related)

Reading different versions of the same story by different authors or further books on the same topic by different authors also develops students' ability to compare and contrast a variety of texts. This becomes more challenging than connections to characters or topics, as we require students to analyze a number of variables across multiple texts. By identifying the similarities and differences between pairs of these books, you will scaffold the thinking processes you require of your students.

The genres that typically present the greatest challenge for making connections are science fiction and historical fiction; both incorporate events and concepts that students have no personal experience with. Beyond genre, text structure is also an important element in scaffolding student connections. Keep this in mind when you are selecting the text for the lesson: Is it in a format that is familiar to the students? Are there text features or a writing style they have not encountered before? If that is the case, it may be best to either read and examine these first and then reread for connections or select a more supportive text.

Preparation

- Copy the reproducible I Can Understand What I Read Strategy Chart (page 100) onto cardstock.
- Copy the reproducible I Can Connect Bookmark (page 151) onto cardstock. Make one for every student.
- Copy of the Comprehension Prompt Card (page 98).
- Have large paper clip or clothespin on hand.
- Select a book (see Reading Materials to Support Making Connections, page 101)
- Optional: Have two to three sticky notes for every student or sticky flags labeled "R."
- Optional: Prepare picture cards for every student representing each type of connection in the lesson.
- Optional: Several plastic math "links" for each student (the kind used for measurement activities).

Tell Me

Present the comprehension strategy chart and place a paper clip next to I Can Connect. Explain what the strategy is and how this helps us as readers:

When we are reading something new, we think about what we already know. Thinking about what we know helps us understand what we read.

Show Me

Display the book and point to the title and any illustration. Describe the steps in your thinking as you activate your "reading brain" to make connections. Point to the icon and statement you use for each type of connection on the chart or bookmark.

Our book today is about _____. Looking at the book, I am thinking, "What do I already know about this topic? What experiences have I had like this? [Or] What books have I read that are like this one?" I know something about _____ because this reminds me of something that happened. [Or] I read a book/ saw something on the Internet/watched a program on TV about _____ . I know _____ .

Prompt for student responses to your think-aloud.

What are you thinking? What might we find out in a book about _____?

Read a short section of the text. Stop and model making a connection. Pinch and use the sentence starters on the bookmark, such as "This reminds me of...." Place a sticky note on the outside edge of the page, and draw a happy face symbol for this or print the letter *R* for this reminds me. If you want students to write a statement during reading, then model by recording your connection on the sticky notes. Repeat for each type of connection you are teaching at this time, such as text-to-self and text-to-text.

Reread a part of the text: *When I read these words this reminds me of ... .*

Show the picture: *When I saw the picture of _____ it made me think about ... .*

This is like something that happened to me... .

Recap your thinking processes.
Notice that as I read I am thinking about experiences I have had that might relate to this book in some way and what I already know about _____.

Prompt students to describe what they heard you say and do. Then prompt them to share their connections so they begin to engage in the thinking process, rather than remaining passive or just imitating your model. Have students share a connection with the group or turn and talk to a partner: *How are my connections the same or different from the connections you made to this? Share a connection you had.*

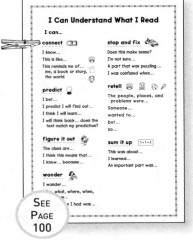

SEE PAGE 100

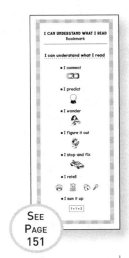

SEE PAGE 151

Guide Me

Set the amount of text you want students to read (2-3 minutes) and remind them of their focus during reading. Distribute sticky notes and ask students to mark the text where they made a connection.

Now it is your turn to read. Read page(s) _____ to _____ on your own and look for things that remind you of someone or something you know. Use a sticky note to mark where you made a connection.

○ **Group Share**

Ask students to pause when they have read to the first stopping point (see above) and have them "turn and talk" (you can call this "push-pause") to share their connections. Extend upon their connections with the following activity.

○ **Connection Cards (Optional)**

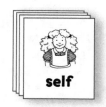

Place the connection cards in three piles, by type (self, text, world). Distribute the connecting plastic "links." Have each student in turn place it on a page in a book where they "connect" to an event or fact. Alternatively, they can simply place their bookmark on it. After they do this, they take a card from the pile that represents the type of connection they have made to this page/event and place it in a collective pile in the center of the table or in a bowl labeled "Our Connections." As they place it on the pile they describe their connection to the text. If you are using masks, pass one around the group, taking turns to share their connections (see Tools for Interactive Learning at the beginning of this chapter).

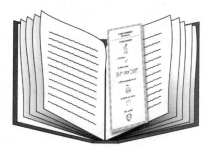

Remind students to use the language on the bookmark that you have modeled. Prompt for responses. Monitor student strategy use. Record their responses and the type of connection (see chart below).

We have read a few pages. Let's stop and talk about the story. Does this part of the reading remind you of something? Did something like that happen to you? Did you ever feel that way? How does this connect to your life? What connections are you making to this?

Does that remind you of something from a book you have read ... a character ... a setting? Describe something you know about that is connected to _____.

How does this connect to the world around you? How does this help you understand the story/ information?

Comprehension in Action: *Bats* by Lily Wood (Scholastic, 2001)

Text	Sharing Our Connections	Type of Connection
Most bats fly at night. (page 3)	I know that bats fly at night because our class talked about that last year.	text-to-self
Bats sleep upside down. (page 9)	That reminds me of something I saw on TV that showed bats hanging upside down in a cave.	text-to-text
Bats live in many parts of the world. (page 10)	This is like when we learned about different animals in Australia.	text-to-world

Review and reinforce how they used the strategy, or demonstrate how they could have used the strategy during this section of the reading.

Coach Me

Ask students to continue reading to the next stopping point. Have them mark two or three more places where they made a connection so they will be ready to share with their partner. Ask individual students to verbalize a connection they have made so far and prompt any students having difficulty.

- Do they link what they already know to something in this text?
- Do they notice when something is familiar to them? Note any difficulties you observe.

    Let's read to _____ and mark _____ more connections so you can share them with your partner.

○ **Partner Think-Pinch-Share**

Ask students to think of a connection, pinch an icon/phrase on their bookmark to share their connections with a partner. Remind them they can use the language on the bookmark to help them, as you did in the beginning of the lesson.

Pinch the word or picture that represents your thinking (self, text, world).

Hold up your bookmark to let your partner know what type of connection you have to this. Share your connection with your partner. What is their connection to this? How is it the same or different from your connection?

○ **Group Share**

Invite students to share one of the partner "think-pinch-share" connections with the group:

What experiences did you share that make this text real for you?

○ **Restate the Teaching Point**

Review how making connections helps us grow as readers:

We have shared all kinds of connections. These will help us understand the message/information the author is sharing with us in [title of book or article].

Reading-Writing Connection

Extend student understanding and strategy use with one of the following writing in response to reading activities:

○ **Reading Response Journal**

Students will now have an opportunity to expand upon their thinking shared during the group and partner discussions. Making connections includes expressing opinions, thoughts, ideas, and personal experiences. Both personal and intellectual connections to the reading are appropriate entries for the reading journal. Journals can be exchanged between reading partners and used as a springboard to more writing as students read and write a reply to each other's journal entries. These provide a basis for further discussion in partner and group shares in subsequent sessions and during independent reading time. Possible prompts for writing and discussions include:

   * Does this remind you of something that happened to you or someone you know?
   * What did you notice in this book that is like real life?
   * How did your connection help you to understand the book?

○ **Sticky Notes (optional)**

Provide sticky notes for each student to use during the reading. Students mark a place where they had a connection. They can draw the type of connection—face, book, or globe on the sticky note for the three levels of connections (self, text, world)—or print an *R* to represent that this reminds them of someone or something (Harvey & Goudvis, 2007). Another easy option is to draw a tally mark on the sticky to represent that this is something "I know." This notation corresponds to the Coding Bookmark and sticky flags described on page 147, which integrates strategies from each of the lessons in this chapter. Sticky flags provide a reusable way to mark locations in the text, with students storing them on a bookmark (see Interactive Tools, page 34). After reading, students locate where they have marked the text and expand upon their thinking in their journal.

○ **Two-Column Format**

Students select a key event, idea, fact, word, or quote from the text and record it on a chart like the one at left in the first column, In the Book, and then note the type of connection to this in the second column, My Connections.

In the book	My connections

Practice at the Comprehension Center

The following activities from *Differentiated Literacy Centers* (Southall, 2007) support the strategy:

- What Do I See? What Do I Know?
- What I Think
- Build a Connection
- Connection Stems
- Read, Relate, Respond
- Tic Tac Connect

The Predicting Strategy

Effective readers anticipate what is going to happen next. Making a prediction requires the reader to think ahead, before and during reading. It also requires readers to pause during reading and think back to check their predictions. Students check and revise their predictions as they acquire more information or clues in the text. A prediction is based on different sources of information in the text and the reader's understanding of the theme, topic, genre, and/or text structure. Like connections (and inferences), predictions will also depend upon the student's background knowledge and experience with this topic.

Predicting and inferring are related processes. The difference between a prediction and an inference is that a prediction can be confirmed in the text, whereas an inference may or may not be confirmed—it depends upon the interpretation of the reader (see Inferring Lessons page 116 and 118). If the students' predictions are neither confirmed nor refuted, they will need to make an inference as to the outcome.

"[S]truggling readers often operate under the misconception that meaning 'will come to them' as they decode words; they do not understand that meaning-getting requires active probing for meaning. These students may need explicit information about how this seemingly instantaneous mental activity works."

(DUFFY, P. 88, 2003)

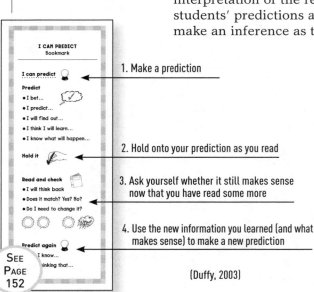

1. Make a prediction
2. Hold onto your prediction as you read
3. Ask yourself whether it still makes sense now that you have read some more
4. Use the new information you learned (and what makes sense) to make a new prediction

SEE PAGE 152

(Duffy, 2003)

Teaching Tips

When we teach predicting, we demonstrate to students that readers actively predict and re-predict continuously as they read. It is not an activity relegated exclusively to the beginning of the reading. Again, the emphasis is on activating strategy use during the reading. The two key concepts we want students to understand about making predictions is that:

- Predicting is a form of self-monitoring
- Predictions change as we read

Initial predictions may be superficial when based on cover clues only. I know some of my students have been led astray or distracted by irrelevant details in cover illustrations. As a consequence, I had to work hard to refocus their predictions. When introducing a book and inviting student predictions, I recommend that you go beyond examining only the title and cover illustration if it is ambiguous and may lead to tangential predictions. Instead, also read the first paragraph or page before inviting predictions. This is typically where we find out the character and setting, or topic statement, upon which to base predictions. In this way you will avoid having to refocus a group of off-track readers. With nonfiction text, examining the table of contents and/or subheadings and captions provides a basis for successfully predicting the information they are likely to learn.

In the following lesson, students are asked to stop at key points in the reading, generate a prediction, read on, and then stop again to check their predictions. By examining the text before the lesson, we can designate critical stopping points in the reading and have students mark these with their sticky notes.

Student Difficulty With Predicting	Teaching Response/Next Steps
Student Is unable to make predictions during reading	**Teacher** ● Selects a text on a familiar topic or theme with supporting illustrations; alternatively, provides background information on the theme or topic and prompts for connections so students can use their prior knowledge to make a prediction (e.g., familiar storyline or character) ● Asks them to generate questions about the book and then turn that into a prediction ● Prompts students to reread a section of the text in which important information is located and use key words to form a prediction: * *Let's read what the author has to say about _____ . Use a word/fact from this to predict what will happen next/you will learn next*
Lists what he/she sees or reads without making a prediction, such as facts about characters, animals, etc.	● Refers to student's retell (information or list of events) and how they support a prediction: * *Now that we know _____ , what do you think will happen?*
Guesses without using clues in the text, resulting in predictions that are not logical or likely to occur	● Prompts for predictions based on the story elements (characters, setting, etc.) or facts learned so far: *What else might the author include in a book about whales?* ● Marks short sections of text and prompts for retelling or provides a retelling; rephrases student retelling and prompts for text-based predictions
Does not integrate new information in the text to revise his or her predictions; sticks to earlier predictions despite a mismatch with the evidence in the text	● Prompts them to examine if the information they just read matches (supports) their prediction: *You predicted _____ . Does it match the text?* ● Probes to find out the clues student is using for his or her predictions; can student justify prediction with evidence? *What makes you say that?* ● Uses Story Structure Sort (I Can Retell, page 142) in which students predict and sort words from the text under story structure headings, such as character, setting and problem; after reading, students return to the sort and may revise predictions by moving words to different category headings

Students share the predictions they made during reading and check if they match the text, or need to be revised.

Student Profiles

This lesson supports students who are under-predictive readers, those who do not anticipate events or information before and during reading. Many students have difficulty adjusting their predictions when they conflict with the evidence in the text. Some over-rely on background knowledge and ignore or fail to integrate new information as they read. It is as if they are saying, "I've made up my mind what is going to happen, so don't confuse me with the facts." Readers who struggle with comprehension may insert words as they read, and tell their own version of the text, without attending closely enough to the author's words. Teaching responses to these profiles of difficulty are listed in the chart on page 107.

Students who are English language learners may not have experience with the concepts in the book that are culturally specific, such as the way a family celebrates a birthday. This will affect the predictions they make and the teacher will need to scaffold success and build background knowledge before reading so that the focus can be upon developing the predicting strategy.

Reading Materials to Support Predicting

Stopping points will be critical to supporting predictions. Look for logical stopping points following the structure of a narrative text: after the basic story elements have been introduced in the beginning of the book; when a problem arises; just before the solution; again before the conclusion or resolution. In non-fiction, we have subheadings and other signals in the text that we have reached an appropriate stopping point. Plan stopping points that invite predictions on the story elements, events, or new information you may learn in the next section.

SEE PAGE 100

LESSON: I CAN PREDICT

Preparation

● Copy the reproducible I Can Understand What I Read Chart (page 100) onto cardstock.
● Copy the reproducible I Can Predict Bookmark (page 152) onto cardstock. Make one for every student.
● Copy of the Comprehension Prompt Card (page 98).
● Have large paper clip or clothespin on hand.
● Select a book.
● Place three 3" x 5" sticky notes at planned stopping points, for example, after the beginning of the story, in the middle, and on the last page. You can also use sticky flags to mark the stopping points on the edge of the pages.
● Have sticky notes or index cards on hand so you can write your predictions and the evidence for your predictions. Prepare two cards labeled "I Predict" and "Because" to serve as category headings (see page 109 in the lesson).
● Optional (for Match-Up Activity): Prepare index cards labeled "Match" and "No Match," plus 10 blank index cards. Alternatively, write these headings across the top of an open file folder ruled into two vertical columns and use as a sorting mat.

Tell Me

Display the strategy chart and place a paper clip next to I Can Predict. Describe the thinking process involved in making a prediction and why it is helpful for the reader to use the language on the strategy chart and bookmark.

When we read a new book, we think about what might happen or what we might learn. This is called predicting, or making a prediction. To make a prediction means we think ahead of what we are reading. We hold the prediction in our head, read some more and check to see if our prediction matches what happens in the book. If it doesn't match, we use the clues in the book ("Now you know") to make a new one. Checking our predictions helps us make sure we understand what we are reading.

Show Me

Display the cover of the book to the group. Guide students to attend to the clues readers use to make predictions.

> *Let's see if I can find any clues about this book in the title and illustration.*

Read the title of the book, a chapter, or a subheading. Examine the illustration.

> *I predict the author used this title to tell us that this book will be about _____. Looking at the illustration and what is happening in the picture I am also predicting _____.*

Activate student background experience with the genre of the book and/or a familiar author. You can focus predictions on the story elements or text features.

> *I'm noticing that this is a story, which means that there will be characters who have a problem to solve or will have something interesting happen to them. I know that [author] wrote another book about _____. So this book might _____.*

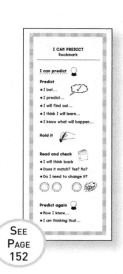

SEE PAGE 152

Model how to skim and scan the text for clues to support predictions. Run your index fingers down each side of the page as you scan the text up to the next stopping point, like moving the cursor on a computer screen. Have students practice this by moving their fingers down each side of the page, searching for clues.

> *Let me show you how I make a prediction as I begin to read. Before reading, good readers skim and scan the text. They look for words that jump out at them and other clues that tell might tell them what they will find out.*

> *I am looking for clues that can help me. Are there any words or illustrations that can help me? I can see _____, so I am predicting _____. I notice the word _____, so I predict that _____.*

Read up to your first sticky note stopping point in the book, just a page or two. Share a prediction you have and pinch the corresponding statement on the bookmark, such as "I predict" or "I bet" (step 1 on bookmark). Model how to hold it (step 2 on bookmark) and write your prediction on the sticky note or index card (or just share orally if students will not be writing during reading). Repeat for each prediction.

> *As I read page __ I find out that _____. Right now I am saying to myself: This means that _____. I will read on and check if that does happen.*

Continue reading to the next stopping point. Model steps 3 and 4 on bookmark:

> *When I get to the bottom of page _, I check to see if my prediction matches what I just read. I think back to the first prediction I made about the title of the book. Now I know that _____ didn't happen, so I need to use what I read to make a new prediction. I predict _____.*

Invite students to comment on what they observed you do and say. Was your demonstration clear to them?

> *What clues did you see me use to make a prediction?*
> *When did I use the book?*
> *When did I use my own thinking about what I already know?*

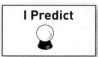

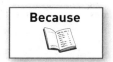

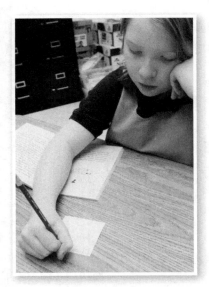

Plan stopping points in the reading where students can pause to write their predictions.

Record reasons for these on sticky notes or index cards and place alongside the predictions (if writing during reading is part of the lesson). Recap the self-monitoring process of confirming or revising predictions:

Did you notice how I ask myself: Does my prediction match what I just read? If it didn't, I used the information to make a new prediction.

Guide Me

Provide a purpose as students read to the next stopping point in the text. Students are to make a prediction when they get to this stopping point.

Now it is your turn to read and make a prediction. We will read to page _____. As you read, think about what might happen next in the story. Use your sticky note to write your prediction so you will be ready to place it on the chart and share it with the group.

○ **Group Share**

Invite students to share their predictions with the group by placing them on the chart under Our Predictions. Remind them to use the language on the bookmark. (If students are just orally sharing and not using sticky notes, then record their predictions on the chart.)

What predictions did you make that helped you understand the story? As a reader, what did you notice that helped you predict?

Take up some of the predictions. Question and prompt students to expand upon their prediction: What evidence did they use in the text to make this prediction? Discuss the evidence for each prediction.

Why do you think that might happen? What do you think the characters will do? Why? What in the book makes you say that?

Ask students to read to the next stopping point. This time they are to check the prediction they made at the first stopping point. Did it occur? If it didn't, they are to make a new prediction.

Read to the next sticky note and ask yourself: Does this match my first prediction? If it does match, write "Yes" on your first sticky; if it doesn't, write "No." Then use what you just read to make a new prediction.

Alternatively, have students mark their sticky notes with a plus or minus sign, instead of "yes" and "no."

Coach Me

Students read to the next stopping point. Ask them to make one new prediction for this part of the story and read on to check the prediction. Remind them to mark the sticky notes with "yes" or "no" (as above).

Let's read to _____ and record our predictions so we will be ready to share them with our partners. Use what you know so far to predict what will happen next. Read and check your predictions.

While the group reads, question individual students on the predictions they have made and the reasoning behind them. Ask yourself the following:

● Are students able to make logical predictions?
● Can they justify their predictions based on evidence in the text?

Comprehension in Action: *Early One Morning* by Greg Lang (Scholastic Canada Ltd. 2001)

Text	Sharing Our Predictions	Match? Because...
Title: *Early One Morning*	This story is about a special day for the girl and her father. They will see all the things that happen in their neighborhood early in the morning.	Yes—title and cover illustration
"Sshh!" he said, "don't wake the others ..." They had something important to do. (page 4)	It is going to be a surprise. *[This matches our prediction that it is a special day.]*	Yes— "Dad says not to wake the others"
As they walked down the sidewalk, Anna and her dad saw the town waking up. They saw ... (page 6)	*[This matches our prediction that they will see what happens in their neighborhood—but now we know it's not just the neighborhood—it's their whole town.]*	Yes—They said it would be "an important day"
But Anna and her dad walked to the bakery. They had something important to do. (page 10)	They are going to buy a birthday cake at the bakery—for a party.	Yes—They "saw the town waking up"
They bought some warm bread and muffins. (page 12)	*[This does not match our prediction that they will buy a cake for a birthday party. We need to make a new prediction.]*	No—they bought bread and muffins
When they got home, everyone was still asleep. "Everybody! Breakfast is ready!" called Anna. (page 15)	The food is for a surprise breakfast. *[This matches our prediction that it will be a surprise breakfast.]*	Yes— "breakfast is ready"
"Happy Mother's Day, Mom!" said Anna. (page 16)	*[We found out that it was for Mother's Day instead of a birthday.]*	No— "Mother's Day"

- Do they recognize that their prediction matched or did not match the text?
- Are they able to form a new prediction when it does not match the text?

○ Partner Think-Pinch-Share

Hold up your bookmark and share your prediction with your partner. What predictions did you make as you read? How are they the same or different from your partner's predictions?

After the partners share, ask students to write the new predictions on the chart or dictate them for you to write on sticky notes. Read through the predictions you recorded on the chart during the group share. As you read each one, ask students to give a thumbs up or down to indicate whether it occurred. Move the sticky notes under "Match? Because" on the chart after each one is examined. Invite students to share how they confirmed or revised a prediction with the group.

Let's read through our predictions and see which ones matched the text or if we needed to revise it and make a new prediction. Are there any predictions we need to change? How could we change them? [For nonfiction:] *Did you learn _____? Did you find out about _____?*

○ Match-Up Activity (Optional)

To make learning concrete, have students sort the predictions they have written or dictated in two piles under cards labeled "Match" and "No Match." If students are not able to write the predictions, record those they shared orally on index cards and write the evidence they cited for each one on separate blank index cards. Shuffle the cards and ask the group or partners to identify which pile or category they belong in. Have students cite the evidence (book and schema) used for each prediction and why this did or did not occur. Give students credit for both columns, as many predictions could have occurred, and the mismatch is a result of the author's plan for the text.

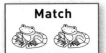

Match

The food is for a surprise breakfast

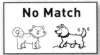

No Match

It is a birthday party

Ask students to review their predictions and identify those that helped them understand the text. *Which of our predictions were most useful?*

○ **Restate the Teaching Point**
Our predictions helped us to think carefully about how each of the character's actions caused further events to happen. [For nonfiction:] *Our predictions helped us find out if this information was new to us or not, and reflect on the new information we learned.*

Reading-Writing Connection

Each of the following reading responses builds upon the lesson activities:

○ **Sticky Notes**
After reading, students use the sticky notes they have marked with a yes or no (or a plus and minus sign) to write about the predictions they made or record them in a two- or three-column chart format (see left) in their response notebook.

I predict	Because...

I predict	Because...	Match... yes or no

○ **Two-Column Format:**
Students record their predictions and the evidence they used from the book and their schema.

○ **Three-Column Format:**
Extend the first format to include a "Yes or No" column and explanation if the prediction did not occur, such as words or events in the text that contradict their prediction.

Practice at the Comprehension Center

The following activities from *Differentiated Literacy Centers* (Southall, 2007) support the strategy:

- What I Think
- I Wonder
- Tic Tac Question #1

I Can Figure It Out: Inferring

Unlike predictions, inferences are open-ended. Authors do not always state key ideas or information directly in the text. They engage their audience by giving them some work of their own to do, some thinking "between the lines." Inferring helps students achieve a deeper level of thinking and gain ownership of their own understanding. We can liken the process of inferring to being a reading detective who gathers all the information and uses it to come up with the most likely explanation.

"In our work with young students, we often note that they do not generate inferences naturally and spontaneously. They can usually deduce information from one segment of the text, but they fail to integrate it with implied information in other parts of the story or in storybook illustrations.... Readers can improve their abilities to infer information when teachers model how to reason, make assumptions, and come to conclusions."

(Richards & Anderson, p. 291, 2003)

Harvey and Goudvis (2007) define inferring as "merging background knowledge with clues in the text to come up with an idea that is not explicitly stated by the author. Reasonable inferences need to be tied to the text" (p. 131). Students need to be able to draw upon multiple sources of information to infer a "reasonable" conclusion. By "reasonable," we mean that they justify their thinking with examples from the text and related personal experiences or connections. In the second inferring lesson, we step students through figuring it out by identifying the clues "in the text" and "in the head." Inferring is often taught in combination with visualizing, as creating a picture in your mind requires that you go beyond the concrete to an image of your own creation. In fact, multiple strategies are used in integration to make an inference. We need to be able make connections (schema), generate questions, predict outcomes, and visualize (Miller, 2002). McGregor (2007) describes this equation as "a dose of schema and a piece of solid evidence" (page 55).

> **Clues + Connections = Inference**

Teaching Tips

There are two types of inferences, causal inferences and relational inferences. The first lesson in this section will address causal, the second lesson relational.

Causal Inferences Causal inferences are based on cause-and-effect relationships, which require readers to infer consequences from a character's actions or an event. For example, in the book *Miss Nelson Is Missing* by James Marshall (1977), the teacher pretends to be a scary witch because her students are misbehaving. In nonfiction text, we may infer information through analyzing cause-and-effect relationships. The first lesson provides a format for supporting students to make causal inferences. To support *causal* inferences:

1. Write the events and their causes on index cards or sentence strips before the session begins. (Alternatively, stop and record the events and causes at stopping points in the reading.)

2. At planned stopping points, display and review the appropriate event card.

3. Ask students to identify the corresponding causal inference(s). Place alongside the event.

4. Conclude by rereading the cards and leading a discussion of how these supported an understanding of the "big idea."

5. As you progress, provide only the events for the "What happened?" or "Then" column and have students generate the "Why Did It Happen?" or "When"— the causes behind each one at the corresponding points in the reading. This supports the development of reasoning skills essential to inferring. For example:

What Happened? (Then)	Why Did It Happen? (When)
Wombat chewed a hole in the door	The people did not give him carrots

Relational Inferences Relational inferences require readers to integrate multiple sources of information across the text and identify the author's message or theme (the big idea). When reading narrative text, we ask students to examine the character as a source of information and to infer their personality traits and emotions by noting the dialogue, action and description the author uses to depict them. The way the author describes *how* characters do or say something is key in making inferences, so we attend to how the author shows rather than tells us *why* something is happening. Themes in literature are seldom explicitly stated in the text; that would take away interaction between author and audience.

This level of inference is more challenging for young readers because it requires sustained attention to clues in the text. In the second lesson, we support students in making relational inferences by integrating multiple sources of information. To scaffold relational inferences:

1. State the main idea or theme. Have students share questions that were left unanswered by the author, e.g., Why did …?

2. Ask students to locate and record the clues in this part of the reading, or throughout the book. Students may role-play being a detective, using a magnifying glass and wearing plastic glasses or a mask, described under Tools for Interactive Learning on page 34, as they "seek and find" clues in the text. Record these on a chart (at left). This helps students hold on to this information and cumulatively integrate the clues as they read further.

3. Prompt for student inferences based on the clues they have found and record these in a statement like the one in the chart at left.

Student Profiles

Inferring is complex and requires higher-level thinking skills. This is typically where struggling and on-grade-level readers alike hit a plateau in their comprehension growth. They respond with literal answers to questions on assessments that require inferential thinking. These are the students who say they cannot "find" the answer to the question. When students do not get it, also consider text-based factors that may present roadblocks to strategy application. Check that they are familiar with the topic or theme, vocabulary, and sentence and text structures.

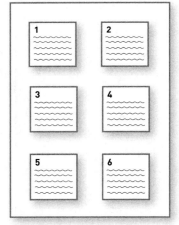

Storyboards Support Both Inferences and Retelling

Illustrations and photographs are often an excellent resource for scaffolding students who struggle making inferences. If you are concerned about the transfer of picture-based inferences to "real reading," have students dictate or write captions and dialogue on sticky notes and place them in the text, numbering each one in sequence. This supports ongoing inferential thinking during reading and the sticky notes form the basis for an oral or written retelling. I have students transfer their sticky notes to the spaces in a storyboard grid (a sheet of paper divided into four to 12 frames) and use this to write a retelling, including dialogue, captions, and other text features used in the text. Both fiction and nonfiction text can be used for this activity.

Reading Materials to Support Inferring

Students need highly supportive text to practice inferring. Limitations of emergent reading materials have always been a challenge when it comes to teaching higher-level thinking. Tales of "the fat cat on the mat," for example, do not always lend themselves to inferring. When students are working with emergent-level text and decodable text, I use the illustrations or photos as a rich source for inferences. For example, examining the expression on a character's face and the way the setting is depicted helps readers infer the mood the author/illustrator is trying to create to convey information. Making text-to-self connections will be an important part of scaffolding the inferences young students make with the text (see I Can Connect lesson, page 103), so familiar topics, themes, and characters that invite connections are also part of our criteria.

Mysteries like the Young Cam Jansen series by David Adler encourage students to make inferential statements, often beginning with "Maybe ..." or "It could be that ...." When you need to connect this strategy to the real world or something students are familiar with, you can always refer to the television series and movie *Scooby Doo* as an introduction to the strategy (McGregor, 2007). I scaffold this strategy with the use of comic strips and graphic novels that rely on carrying the message through illustration. The Owly series by Andy Runton is almost wordless and supports emergent readers, while other titles, such as Raymond Briggs's humorous tale *Ug: Boy Genius of the Stone Age* (2001) are more challenging and contain a range of text features. Those who enjoy mysteries will find graphic versions of these as well, including the Nancy Drew graphic novels by Stefan Petrucha and Sho Murase.

Student Difficulty With Inferring	Teaching Response/Next Steps

Student
 	
 Is unable to make inferences
	Teacher
	
	 • Provides concrete examples to demonstrate the strategy, such as a type of shoe/boot or hat that reflects an occupation: *Who might wear this hat? How do you know?*
	
	 • Uses examples from familiar stories, such as "Goldilocks and the Three Bears: *There were three bowls of porridge, three beds, so how many lived in the house? How did Papa Bear know that someone had been in their house while they were away?*
	
	 • Selects a supportive book that has:
	     * a familiar character, so students can use what they know about this character to infer how the storyline may unfold
	     * a familiar theme or experience that the student can make connections to
	     * a familiar topic
	     * a familiar text structure
	
	 • Has the student quickly sketch the clues (+) and what they think is happening (=) in a + __ + __ = formula for an inference, describe their drawing, and provide a caption or speech bubble

Does not make logical inferences based on text clues and background knowledge	• Points out sources of information in illustrations: *What is in the picture to help you?* • Draws attention to what the student already knows about the character, setting, events, theme, or topic: *You know about ___. How is this like ___?* • Takes specific examples from the text, such as dialogue, action, or description, and reads to student, prompting them to think about what this reminds them of (connections): *What did they do and say? Why? What might they be thinking when ___? What would you do if that happened to you? Why?*
Gives a text-based answer to a question that requires reading between the lines	Supports visualization with picture cues for the five senses: *As you read this part, think about what you can see, hear, feel, smell, and taste. Imagine a picture in your mind. Tell me what you see.* (See further suggestions for inferential thinking in the chart with the I Can Wonder: Inferential and Evaluative Questions lesson page 129)

Riddle books, where getting the joke requires making an inference, are also a useful source for student practice and illustrate the relevance of this strategy in our lives. Poetry that requires visualization and interpretation is also an appropriate context for practicing the strategy of inferring. Finally, we don't always have to read the 16- or 36-page book; short texts—and lots of them—provide meaningful practice for this and all comprehension strategies.

Remember, when the student reading goal is developing comprehension—not decoding—the guiding principle is to select text that every student in the group can read at their independent level (95% +). Easy text is a good thing when practicing this strategy! If you need to read the text with them first to make it accessible—that is okay, too. I do teach word solving (see Chapter 4), but not in combination with a comprehension strategy that requires higher-level thinking, especially when it is challenging for so many of our students (see Chapter 2 for more detail on selecting text for the lessons).

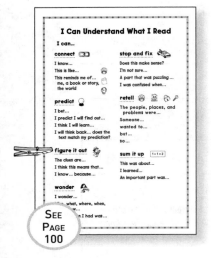

SEE PAGE 100

LESSON: I CAN FIGURE IT OUT: MAKING CAUSAL INFERENCES

Preparation

- Copy the reproducible I Can Understand What I Read Chart (page 100) onto cardstock.
- Copy the reproducible I Can Figure It Out Bookmark (page 152) onto cardstock. Make one for every student.
- Copy of the Comprehension Prompt Card (page 98).
- Have large paper clip or clothespin on hand.
- Write three to four events and their causes from the text on index cards or sentence strips. Prepare two category headings on separate cards: "What Happened?" or "Then" and "Why Did It Happen?" or "When."
- Optional Match-Up Activity: blank index cards.

Tell Me

Display the strategy chart and place a paper clip next to "I Can Figure It Out." Introduce the inferring strategy using the language on the strategy chart and bookmark:

Authors don't always use words to tell us why something happens, so we can use the clues to figure it out. Just like a detective, we look for clues in the words and in the pictures. There is always a reason why something happens. We think about what we know and what makes sense to figure it out.

Show Me

Read up to the first event and cause (inference) you recorded on the index cards.

Display and review the event card. Place it under the "What Happened" category heading. Select the corresponding causal inference(s). Place alongside the event under the heading "Why Did It Happen?" Reread the event and cause cards. Discuss how you used the clues in the text to support your inference. Demonstrate the use of clues to figure it out and pinch the corresponding statement on the bookmark, such as "I can use the clues in the words" or "I can use the clues in the pictures." Use a think- aloud to demonstrate how you arrived at the cause. For example:

What Happened?	Why Did It Happen?
Wombat chewed a hole in the door	*The people did not give him carrots*

Text: *Diary of a Wombat* by Jackie French (2002)

The author, Jackie French, doesn't say why Wombat chewed a hole in the door. I will search for clues in the words the author used to tell the story. I know that Wombat likes carrots, because he said, "The carrot was delicious." I also read that he "demanded more carrots" but there was "no response." I can use clues in the pictures. When I look at this picture, I see he has a sad look on his face, so I am figuring out that this means he is not happy that they have not given him any more carrots. On the next page, I see Wombat after chewing a hole in the door. He is looking hopeful. I think that Wombat chewed the hole to get the people's attention, and more carrots. And look—it worked!

Ask students to give you feedback on what they observed and their own thinking about what happened in the story. Are there any clues that you missed? Repeat with a second example.

How did I figure that out? What clues did I use? Did I miss something? What connections are you making to what has happened so far? Do you see a picture in your mind of why this happened? Describe your picture.

SEE PAGE 152

Guide Me

Students read to the next stopping point in the text. Students are to look for clues that will tell them the reasons why the characters act the way they do, why events occurred.

○ **Group Share**

Ask students to retell the events up to this point. Display (or write) the corresponding event card and place under the "What Happened?" (Then) category. Prompt students to think of reasons why this happened. Refer to the strategy chart and/or bookmark statements and guide them to look for clues in the words, in the pictures, and in what they already know.

Think about the clues in the book and what you know that will help you figure it out.

As a reader, what did you notice in the book that helped you to figure it out?

On page ___ the author says ___. What does that tell you? What does the author mean? How do you know?

Does this remind you of someone or something you know?

What did the character do and say? This caused something to happen. What was it?

Discuss and record their responses on cards and place under the "Why Did It Happen?" (When) category heading. You can use cards (or record the information at each stopping point on a two-column chart like the one below). Conclude by rereading the cards and leading a discussion of how these supported an understanding of the "big idea."

Coach Me

Ask students to read to the next stopping point and see if they can find clues to the main event.

Let's read to ___. Use what's in the book and what you know to figure out why these events happened.

Prompt for strategy use and probe the reasoning behind the inferences they make.

Why do think ___? What in the story makes you think that? How do you know? What are the clues?

○ **Monitor for Strategy Use**
  * Are students able to make and support inferences?
  * Do they notice the clues in the text?
  * Are their inferences reasonable?
  * Can they create a picture or movie in their mind?

○ **Partner Think-Pinch-Share**

Have students share their thinking with a partner. Invite partners to share an example from their discussion with the rest of the group. Add these to the chart.

Use your bookmark to talk about how you figured out something in the story.

Comprehension in Action: *Diary of a Wombat* by Jackie French (2002)

What Happened? (Then)	Why Did It Happen? (When)
Wombat bashed up the garbage bin.	He wanted to get more carrots.
The people did not give him rolled oats when he wanted them for dinner. He was amazed that humans were so dumb.	Wombats can't talk. The people didn't know what he wanted.
He chewed up the people's boots, flower pots, and garden chair.	He wanted to get their attention so they would give him something different.
Wombat called the humans his "pets."	He has trained them to do what he wants.
Wombat dug a hole under their house to live in.	He wouldn't have to go far to get his food. He likes being near them.

○ **Match-Up Game: Events and Causes (Optional Activity)**
As a review, the statements on the chart can be written on index cards, shuffled, and then displayed for students to match each event with the cause.

○ **Restate the Teaching Point**
Today we read like a detective. We used the clues in the book and what we know to figure out what happened, and why it happened. Now we know why Wombat did all those naughty things and why the people acted the way they did.

Reading-Writing Connection

Reading Response Journal

The following writing in response to reading activities can be completed in students' journals.

- **Two-Column Chart:** Have students record their own chart based on the model you constructed during the lesson.

- **Connections:** Students can describe how they figured out the cause of the events by using experiences and prior knowledge—what they already know about characters, events, and facts similar to these.

Practice at the Comprehension Center

The following activities from *Differentiated Literacy Centers* (Southall, 2007) support inferring:

- I See, I Wonder
- Who or What Am I?
- Character Close Up
- Tic Tac Question #2 and #3

LESSON: I CAN FIGURE IT OUT: MAKING RELATIONAL INFERENCES

Preparation

- Copy the reproducible I Can Understand What I Read Chart (page 100) onto cardstock.
- Copy the reproducible I Can Figure It Out Bookmark (page 152) onto cardstock. Make one for every student.
- Copy of the Comprehension Prompt Card (page 98).

- Have large paper clip or clothespin on hand.
- Optional: Have three or four sticky notes for each student.
- Optional: Index cards labeled "I Figured Out," "Book Clues," and "My Clues"; sorting mat divided into three columns; blank index cards

Tell Me

Display the strategy chart and place a paper clip next to "I Can Figure It Out." Introduce the inferring strategy using the language on the strategy chart and bookmark.

Authors don't always tell us why or how something happens in their story, but they always give us clues to help us to figure it out. So, just like a detective, we look for clues in the words and in the pictures. We also think about what we know that will help us figure it out.

Show Me

After introducing the book, read a short section of text. Recap what you have read and share a question you have that is not answered in the book. Demonstrate the use of clues to figure it out and pinch the corresponding statement on the bookmark, such as "I can use the clues in the words" or "I can use the clues in the pictures."

When we read we ask ourselves, how does this all fit together to make sense?
I am thinking about what I know so far. I know that _____, but the author doesn't say how/why_____.
I wonder _____? How will I figure it out? I can figure it out using what I know and what is in the text.
I will search for clues in the words and pictures. Here it says that _____. I know something about _____ because we read another story where _____, so I am figuring out that this means _____.

Write clues (book clues, my clues) and inferences (I figured out) on separate index cards if you are going to sort them by category in the activity below.

Repeat with a second and third example, using different sources for clues.

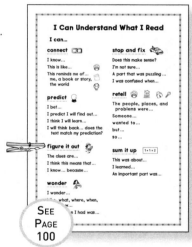

I will look at the pictures and see if they help me. I can see _____ and this tells me that _____.
If I put this together I can make a picture in my mind of what is happening. I see _____. I think _____. The author doesn't tell us much about _____. I am questioning how _____. I will read and use the clues to figure it out.

Recap the think-aloud.

I used the clues to figure out that _____.

Ask students to give you feedback on what they observed and their own thinking about what happened in the story. Are there any clues that you missed? Which clues do they think were the most important? Which ones give a hint or tells us the big idea or theme or author's point of view?

How did I figure that out? What clues did I use? Were these clues in the book or something I already knew?

Record student input on index cards. Place the clues under the correct category heading as you identify what type of clue it is.

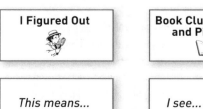

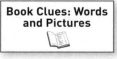

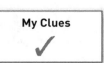

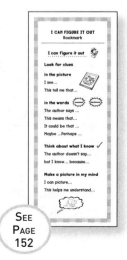

SEE PAGE 100

SEE PAGE 152

Did I miss something? Which one do you think is going to be important for us to know to understand the story? What connections are you making to what has happened so far?

Guide Me

Provide a purpose as students read to the next stopping point in the text. Present questions or have students generate a detective question. Students are to generate a detective question that requires the group to use the clues to figure out the answer. You may have them mark the places where they found clues to a question with sticky notes.

What question would you like to ask that is not answered in the book?
Think about the clues in the book and in your head that will help you figure out the answer.
Does this remind you of someone or something you know?
Make a picture in your mind of what it would look like.

○ **Group Share**

Begin by having students retell or summarize what they have just read. Invite students to share their questions. You may have them turn and quickly share one question with a partner before sharing with the group. Record their unanswered questions on the chart (see below) under "It Doesn't Tell Us."

Read each of the questions and ask students to think what might be a possible answer. Explain that there is no "right" answer. Write their inferences under "But We Figured It Out."

Ask students to locate the places in the text they marked with sticky notes and share the clues they found to answer the question. Probe for the reasoning behind student inferences and record these under "Because." If there is more than one answer under "We Figured Out," read through the reasons and come to a consensus on the most likely answer; and a star next to it. Prompt students for their inferences:

What do we know so far? Are you picturing what has happened in the story? Can you see _____?
What does it look like? What did you wonder about when you were reading?
As a reader, what did you notice in the book [picture, words] that helped you to figure it out?
How does knowing [events and information in retelling] help you figure it out?
How are you connecting to this? Did _____ remind you of something or someone you know?
We learn about characters by what they say and do. Notice the expression on _____'s face.
What do you think _____ might be thinking?
How do you think the character felt when _____? Why? What were the clues?
On page ___ the author says _____. What does that tell you? What does the author mean? How do you know?
The author didn't tell us _____, but we figured out/think _____ because _____.

Record questions, clues, and inferences cumulatively in a three-column chart.

Comprehension in Action: *Yo! Yes?* by Chris Raschka (1993)

It Doesn't Tell Us	But We Figured Out	Because
Why does the [second] boy talk so quietly?	He is afraid to play with the other boy. He is lonely.	He has his hands behind his back. He says "Who? Me? No fun. No friends."
What happens to the boys? What will they do next?	They will be good friends. The second boy won't be lonely anymore.	The boy is smiling. He says, "Yes!" in a big voice. They say "Yow!" And jump into the air and do a "high five."

To focus on a single inference that is central to understanding, use the alternative format at right. Record the most common or "important" unanswered question that students share using the format at right. List the clues they located and then the inference they made based on these in a statement.

○ Detective Game Activity (Optional)
Use the index cards labeled Book Clues and My Clues/I Know as category headings. On blank index cards record student inferences and the clue(s) they used. Read each inference aloud to the group and have students identify if the clues they used were based on information the author provided in the book or what they already knew, and place the card under the appropriate heading.

Inferences based on clues:

Our Question:
_____

Clues:

1. _____

2. _____

We think
_____

because
_____

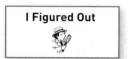

I Figured Out

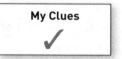

Book Clues: Words and Pictures

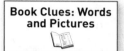

My Clues ✓

Coach Me

Ask students to read to the next stopping point and see if they can find any more clues to support an answer (inference) to a question on the chart. Alternatively, they can generate a new question and search for clues.

Let's read to _____. Use what you know in the book and your connections to figure out the answer to a question you have about the story.

Prompt for strategy use and probe the reasoning behind the inferences they make.

What in the story makes you think that? How do you know? Why do think _____? Did you connect this to something that you know about _____?

How do you know _____? What are the clues?

What makes you think _____?

○ Monitor for Strategy Use
  * Is the student able to make (and support) inferences?
  * Do they notice the clues in the text?
  * Do they integrate clues to make an inference?
  * Are their inferences "reasonable"?
  * Do they make connections to the characters, events, or information?
  * Can they create a picture or movie in their mind?

○ Partner Think-Pinch-Share
Have students share their thinking with a partner. Invite partners to share an example from their discussion with the rest of the group. Add these to the chart.

Use your bookmark to talk about how you figured out something in the story.

○ Restate the Teaching Point

Sometimes we have to read like a detective and use the clues in our head to figure something out that we don't know.

We used the clues the author gave us in the book and put it together with what we know about _____ to figure out the answers to our questions.

Reading-Writing Connection

Extend the learning with the following responses:

Fiction: Students can make a character web listing traits of the protagonist. Support this by restating the actions and dialogue associated with the character and asking students to think of a word that would describe someone who does or says that.

Nonfiction: To respond to an informational text, have students describe how the information might be used by a scientist (or other related occupation) or why the author wrote about this topic.

Visualization: Students can draw a thinking bubble. Inside the bubble they can sketch the events or information as they "see" them.

Practice at the Comprehension Center

The following activities from *Differentiated Literacy Centers* (Southall, 2007) support inferring:
- I See, I Wonder
- Who or What Am I?
- What Kinds of Questions Do They Ask?
- Character Close Up
- Tic Tac Question #2 and #3
- Partner Quiz Cards

Generating and Answering Questions

Questioning is where we often spend the most time in comprehension instruction, particularly on the questions that require higher-level thinking. When we see readers skim the surface of the text without generating questions, we know their understanding will be negatively impacted. However, the purpose of teaching questioning reaches far beyond an effort to engage the reader; student questions are the raw material we need to build upon in order for students to infer, clarify (self-monitor for meaning), and retell. When reading expository text, students can easily become overwhelmed with factual information. Questioning provides a way for them to self-check their understanding as they read and then determine what is important to remember.

Teaching Tips

We incorporate questioning into the text activities before, during, and after reading so our readers will be able to apply higher-order processes when the text demands it. The first type of question we teach is the open-ended "I wonder" question, where no specific question words are required and where there is no right answer. This is a "safe" type of question for young readers who may have already developed an awareness of their own lack of success on assessment questions. Open-ended questions are appropriate throughout our comprehension lessons; however, for students to continue to develop as readers and to be able to understand and respond to assessment questions successfully, we introduce sentence starters that familiarize them with the language and thinking behind specific types of questions.

The I Can Wonder bookmarks on page 153 provide supportive picture cues and sentence starters for questions and personal responses to the reading. In the first lesson, the bookmark for literal level, or "*seek and find*," questioning focuses on the story structure in fiction or the facts in informational text. Each student is accountable for supporting their answers with evidence in the text, to seek and find the facts or quote. The second bookmark, at the "*think and feel*" level, targets higher-level questions, with readers sharing their thoughts, feelings, and opinions about what they have just read. This requires inferential and evaluative thinking.

Body or kinesthetic cues are also incorporated in the language of the lesson and bookmarks (see chart below) to represent the thinking processes (Willner, 2003). In both lessons, students retell, reflect upon, and then question the text. This provides a three-step scaffold for students who might not otherwise be successful in generating and answering questions.

As students progress from the literal to the inferential and evaluative tasks, you can copy the two bookmarks onto both sides of the cardstock so that students can then have the flexibility to select the response that best fits their thinking.

Question Types

Question Type	Character Cues	Body Part Cues	Key Words
Literal (reading the lines) Questions that can be answered by identifying or touching information in the book	Reporter or game show host	Hand	Who, what, where, when, how
Inferential Questions you can figure out by using the clues in the book and what you already know	Detective	Head	How do you know? Why did ___? Figure it out. The author doesn't say, but I know because ___.
Evaluative Questions that ask the reader to form an opinion or make a decision about the actions, ideas, or information in the text	Me	Heart	What do you think? How do you feel about ___? What is your opinion of ___? Should ___? I believe ___. I feel that ___.

(Based on the work of Raphael et al., 2006; Boyles, 2004)

Student Profiles

When a student struggles to generate or answer a text-based question, first we need to determine whether the issue is word recognition or lack of familiarity with the sentence/text structure, writing style, vocabulary, or concepts. All of these can interfere with processing the text sufficiently to come up with a question or to respond to one. Students who struggle with questioning an informational text may rely on background knowledge and ignore new information.

Some students demonstrate avoidance tactics and "shoot from the hip" with answers that require the least thought and time to provide. This may be because they associate questioning with testing and pass/fail answers. Open-ended questions that invite personal responses, such as observations (*I wonder why*) and opinions (*I think … What do you think?*) are an important place to begin, as these are not "teacher questions." My students enjoy asking *other* students in the group questions when this is presented in a role-play format: Each student in turn can be the quiz show host, passing the plastic microphone around the table.

From open-ended questions we progress to providing specific types of question starters that require literal, inferential, or evaluative responses (see bookmarks on page 153).

Student Difficulty With Questioning	Teaching Response/Next Steps
GENERATING QUESTIONS **Student** Struggles to generate questions about the text	**Teacher** ● Incorporates student "I Wonder" questions within literature study, social studies, and science activities and records and displays student questions on a class bulletin board; encourages individual research for answers ● Invites open-ended questions based on personal connections before reading so that there is not an emphasis on one "right" type of question (and answer) ● Focuses students' attention on what they notice in the illustrations: *What do you wonder about what you see?* ● Provides picture cues and question starters (see bookmarks on page 153) ● Includes a game show format during which a toy microphone is passed around the table and each student role-plays being a game show host by asking the group a question ● Incorporates board games in which students use picture-cued story element cards as the basis for generating questions (see I Can Retell lesson cards, page 155)
Asks questions that are not logical or are unrelated to actual events or information; questions focus on details rather than main ideas or important information	● Supports memory of important ideas and events by pausing after short sections of text for students to retell and question ● Provides multiple think-aloud demonstrations and encourages building upon the responses of others: *Piggybacking off* [student's response], *I wonder* _____
Difficulty generating inferential and evaluative questions	● Incorporates kinesthetic questioning to make the concept concrete by using the "Body Parts" approach—hand, head, and heart (see chart on page 123)
ANSWERING QUESTIONS **Student** Does not volunteer answers to teacher questions	**Teacher** Ensures responding to teacher questions is a safe activity: ● Allows at least an eight-second wait time before inviting a response and may cue by counting down with fingers one at a time ● When one student volunteers an answer, teacher asks a second student to locate/read the part that supports the first student's answer so that the first student is not put on the spot to read aloud in front of peers; this is especially important for disfluent readers and students with low self-esteem as a reader ● Includes partner questioning before sharing with the group ● Provides positive feedback to all responses ● Invites responses from all students without spotlighting individuals
Is unable to answer the question	● Rephrases the question; allows wait time (see above) ● Retells the part of the text related to the question ● Prompts for connections to the information or event ● Changes the question into an answer statement to model an appropriate response for literal questions; thinks aloud for inferential and evaluative questions

Student Difficulty With Questioning	Teaching Response/Next Steps
Retells accurately and responds to literal questions with success, but is unsuccessful with questions requiring higher-level thinking; provides text-based literal answers to inferential questions and may respond to probing by the teacher with comments such as *The book said that _____, That wasn't in the book*; or *It didn't tell us about that*	• Models and provides supported practice answering questions that require integrating information and personal reflection • Demonstrates the difference between literal, inferential, and evaluative questions with examples and picture or body part cues; reaffirms personal responses are appropriate with inferential and evaluative questions • Focuses on making connections to the theme or topic in the prereading activities; points out how these are related to students' lives and validates their ideas • Highlights the "markers" or key words in the questions on the group chart that indicate which type it is (for student- and teacher-generated questions) • Supports students in discriminating between literal and inferential or evaluative questions with a sorting activity in which the group identifies the questions that require them to *seek and find* (literal) or *think and feel* (inferential and evaluative); records these and has students place the cards under the appropriate categories • Provides time for journal writing and partner dialogue journals during which partners (or teacher and student) exchange journals to ask and respond to each other's "I Wonder" statements • Incorporates regular sharing of book reviews in which students give their evaluation or opinion of the book in "sharing circle" format (see Scheduling in Chapter 3)
Responds to higher-level questions with vague and/or ambiguous answers full of general statements and weak descriptors; is unable to explain what they mean; says *I don't know*	• Focuses on story or text structure and cause-and-effect relationships, such as chain (sequence) of events, two-column "This Happened/Because" formats, story maps, story structure sorts (see I Can Retell lesson, page 141), character analysis to identify the theme or main idea in fiction, and summarizing activities with nonfiction to determine important information (see I Can Sum It Up lesson, page 145) • Includes compare-and-contrast activities using Venn diagrams or two-column charts to clarify students' thinking • Highlights key words in the text such as *before, after*, and *because* that indicate a relationship between events and ideas (see inferring lesson, page 129) • Integrates vocabulary development in the prereading activities so students are able to understand and use these words or concepts they represent to express their thinking (See Story Structure Sort in I Can Retell lesson, page 142)
Provides brief responses that lack sufficient detail to be "correct" answers; for example, when asked to describe how a character might be feeling at this moment in the story, responds *bad* and when asked to expand says *very bad* or *That's all I can think of*	• [see vocabulary development above] • Provides guided practice on cumulatively integrating multiple sources of information across the text by breaking text into short sections and analyzing the clues available to the reader so far. *What do we know so far? How does this help us figure out ...?* • Suggests students sketch a visual representation of their understanding in their response journal before reading, then add more details to represent new information, during and after reading • Supports understanding through concept maps
Neglects the information in the text	• Provides categorizing information activities such as sorting facts under subheadings or doing a story structure sort (see I Can Retell lesson) • Incorporates visualization activities (see "I can make a picture in my mind" on the Stop and Fix Bookmark, page 154) • Provides vocabulary from the text before reading so that students use the words to generate their prediction; after reading they compare their predictions to the actual events or information in the text • Asks "How do you know?" and prompts students to locate and read the evidence in the text and/or give reasons for their thinking
May appear to be anxious during questioning activities and have a fear of being *wrong*, asking *Did I get it right*?	• See under the first category for "Generating Questions"

Reading Materials to Support Questioning

To encourage student participation, we look for reading materials that are likely to evoke questions. For narrative, a clear story structure supports literal questioning, the "seek and find" strategy in the first lesson. We also integrate nonfiction content reading about our social studies and science topics, where questioning will support recall of important information. By pausing and inviting student questions, we give them a chance to note what is familiar and what is new and to ask "teacher questions" of the group.

Only certain books have the necessary content for generating inferential and evaluative questions in the second lesson, the "think and feel" question types. The types of reading materials suggested for making inferences with the I Can Figure It Out lesson on page 116 are those that also support both generating and answering inferential questions. For evaluative questions, select reading materials that have a theme students can relate to and express opinions about, such as friendship, loyalty, bullying, and overcoming challenges, where students are likely to evaluate the character's actions through the connections they make to them. Nonfiction text that describes larger issues in the world around them, particularly those written in a persuasive style, will engage the critical thinking skills that support evaluative questions. I often use nonfiction articles in children's magazines as a source for generating these types of questions, as they reflect the current "hot topics" of interest to our students. For example, magazines such as *National Geographic Explorer* (available in two reading levels on the same topic), *Time for Kids*, and *Scholastic News* are popular choices.

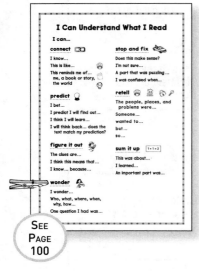

SEE PAGE 100

LESSON: I CAN WONDER: GENERATING AND ANSWERING LITERAL QUESTIONS

Preparation

- Copy the reproducible I Can Understand What I Read Chart (page 100) onto cardstock.
- Copy the reproducible I Can Wonder Bookmark (page 153) onto cardstock. Make one for every student.
- Copy of the Comprehension Prompt Card (page 98).
- Have large paper clip or clothespin on hand.
- Have on hand two to four sticky notes of two different colors for each student, or reusable page markers or flags (see Integrating Multiple Strategies—I Can Code My Thinking lesson page 149)

Tell Me

Point to the icon for "I Can Wonder" on the I Can Understand What I Read Strategy Chart. You may place a paper clip or clothespin alongside the icon for the reporter as you introduce "seek and find" questions.

Readers ask questions about what they are reading. We read to find out the answers to our questions. Often we ask about something we don't know yet. Today we are going to learn about questions that you can seek and find in the book. You can touch the answer on the page with your hand. These are questions that tell us who this is about, what it is about, where and when something happened.

Show Me

Pose focusing questions before reading. Point to the question words on the bookmark.
What can you tell me about [topic or theme]?

Why do you think the author wrote this book? Why might we want to read this book?

What do you want to find out about? [Record answers on chart paper.]

Demonstrate the seek-and-find strategy:

Looking at the title and cover of the book, I wonder _____.

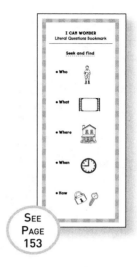

SEE PAGE 153

Invite student questions before reading. List these on your whiteboard or on index cards with student initials beside each one (optional).

What are you wondering? Let's read and find out if any of our questions will be answered.

Model asking a main idea question or a question about a story element or important fact on the topic:

I am going to read the first part of the book and see if I can find the answer to _____.

After reading the part about _____, I wonder, _____?

Guide Me

Students read to the first stopping point.

Read to page ___. Put a sticky note where you have an "I wonder" question.

○ **Group Share**

Ask students to retell what they have just read.

If it is fiction, ask questions about the characters, setting, problem, and sequence of events or plot.

If it is nonfiction, pose questions about important information that represents the main purpose of the text. Refer to information from any illustrations or graphics as well as the text to support integration of information. Record the facts or events under the first heading on the chart "We Read."

[Ask the first student] *What have we learned so far?* [Ask the second student] *Show me in the book where it says that. This part was about _____.*

Have students use the retelling to generate a question. Ask them to quickly "turn and share" a question they have about this part of the reading with a partner.

Students use the information in the first column together with the question starters on the bookmark to compose a question for the group, in a game show format. They may pass around a toy microphone or wear the mask of the questioner to "get into the role" of the game show host.

Ask the rest of the group a quiz question that can be answered in the book. Use the question words on the bookmark to help you.

Record these under "Seek and Find Questions" on the chart. Support with prompts and model as necessary.

Prompts:

I have a [where] *question: _____?*

Who are _____? What does _____ mean? What did _____? How many _____?

What kind of _____? Where did _____? How many _____? What happened before/ after to _____? How do you _____? What examples can you find?

Note: "How" questions can be literal when they refer to how many or how much or how something occurs. Students do not have to use the bookmark starters if this constrains their questioning.

Read to the next stopping point and repeat the process, adding to the group chart.

Comprehension in Action: *Mountain Gorillas* by Julie Connal (1995)

📖 We Read	☞ Seek and Find Questions
Zaire is in Africa.	Where is Zaire?
Gorillas build a nest from branches and foliage to sleep in at night.	How do mountain gorillas sleep at night?
Park rangers guard the gorillas in the parks.	Who protects the gorillas?

Coach Me

Students read the selected passage, as you monitor and provide feedback. Students generate a question(s) from the reading and mark the places where a question occurred to them and where the question is answered, using two colors of sticky notes or flags.

As you are reading, think about the questions that come into your mind. Mark the places you have a question with the [yellow] sticky notes. Seek and find the answers to your question. Place a [green] sticky where you find the answer.

Prompt students to use evidence from the text to support their answers:

What did you wonder about _____?

Show me the part that supports your answer.

○ **Monitor for Strategy Use**
   ∗ Are students able to generate questions that are related to the main idea or only asking detail questions? Are they logical questions?
   ∗ Do they locate evidence in the text and use this to answer the question?
   ∗ Can they integrate information in more than one place in the text?

○ **Partner Think-Pinch-Share**
   Each student presents their question to their partner. Partners need to both answer the question and prove it by locating the evidence that supports it in the book. If they are unable to find the evidence, then their partner supports them by pointing to this in their book (they have marked the answer in the book with a sticky note). Then students switch roles.

   Read page(s) ___. Think of a question you have about what the author just shared.
   Use your bookmark to help you think of a question.
   Pinch the question word (so your partner knows the type of question it is).
   Ask your partner a question and to show you the evidence in the book that proves her answer.

   Ask partners to share a question they had with the rest of the group. Add these to the chart and invite sharing of possible answers.

○ **Restate the Teaching Point**
   Readers ask themselves questions as they read. We shared questions that could be answered in the book and this helped us to remember important information.

Reading-Writing Connection

Students record their opinions and other personal responses to the reading. Provide the prompts on the bookmark along with others that are appropriate to the text:

Practice at the Comprehension Center

The following activities from *Differentiated Literacy Centers* (Southall, 2007) support:

- I Wonder
- Who or What Am I?
- I See, I Wonder
- Tic Tac Question #1, #2
- Picture Question Cards

SEE PAGE 153

LESSON: I CAN WONDER: INFERENTIAL AND EVALUATIVE QUESTIONS

Preparation

- Copy the reproducible I Can Understand What I Read Strategy Chart (page 100) onto cardstock.
- Copy the reproducible I Can Wonder Bookmark (page 153) onto cardstock. Make one for every student.
- Copy of the Comprehension Prompt Card page (page 98).
- Have large paper clip or clothespin on hand.
- Have two to four sticky notes or reusable sticky flags for each student.
- Optional: Create category cards labeled Head and Heart; provide blank index cards.

Tell Me

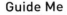

Point to the icon for I Wonder on the I Can Understand What I Read Strategy Chart. Put a paper clip or clothespin next to the icon for the "What I think and feel" questions.

> *Using your head and your heart is part of being a reader. Authors can write stories and information that make us laugh, cry, even feel angry. They know that if we think about it and not just read the words on the page we will understand their message even more. For example, when we read about how a character behaves in a story or something that happened, we usually have opinions about it. Remember, an opinion is how you feel about something; it does not have to be a fact.*

Show Me

Engage students' thinking on the topic or theme:

> *What do we already know about [topic or theme]?*
> *Why do you think the author wrote this book? Why would we want to read this?*

Demonstrate the strategy by sharing your inferential and evaluative thinking:

> *I think _____ because on page ____ it says that _____ and _____.*

Guide Me

Students read to the first stopping point. Have them mark places in the text where something made them think more about it (connect, predict, question) or have an opinion. They can sketch a head or heart on their sticky note to indicate the type of response.

> *Read to _____. What are you thinking and feeling as you read?*
> *Place a sticky next to a part where you had a response with your head or heart.*

○ **Group Share**

Ask students to retell what they have just read. Record on the chart under the heading "We Read." Students then ask the group questions that require them to share their opinions and feelings, using the bookmark as a support. List these under "Think and Feel." Have students turn to the part in the text that is being discussed.

Prompt students to include references to the text and their life (connections) in their responses.

> *Ask the group a "think and feel" question. Use your bookmark to help you.*
> *Let's hear a thought that you are having.*
> *How do you feel about _____? What do you think about _____? What is your opinion of _____?*
> *Why do you think they said/did that? Do you think _____ should _____? Why or why not?*
> *What in the book or your life makes you feel/think that way?*

Comprehension in Action: *Hit by a Blade* by Brian Beamer (2000)

📖 We Read	🙂 ❤️ Think and Feel Questions
Jessie and Juan went on motorboat trip with their granddad. The boat hit a manatee and the propeller hurt it.	*Why didn't they look where they were going?* *I feel worried that the manatee won't be all right.* *I feel angry with the people.*
They took the manatee to a place for sick sea animals.	*How will they take the manatee to the hospital?* *I hope the manatee gets well again.*
The vet told them that the manatee would get better.	*How could we stop this from happening to other manatees?* *Should people be allowed to use motorboats where manatees live?* *What if we could have some places for the manatees where people aren't allowed to have motorboats, just sailboats?* *I think there should be speed limits for the boats so they can see the manatees better.*

Rephrase what students say. Probe for an explanation of their thinking:

> *What in the book and in your life makes you think/feel that? What does it remind you of?*

Invite students to piggyback off the responses of others to extend and clarify their thinking.

> *I hear _____ feels that _____. Let's piggyback off what _____ just said and add our own thoughts and feelings.*
> *Who would like to add to that?*

Read to the next stopping point and repeat the process, adding to the group chart.

○ **Head and Heart Question Sort (optional)**

Record student questions on index cards. Shuffle and pass out to the group. Students take turns placing them under the appropriate categories and justifying why a particular question requires a particular type of answer.

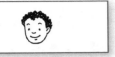
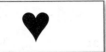

| *How could we stop manatees being hurt by motor boats?* | *Should people be allowed to use motor boats where manatees live* |

Coach Me

Students read the selected passage, as you monitor and provide feedback.

What do you think and feel about what you just read?

Where did you place a sticky with a head or heart response?

[Prompt students to explain and expand upon their responses.]

How did you feel about the part where …?

Do you agree with what the author has to say about ..?

What would you do if …? If you were going to …? If you could …?

○ **Monitor for Strategy Use**

　＊ Do they support their statements with examples from the text and their own life?

　＊ Do they synthesize information to come up with their own ideas or do they simply retell?

　＊ Are the statements related to the theme or purpose of the text?

○ **Partner Think-Pinch-Share**

　Students use their bookmarks to share a response.

　　Share a thought you had with your partner.

○ **Group Share**

　Ask partners to share a response they discussed with the rest of the group. Provide feedback and probe with "think and feel" questions that require them to extend beyond the information in the book.

　　Let's hear a thought that you shared.

　　What would have happened if …? What if ….? What might…?

　　Why would the author write this way about …? How could someone use this information?

　　What would you tell a friend about this book?

○ **Restate the Teaching Point**

　　By using your head and your heart you were able to think deeper into the author's message and gain a greater understanding of what you read.

Reading-Writing Connection

In their reading response journals students can:
- record their responses in a two-column chart in their notebook: I Think/I Feel
- chart their responses and questions under a "body parts" three-column chart
- write their thoughts and opinions and then exchange journals with a partner
- write a book review that will be shared with a group of students

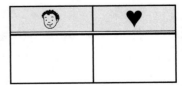

Practice at the Comprehension Center

Center activities include those from *Differentiated Literacy Centers* (Southall, 2007):

- What I Think
- Talk to the Author
- Critic's Cube
- Connection Stems
- Read, Relate, Respond

I Can Stop and Fix: Self-Monitoring and Clarifying Strategies

Clarifying is when we first identify and then resolve problems in compre-hension by using specific strategies. Clarifying or fix-up strategies are important for every student, not just struggling readers. Understanding can break down for a number of reasons, including an unfamiliar writing style or a point that is not clearly made. We may also lose track of information and how it is related to what we are currently reading over a stretch of text, such as relationships between different characters, or cause-and-effect rela-tionships. Clarifying strategies are different from questioning strategies (see I Wonder lessons) in that these are questions we ask ourselves as a reader to help our understanding of the text.

Teaching Tips

Teachers model how to stop and ask themselves self-monitoring questions as they read, such as:

- *Does this make sense to me? How does this part fit with what I just read?*
- *Am I following what is happening? Can I make a picture in my mind of what I just read?*
- *Am I getting the main idea?*
- *Do I know what this word means?*
- *How can I fix this problem so I understand what I am reading?*

When we stop to question our own understanding during reading, we can then demonstrate how to apply several fix-up strategies including the following.

- **Reread the sentence and look for key ideas.** Model how much rereading is necessary—whether it's on the same page or earlier in the text. This requires us to scan the text for the needed information. Demonstrate the different ways to reread, always keeping a specific purpose in mind, and looking for something that will answer our question/solve our problem, such as searching subheadings, illustrations, and captions.

- **Reading on.** Show how to read the next sentence or two to see if new informa-tion is provided that solves the puzzle.

- **Creating a picture in our head.** When we read fiction, we see an ongoing movie in our mind, as the camera in our head captures/interprets each scene. For nonfiction, it is more like a slide show of facts, as if we were watching the news on TV. New information keeps coming as each new slide appears. If the picture screen in our mind goes blank during reading, we stop to think about the character or topic and what the author's purpose was in writing.

- **Thinking about what we know:** our connections with this experience or topic; what this story or topic is about; the big picture and how what we've just read relates to this.

- **Breaking the word apart, looking for parts we know and saying each part.** For students who have had instruction in roots and affixes, this would include meaningful parts of the word (morphemes such as *sand* in *sandstone*). Lastly we coach students to try another word that would make sense.

● **Older students:** Looking for commas in the sentence since an explanation is often between commas; scanning the sentence or next sentence for words that tell us there is an example, e.g., *such as, for example.*

The stoplight visual is a color-coded self-monitoring tool. Students can use the color sequence of the stoplight as a barometer of their understanding, touching the color as they read that best represents their level of understanding for this part of the reading. For example, they touch green when they understand, yellow when it's getting confusing and they need to slow down to process the text more carefully and use all available clues, and red when they need to stop and use a fix-up tool. Another option is to provide students with a color wheel such as those found at paint stores, where colors are displayed in a gradient from green to red (McGregor, 2007).

Student Profiles

Some students read at a brisk pace but do not notice or pay any attention to something they don't understand. A fast pace of reading without adjusting reading speed at any point is not conducive to self-monitoring. I use the analogy of driving a car to explain why they need to monitor their reading or keep their "navigation screen turned on" (Marcell, 2007). They need to slow down (I use a colored flag made out of colored paper) for the curves in the road—such as new information, text that is dense in information, complex sentence structures, and figurative language—which is where we often have to stop and repair our understanding, just like racing car drivers pull in for a pit stop.

To ensure all students participate in the self-monitoring activities and internalize this strategy, we need to be very aware of the prompting language we use—it needs to keep students' self-esteem intact and encourage sharing of strategy use. Students who lack confidence as a reader are especially sensitive to identifying something they do not understand and may remain passive rather than share a part that was puzzling to them or seek help during reading. I never say: "Is there something you didn't know?" They do not want to be seen by their peers as not knowing something. Instead I say something like: "Is there something you found puzzling or confusing or would like to ask the author about?" Or the driving analogy: "Did your navigation screen go blank at some point and you had to turn it on again?" or "Did you need to have a pit stop and fix something along the way?"

Reading Materials to Support Self-Monitoring and Clarifying

Reading materials that are useful for practicing this strategy include those that contain a few words that students are unlikely to be familiar with and that represent useful vocabulary (i.e., not technical terms they are unlikely to encounter again). Many expository texts such as the Magic School Bus series (Joanna Cole) provide practice using text features such as sidebars and diagrams to clarify important information.

When new vocabulary poses a roadblock to understanding, students record the word on a card to share and discuss with the group.

Even the simplest fiction or nonfiction emergent text can provide practice in using context clues to gain meaning. Narrative texts with twists in the plot develop self-monitoring. For young readers, I use many of the books by Joy Cowley, which typically have a twist at the end. Literary devices such as flashbacks are another source for clarifying practice; the author provides plenty of clues—phrases such as "I remembered when" or "only yesterday"—found several times within one part of the text.

Student Difficulty With Self-Monitoring and Clarifying Strategies	Teaching Response/Next Steps
Student Does not notice when something does not make sense	**Teacher** • Provides a self-monitoring tool with visual cues, such as the bookmark and traffic light, which are a concrete reminder of clarifying strategies available to them; the traffic light visual can also be used as a color-coded indicator of their understanding that they touch as they read in order to self-monitor understanding (see Teaching Tips on previous page) • Models self-questioning, asking why and how questions throughout the reading • Poses questions for each short section of the text
Keeps on reading even when they recognize they do not understand; does not pause to self-monitor for meaning	• Provides short, easy text read with frequent stopping points; has student stop and mark with a sticky note, retell with partner, and check for understanding • Models fix-up strategies (see following lesson) • Suggests visualization activities (see Inferring) • Prompts to adjust reading speed, going slower in parts with new information, important events and marks places in the text with a sticky note to show they need to slow down and watch for/integrate new information (see Monitoring and Responding to Student Difficulty section in I Can Retell lesson, page 139)
Is unfamiliar with concept and lacks background knowledge	• Refers to supporting text features such as photos and diagrams. Explains the author's purpose for including them and how it fits with the information in the text
Is unable to see how information is related	• Uses graphic organizers, such as concept webs, cause-and-effect two-column charts
Loses track of pronouns; doesn't know who or what is being talked about	• Asks student to highlight pronouns in text (with highlighter tape), read sentences before to find point of reference and highlight it; write noun on sticky note and use this to replace the pronoun (place it in the text - they can move this sticky as they read where necessary) • Lists characters, facts, and corresponding pronouns in a two-column chart
Is able to pronounce the word and understands one meaning for the word, but it does not fit the context	• Incorporates a multiple-meaning web activity in which students are asked where they have seen and heard this word before. Responses are used to construct a mind map, where the word is written in the center and then student examples are recorded in a web around it • Presents word in context of a sentence where it represents a different meaning

LESSON: I CAN STOP AND FIX

Preparation

- Copy the reproducible I Can Understand What I Read Strategy Chart (page 100) onto cardstock.
- Copy the reproducible Stop and Fix Bookmark (page 154) onto cardstock. Make one for every student.
- Copy of the Comprehension Prompt Card (page 98).
- Have two to four sticky notes or reusable sticky flags or highlighter tape for each student.
- See Reading Materials to Support Self-Monitoring and Clarifying page 133.

Tell Me

Point to the icon for I Can Stop and Fix on the Comprehension Strategy Chart.

All readers have times when something they are reading does not make sense to them. When I am reading, I often come to a word I have never seen before—and I'm not always sure what it means. Other times I am confused about what the author is talking about; it is not clear to me. I stop reading and use one of my fix-up tools so I can understand what I am reading. Have you ever talked to yourself when you are doing something, talking through each step? Today we will talk our way through using three fix-up tools.

Show Me

Use the bookmark traffic light visual as a reference when you demonstrate the clarifying strategies.

This part I just read on page _ doesn't make sense to me/is not clear to me. I don't understand ___. Which fix-up strategy will help me?

First I will reread. [Point to first picture cue, for rereading, in traffic sign visual.] *No, that still doesn't make sense. I will try another fix-up tool, read on to the next sentence or two.* [Slide the moving piece across to show second picture cue.] *Oh, now I get it. The next sentence explains ___.*

But I don't know what this word means. This is a tricky word because ___. Let's see if one of my fix-up tools will solve the problem. [Slide to third picture cue.] *I will break the word apart and look for parts I know.*

Guide Me

Read to the first stopping point.

Provide sticky notes or red/pink highlighter tape for students to mark the text where there is a word, fact, or idea they find puzzling or confusing.

Mark the places where something doesn't make sense or is confusing. Think about the strategies you can use on your bookmark to stop and fix it. Remember, as you read, keep a picture in your head. If your navigation screen goes blank, use a fix-up strategy.

○ **Group Share**
  Have students briefly turn and share these puzzling parts with a partner. Then, each pair shares one with the group. Record these on a chart like the one below.

  Were there any words/idea/facts you found puzzling or confusing? That you had questions about? Did your navigation screen go blank at one part of the reading?

  Ask students to share with the group how they fixed the problems and record these solutions in the second column.

  What do you think the author meant when he said ___? Which fix-up strategy did you use? How did you use it? Were there any clues that helped you?

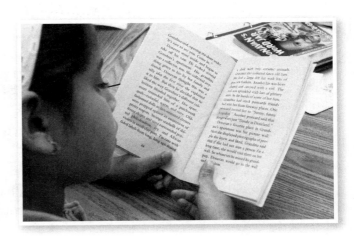

Students self-monitor their understanding by highlighting puzzling words, ideas or facts in the text during reading. The group will practice applying fix-up (clarifying) strategies to solve these roadblocks to comprehension, and repair their understanding.

Comprehension in Action: *Dogs* by Gail Gibbons, 1997

We Stopped	And Fixed
The first <u>ancestors</u> of wolves and dogs ...	Used <u>parts we know</u>: an_ est__or Put the parts together to say the word
Four of their teeth are called <u>canine</u> teeth, or fangs.	<u>Looked at picture</u> with caption "canine teeth, or fangs"
Inside the nose are about 400 million cells that help identify <u>odors</u>.	<u>Reread</u>: "Smell is a dog's sharpest sense"
It is learning to be a <u>social</u> animal.	<u>Reread</u>: "A puppy will become a good pet if it is around people"

Coach Me

Students read the next part as you monitor, prompt, and provide feedback.

- ○ **Monitor for Strategy Use**
  - ∗ *Show me a spot in the reading that was puzzling or confusing to you. Were there any parts that were messy or seemed to be mixed up?*
  - ∗ *Which fix-up tool did you use? Did it work? What else could you try? What do you know about* [the story or topic] *that could help you?*
  - ∗ *What questions did you ask* [the author] *as you were reading?*

- ○ **Partner Think-Pinch-Share**
  - *Share with your partner how you stopped and fixed something that did not make sense.*
  - Ask partners to share one of the responses they discussed with the group and add each to the chart.

- ○ **Restate the Teaching Point**
  - *We noticed that there were some tricky parts in the reading today that were not clear to us/ where we lost understanding. We stopped and used three fix-up tools so we could understand what we read.*

Reading-Writing Connection

Students:
- Draw and describe a picture they had in their mind as they read
- Record the questions they would like to ask the author
- Describe how they used a fix-up tool to clarify a part that was puzzling

Practice at the Comprehension Center

- In the Driver's Seat activity from *Differentiated Literacy Centers* (Southall, 2007)
- Students read independent level text and use the bookmark and a corresponding checklist to mark the tools they used to stop and fix something confusing in the text

Retelling and Summarizing

Retelling of a narrative text requires students to recall important events in sequence and notice causal relationships between characters and events. A summary of a narrative demands the reader synthesize the events, identify the theme, and state this in her own words, rather than regurgitating the text verbatim. An expository retelling requires students to accurately recall facts, while a summary also requires that they determine which information is important to remember and then paraphrase this to make a "main idea" statement. Main ideas may be stated in the topic sentence, or students may need to infer. Summarizing requires an understanding of what you have read; it is not just rote recall.

Teaching Tips

The first lesson focuses on retelling. When students are able to retell, they are then able to progress to the next lesson, which scaffolds the summarizing strategy. The lesson on retelling integrates story structure, predicting, and examining the meaning of story vocabulary. Students are asked to predict which vocabulary word belongs with each story element or which words they think the author will use to tell them about the people, problem, and places in the story. Students will need to check that their predictions are justified, or revise them by moving the Retelling Cards (page 156) used as props in this lesson (Richek, 2001). When the vocabulary is linked to the story elements, students have the building blocks for a retelling.

You may use the language in the lesson of People, Places, and Problems that is on the bookmark (page 155), the terms on the Retelling Cards (problem, events, solution, ending) or the question cards from the I Can Wonder: Literal Questions lesson (who, what, where, etc.), depending on what is developmentally appropriate for your students. To explain the concept of retelling, I use an example of a classroom scenario in which a student was absent and we need to fill him in with all the details of what happened on the day he was out. Some teachers use the cell phone conversation analogy, in which the speaker is describing an event to someone who is not there.

In retelling, we model and guide students to successfully do the following (in order of complexity):

1. Identify the beginning, middle, and end, e.g., What happened in the beginning/first part?
2. Describe the character and setting, e.g., Who is the main character? Where did the story take place?
3. Identify the problem and resolution.
4. Retell events and facts, e.g., What happened in the story?
5. Make inferences to link events and information, e.g., How do you know?
6. Identify what caused the actions or events and the effects that resulted, e.g., Why did _____?
7. Evaluate the actions of the characters in the story, e.g., Was this good or bad? Why?

In the second lesson on summarizing, we help students determine important information from the list of facts they recall from the reading and then use these facts to compose a summary statement. We support students to provide a summary that:

- Is accurate

"Teachers and students often confuse retelling with summaries. Retellings are oral or written postreading recalls during which children relate what they remember from reading or listening to a particular text. Conversely, a summary represents a short, to-the-point distillation of the main ideas in the text. When students retell, they attempt to recall as much of the information in the text as possible, not just the main points. Retellings are an important precursor to helping students develop summarization skills, both oral and written. Students who are unable to retell will find it difficult, if not impossible, to summarize effectively."

(Moss, p. 711, 2004)

- Includes important information
- Contains the main idea (in 10 words or less, one word on each finger as they summarize)
- Is in the student's own words

I explain (and demonstrate) the principle of summarizing with the analogy of a funnel, where we take a lot of information and narrow it down to a short summary. I may also use a strainer (such as the kind for draining salads and pasta) to show that when we remove the extra water we are left with the key ingredient. In the same way, when our brains remove all the unimportant details we are left with the "big idea." A further, less messy analogy, is one involving packing for a holiday and only being able to take one suitcase, thus needing to decide what is going to be most important to take and why. A student backpack or your purse could be used to illustrate in the same way: What do we really have to have with us each day, what is most important? (McGregor, 2007). Together we brainstorm a list of possibilities and then narrow them down in the prioritizing process described in the lesson I Can Sum It Up.

Student Profiles

Here we may find our "minimalists," who demonstrate a "shorter is better" approach to oral retellings. That might be acceptable in summarizing—if in fact they do determine what is important—but these students will not meet the requirements of a complete retelling that assessments typically require. We also find here students who are "lost in plot" and unable to provide a logical and sequential retelling.

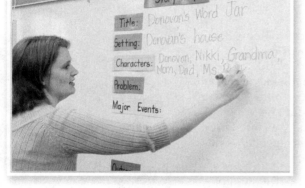

A story map outline provides a supportive structure for students, allowing them to expand upon each of the key elements

Often students view stories as a series of random events, and this perpetuates the problem of disjointed retellings. In a narrative, the character and their motives drive the plot: How they respond to other characters and situations as they strive to achieve their goal or overcome a challenge forms a chain of events or roadmap for a retell. When students are confused, I bring them back to the characters—their goals, what they say and do as a consequence, how one thing leads to another or the causal relationships discussed in the second lesson on making inferences on page 129. I often use a story analysis chart (see Reading-Writing Connection in the I Can Retell lesson) to present this concept visually to students.

Visual aids, such as the Retelling Cards on page 156 will be an important scaffold to understanding the text structure that determines the retell.

Reading Materials to Support Retelling and Summarizing

Supportive reading materials for fiction include stories with a familiar structure, such as the following:

- Circular stories, like the If You Give ... series by Laura Joffe Numeroff (1991)
- Linear stories, such as *The Grouchy Ladybug* by Eric Carle, that have a time sequence
- Cumulative text that repeats the events in sequence several times throughout the reading

(continued on page 141)

Student Difficulty With Retelling and Summarizing	Teaching Response/Next Steps
Student Is unable to retell	**Teacher** ● Connects theme or topic with child's prior knowledge and personal experience ● Uses concrete analogies, such as a cell phone conversation or dialogue from a familiar TV show (see Teaching Tips, page 137) ● May provide a prop such as a cell phone for students to use as they role-play ● Implements sharing circles during which students share personal news, book reviews, and their work to provide oral practice retelling events and information (see Scheduling in Chapter 3) ● Provides tactile learning aids, such as the Retelling Cards on page 156 made of poster board; students touch each card as they orally retell the story ● Integrates retelling with writing instruction in which students write a play script for the characters in the story (as with Readers Theater) ● Invites student questions about the theme or topic ● Models "look backs" by rereading and focusing student attention on the section they are unable to retell ● Provides key vocabulary (see activity in the I Can Retell lesson) ● Introduces the vocabulary cumulatively—before each part of the reading; students use the vocabulary in their retelling of each section and in the final retell ● Focuses on developing understanding of the concept of "event" as something that happens in a typical day at school, or in a TV show (Caldwell & Leslie, 2005) ● Explains the parts of a story—or the text structure (character, setting, goal, problem, events, solution/resolution) —using a highly structured text and picture cues (see Retelling Cards page 156) ● Uses examples from videos of classic children's novels to illustrate the importance of setting, actions, and dialogue of the characters ● Includes story mapping activities or graphic organizers for expository text for the students to represent the information with a visual; students can use this as a springboard for oral retells when they require additional "think time"
Is unable to summarize	● Relates the principle of summarizing to personal experience by asking: *What happened to you today that was important? What do you bring to school each day that is important to remember?* ● Uses concrete analogies, such as a funnel, strainer, or suitcase to demonstrate the process of reducing a list of events or facts to only the most important (see Teaching Tips, page 137) ● Supports the student by prompting with a short section of text to identify the subject and what it is about: *What or who is this about? Why? Where? When? How? (is something done or looks)* (See also "struggles to integrate new information" (on the next page)
Echoes the child next to him/her when asked to retell	● Uses the round-the-table retelling (see Reading-Writing Connection), distributing picture cues for the story elements that each student is responsible for recording on their whiteboard or marking the text information on one of the story elements (in addition to I Connect and I Wonder responses); students then cumulatively retell—repeating what the students have shared before them and then adding on their information from the notes they made or marked in the text

Student Difficulty With Retelling and Summarizing	Teaching Response/Next Steps
Student Provides an incomplete two- or three-word retelling	**Teacher** • Relates retelling to having a cell phone conversation where you want the other person to know all the details of what just happened • Focuses student attention on the dialogue between characters as an aid to recalling events • Refers to graphic features in nonfiction text, illustrations in fiction, and demonstrates how these add additional information to the running text • Cues retelling of each story element with a picture-cued five-finger retelling glove (attach picture cards with Velcro to fingers of a gardening glove); cues retelling of nonfiction using topic, three details, and "big idea" as the five fingers; for nonfiction, students pinch their thumb and baby finger together as they sum up the topic and concluding sentence, the other three fingers represent three facts with details • Provides the icons and/or question words (see Retelling Cards, 156) • Displays picture cards representing each story element vertically on the table in front of the student (number them in order of the retelling sequence), and prompts them to slide these across the table or magnetic board one by one as they retell the information related to each icon (Caldwell & Leslie, 2005) • Incorporates graphic organizers (see "Is unable to retell," above) • Models embellished retellings by including personal connections, evaluating character actions, expressing opinions (connecting, evaluative questioning, inferences)
Struggles to integrate new information into their retelling or summary, relying on prior knowledge only	• Prompts to adjust reading speed, going slower in parts with new information, important events, and includes frequent stopping points for student to retell and check their understanding of the part of the reading; may place color-coded sticky notes in the text to show parts where they need to slow down (yellow or orange) • Has student record information on two colors of paper strips, what they know on green, new information on yellow or orange • Asks student to stop and jot or sketch each short section, cumulatively adding details onto the same sketch as they read the next section or adding more details to their writing • Includes characterization activities that focus on why and how the character acted in a certain way, demonstrating how characters drive the plot and how their responses to others and to situations cause the next event • Prepares concept sorts to support summaries in which students list the facts after reading and then identify possible categories; alternatively, provides the words before reading for students to sort under subheadings in the text based on their predictions, then checking the sort during and after reading and asking, *Do they still belong in these categories?* (See I Can Retell lesson)
Does not include key elements of the story or key information	• Supports students in a story element match-up activity where they sort character names, events, etc., under cards depicting each of the elements (see I Can Retell lesson) • Highlights words and phrases in the text that indicate when new facts or details are being introduced (another, for example), so that students can identify new and supporting information; displays these on cards or a chart for student self-monitoring
Responds with a retelling that is not in logical sequence	• Writes the events on a chart (may be student-dictated) and cuts apart or prints on index cards, with the student sequencing these to retell; teacher provides the book as a model for student self-checking, gradually removing this scaffold in following sessions • Has student complete a four-frame comic strip version of a familiar story in a shared writing format ("freeze frames" in a movie), listing events on sticky notes or sentence strips and placing them in the order they occurred, using the text as a reference • Has student create a storyboard using a sheet of paper divided into 4–12 frames, depending on the length of the text and student need, sketching the events in sequence, completing the beginning and ending first to ensure a logical and linear sequence (for shorter text, each frame may represent a page they read); this same format can be used as a draft for writing their own innovation to the story in a Reading-Writing Connection activity • Highlights transitional phrases, such as *first, then, after that, next, finally* that indicate to the reader that another event or new information is coming; has student use these in oral and written retellings (see Reading-Writing Connection in the lesson)

- Character/problem/solution narrative structure of so many familiar fairy and folk tales, like the "Three Billy Goats Gruff," and series that center on a character, such as the books about Arthur written by Marc Brown (Scholastic). These have a clear sequence of events with cause-and-effect relationships and support plot analysis as they emphasize the main character and the steps they take to solve a problem, and how they grow and change as a result. These can usually be easily divided into beginning, middle, and end.

Nonfiction retelling and summaries are supported by text with features that provide signposts to new information such as:
- Table of contents
- Subheadings
- Key words in bold
- Diagrams and photos with captions and labels
- Signal words that indicate the text structure: *because of, so that* in cause-and-effect text structure; *compared to, different from* in compare-and-contrast text structure; and words such as *first, then, finally,* which tell us that section of the text or entire text is a sequence structure

LESSON: I CAN RETELL

Preparation

- Copy the reproducible I Can Understand What I Read Chart (page 100) onto cardstock.
- Copy the reproducible I Can Retell Bookmark (page 155) onto cardstock. Make one for every student. Option for nonfiction: Copy the I Can Wonder bookmark (page 153).
- Copy of the Comprehension Prompt Card (page 98).
- For fiction, print words from the text that represent the main character, setting, problem, and solution on index cards. Prepare category headings for these (see illustration in the lesson). For nonfiction, print the headings or subheadings in the text on cards, or entries from the table of contents and words from the text related to them.
- Optional: Copy Retelling Cards, page 156, onto cardstock and cut apart.

Tell Me

Point to the icon for I Can Retell on the Comprehension Strategy Chart. If you are using the Retelling Cards, substitute the language on the cards in the teacher dialogue below.

○ **Fiction Retell**

When we are telling a friend about something that happened to us, we tell them what happened and how it happened—enough detail to give them a picture in their minds, so they can understand what happened. We tell them who was there: the people, where it happened, and what happened. Sometimes there might have been a problem, like the dog running away, that we had to solve. Before we stop talking, we always tell them how it all ended.

As a reader, it also helps you understand a story when you think about all the people (characters), places (settings), and problems. [Point to the icons on the bookmark.]

○ **Nonfiction Retell**

If you are reading a book with lots of facts, then retelling will help you to remember them. We want to know what the book is about, where and when it happened, and why or how (4 W's and an H).

Show Me

○ **Before Reading**

Introduce the title or topic of the text. Invite connections and questions in a brief discussion. This may be a partner "turn and talk" activity only.

○ **Story Structure Sort**

Explain the category headings and introduce the vocabulary words or phrases you have printed on cards one by one (see Preparation). Briefly discuss the meaning of each word, where necessary.

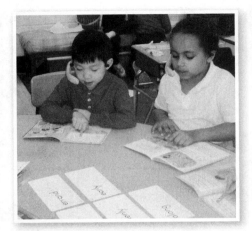

Students read the vocabulary words in context to determine if the author used them to tell about the people, places or problems in the story. Next they will sort the word cards into the corresponding categories using the Retelling Cards as category headings (p. 156)

Authors choose certain words to tell us about the people, places, and problems in their story. In our story today, we will find these words [Show and read the word cards.]

I am going to read the first part of the story and see if I can find how the author used these words. I will ask myself if they tell me about the people (or animals), the place where the story happens, or whether they describe a problem that one of the people has.

Read a short section of the text and identify the category on the Retelling Cards for two to three words, leaving some for students to sort. Model the reasoning behind identifying the category:

Tiger belongs under People/Who, because we know the story is about "my sloppy tiger," and we have read other stories about Sloppy Tiger.

The word room *belongs under Places/Where because it tells us where the action happened.*

Comprehension in Action: Before Reading: *My Sloppy Tiger* by Joy Cowley (1987)

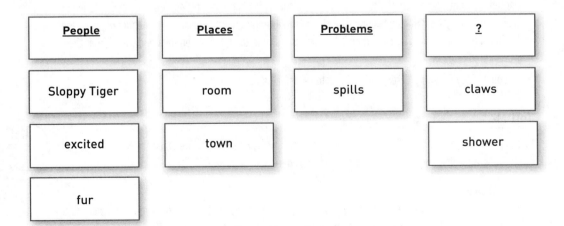

People	Places	Problems	?
Sloppy Tiger	room	spills	claws
excited	town		shower
fur			

Guide Me

Challenge students to help you identify where the rest of the words should be placed, which category they belong in. You may move the card along under the categories, pause under each one and ask students to indicate whether you should place it here with a show of thumbs (up or down). When the word could belong in more than one category or when there is not consensus among the group, place the word under the question mark header.

Shower could be just a place or it could be a problem if S.T. gets into trouble with it. The word claws *could be telling us about a part of S.T.'s body or it could be a problem. We will read on to find out.*

Ask students to read the next section of the text and be watching for the vocabulary words from the sort and check that they really tell us about the same story element.

Let's read to check our story sort. Did the author use this word to tell us about people, places, or problems?

○ Group Share

Pause and have students retell what they have read with a partner in a quick one-minute retell. Invite them to share this with the group. Model and support student retelling as necessary.

What did we find out first/What happened in the beginning? What happened after that?

Let's check our story sort. What words have we read so far in the story? Did ___ tell us about ___? Show me that part. How does the author use that word?

We still haven't read the word __. Keep reading and see if they really do tell us about people, places, or problems.

Coach Me

Students read on to the end of the story. Prompt and listen to individuals retell what they have read.

Tell me about _____.

In the story, why did _____ happen?

Can you tell me more about that?

Tell about this book as if you were telling a kindergarten student.

Review the story vocabulary sort with the group. Reread the words under each category and ask students to indicate whether they still match. If not, why?

Now we have read the story, we need to check our sort and see if it still matches the story.

We need to revise our predictions for words that tell about the problem because [when we read this page], *we found out _____.*

Example: *Sloppy Tiger made a mess in the shower, so the word* shower *was part of the problem. He ripped up the T-shirt with his claws. The word* claws *was not just telling about parts of the body of the tiger; it was part of the problem.*

○ Step 2: After Reading

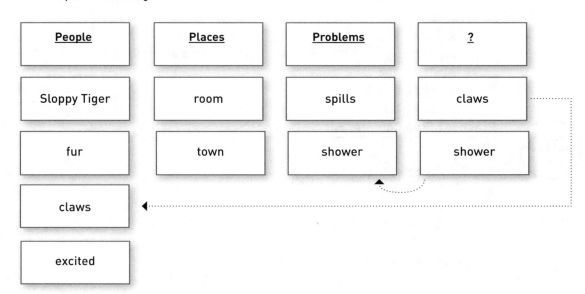

○ **Partner Think-Pinch-Share**

Tell your partner what you remember about the story. Use your bookmark to help you tell about each part.

Who was the most important character and why were they important?

How do they solve their problem in the story?

Retell what happened. Use the words in our sort to help you.

○ **Group Share**

Invite retellings from the partners within the group.

What can the next partners add on to what we just heard? What else do we remember?

Let's use the words in our sort to retell all the things that happened in the story. What happened in the beginning? In the middle? At the end?

What else can you remember?

What do you think the girl would tell a friend about what happened that day?

Optional: Write on a whiteboard as a shared writing activity.

What might the girls have written in their diary after this happened?

○ **Restate the Teaching Point**

When we retell what we read, it helps us understand more about the people, places, and problems in the story.

Reading-Writing Connection

To support students in processing all the information in the text, have them complete one of the writing in response to reading activities:

○ **Round the Table Retell (During Reading)**

At the Coach Me step in the lesson, distribute a whiteboard and a different story retelling card (page 156) to each student. Have students place their card at the top of their whiteboards. Students stop and jot the information for their Retelling Card on their whiteboard during the reading of the next section/text (e.g., one student is responsible for recording the main characters, another the setting(s) and so on). After reading, go around the table and have each student read what they have on their whiteboard; this is recorded in a shared writing format for a complete written retelling.

○ **After Reading**

Students may:

＊Write dialogue that could have taken place in the story (such as a cell phone conversation)

＊Write a news report on the information

＊Sketch the main event

Practice at the Comprehension Center

These activities are from *Differentiated Literacy Centers* (Southall, 2007):

● Retelling Flap Book
● Retelling Cube for Stories
● Tic Tac Tell for Facts
● Retelling Cube for Facts
● Tic Tac Tell for Stories
● Stop, Draw, and Write

Preparation

- Copy the reproducible I Can Understand What I Read Chart (page 100) onto cardstock.
- For fictional text: Copy the reproducible I Can Sum It Up Bookmark (page 155) onto cardstock. For nonfiction, copy the Summary Cards and I Can Sum It Up bookmark for each student.
- Copy of the Comprehension Prompt Card (page 98).
- Choose a short text (passage or article).
- Gather three to four sticky notes for each student.
- Chart paper.
- Optional: Provide three star-shaped sticky notes.

Tell Me

Point to the icon for I Can Sum It Up on the Comprehension Strategy Chart.

When we read a book that has a lot of information, we can't remember everything the author said. We can only remember what we absolutely have to know. Just like packing a suitcase for a holiday, we can only take what we really need [see Teaching Tips]. *So we have to decide what is most important—and we use our own words to sum it up in one or two sentences.*

Show Me

Read a short passage or article. Model the process of summarizing, using the bookmark as a guide.

I know _____.
I learned _____.
An important word was _____.
Three important facts were _____.
This was about _____.

Introduce the new text. Invite student predictions about the content to provide a purpose for reading.

What do you predict you will learn in a book about kangaroos?
What information do authors typically share with us in a nonfiction book about an animal?

Guide Me

Students are to read the text and mark the places where they find important information. Provide sticky notes for each student. Remind them they only have so many sticky notes, and there are more facts than that in the book. They will need to decide which ones are important. Students can change their mind and move a sticky if they come to a fact they think is more important.

Find [1–3] important facts the author wants us to remember. Use your bookmark to remind you to look for important words and facts. Put your sticky note on the edge of the page next to it.

Think of your purpose for reading this book. What are you trying to find out?

Have more advanced readers/writers write a fact on the sticky note at each stopping point in the reading.

○ **Partner Share**

Read your facts to your partner. Are they the same or different from yours?
Can they explain to you why they chose those facts?

○ **Group Share**

Have students tell as many facts as they can remember and record on a chart like the one on the following page.

mammals	warm-blooded	joeys are baby kangaroos
tails help them balance	short legs for scratching	there are lots of different types of kangaroos
bettongs, potoroos, wallabies, and wallaroos are kangaroos	the largest are red kangaroos	all kangaroos eat plants, like grass, leaves, and bark
kangaroos live only in Australia, Papua New Guinea, and Indonesia		

Interesting

Tails help them balance

Important

Kangaroos are mammals

Review the list of facts, reading them one by one. Each time, ask students if this is a very important fact.

They can choose one to three depending on how many facts you have listed.

Allow flexibility, as students may change their minds as you read further on the list; this supports the prioritizing process involved in determining importance.

Place sticky notes alongside these important facts.

> *Remember, you only have three sticky notes, so we have to decide what the author really wants us to remember about kangaroos.*
>
> *Were there any facts that the author repeated or gave us more information (details) about?*
>
> *Which are our all-star facts (the most important)?*

You may need to talk briefly about what is interesting as students may be sidetracked by startling facts or personal interests. We code those facts that are merely interesting with and a little *i* for interesting, and those that are more important with a big *I*. You can also sort the facts on cards in two columns under these headings to make this process more concrete and support the discussion that is necessary so students can talk, think, and reason through the prioritization process.

Coach Me

Support students during reading to mark important facts or events. Ask them to explain their rationale for the decision they made.

> *Look for facts that are repeated in more than one place; they are usually important*
> *What was this part about?*
> *Why was this an important part?*

○ **Partner Think-Pinch-Share**

Ask students to use these facts to sum it up for their partners, using the bookmark phrasing "this was about _____" or "I learned _____."

Listen in to the partner discussion, and prompt, support, and provide feedback.

> *If you were telling someone about kangaroos and you had to say it in two sentences, what would you say? Which facts would you use?*
>
> *If you had only one minute to tell a friend (or younger sibling) about this, what would you tell them that would sum it up?*

What words from the chart would help you to sum it up?

○ **Group Share**

Have partners share their summaries. Optional: You may have them compose and write a cooperative summary, each student using a strip of paper, so it has to be short.

In a shared writing format, compose one or two sentences that sum it up:

This was about _____.

We learned _____.

○ **Restate the Teaching Point**

When we sum up the important parts, it helps us to understand and remember.

Reading-Writing Connection

Students can record important information using these simple graphic organizers:

Two-column chart formats:
- Picture/Why it is important
- Words/Why they are important
- Interesting/Why
- Important/Why
- Sketch and label a picture that represents the theme or "big idea"
- Round the Table Summary: Use the same format as page 144, using the Summary Cards on page 157

Practice at the Comprehension Center

Provide independent practice with these activities from *Differentiated Literacy Centers* (Southall, 2007)

- Pyramid Summary
- Critic's Cube
- Roll and Respond Cube
- What's Most Important?
- Partner Quiz Cards

I Can Code My Thinking: Integrating Multiple Strategies

My students love coding, a hands-on approach to reading! Many colleagues across the country have given me positive feedback after workshops during which I shared this idea—telling me how their students have taken off in their comprehension strategy use with the coding technique. They use it continuously throughout the year in small-group, partner, and independent reading contexts.

The codes are simple notations, such as a star, printed on to sticky notes or flags to represent a comprehension strategy or self-monitoring behavior. These are the same strategies from the previous lessons and on the comprehension strategy chart at the beginning of the chapter (see page 100). Students use these coded flags to mark the text with their thinking, and in doing so apply multiple comprehension strategies. The power of these coded flags is that every student is accountable for interacting with the text using a strategic focus (Harvey & Goudvis, 2007; Hoyt, 2002). These are prepared before the reading and distributed to the students, who keep them on their bookmark alongside each code (see Teaching Tips).

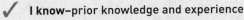

✓ **I know**–prior knowledge and experience

❓ **I wonder**–all levels of questions

★ **I learned**–events, facts, or information that are new to me

☺ **This reminds me**–connections to self, text, and world

🧩🧩 **I am puzzled**–this does not make sense, I need to stop and fix

💡 **Aha! Now I get it!**–a number of strategies are used to clarify understanding, such as the ones listed in the I Can Stop and Fix It lesson, as well as inference, synthesis

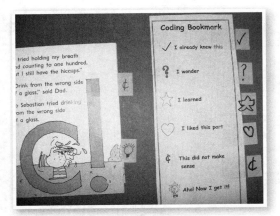

Sticky flags labeled with the codes are stored on a strip of card. Students place these in the margin of the text to mark their "thinking spots." The evidence for their thinking is now easy to locate after reading and will support both their oral and written responses.

Teaching Tips

The codes are introduced and practiced one by one, then cumulatively across a series of lessons. For example, after you have introduced the first and second codes, students use both to mark the text. When I am teaching connecting and questioning, we use the first three: know, wonder, learn. Then I take up student responses and record them on a KWL chart. At first, students practice the codes in lessons where the teacher identifies which one to use, but after sufficient practice, students will be able to self-select the appropriate response at different points of the reading. At this point, the activity has become a student-driven form of self-monitoring.

I prefer to use sticky flags and print the codes with a permanent marker. Each student has his or her own bookmark with the sticky flags that are appropriate for the lesson on the bookmark. You will find that if you laminate the bookmark, the flags will last even longer. I keep a group set of coding bookmarks with flags in my reading toolbox on the teaching table. You may provide more than one for a strategy you are focusing on, for example, three question mark flags when you want them to mark three places where they had a question. If you find students use all their flags on one page and you want them to interact at different points in the reading, chunk the text into short sections and specify the number of flags for each section, such as, "Read pages 6 to 8 and find one connection you have and one question." You can also divide books into beginning, middle, and end with specific requirements for each part.

Student Profiles

This activity is successful with students who are passive readers and/or apply strategies in isolation rather than integration. We know that to be effective readers, students need to be able to apply comprehension strategies to the text simultaneously. Predicting alone is not enough; you also need to question, infer, and so on. We may teach each strategy one at a time and explicitly, but we also continually model and practice how they build upon each other. Our goal is for students to become strategic readers who use multiple strategies in a flexible manner.

Reading Materials to Support Integrating Multiple Strategies

Any text is appropriate for coding, fiction and nonfiction of all genres. Nonfiction may generate more "I wonder" and "I learned" responses, while narrative text often supports personal connections with students using the "This reminds me" sticky flags.

Preparation

- Copy the reproducible I Can Understand What I Read Chart (page 100) onto cardstock.
- Copy the reproducible I Can Code My Thinking bookmark (page 158) onto cardstock. Make one for every student.
- Copy of the Comprehension Prompt Card (page 98).
- Prepare the coded sticky flags: Print the code(s) you are using in this lesson on sticky flags and place on the bookmark alongside the code.

Tell Me

Point to the Comprehension Strategy Chart and review the strategies that are related to the codes you are using in the lesson.

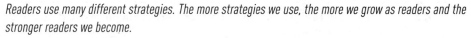

Readers use many different strategies. The more strategies we use, the more we grow as readers and the stronger readers we become.

Point to the codes on the bookmark as you describe how to use each one.

Today we will use the strategies we practiced as we read about [title, topic of the book].

I will show you how we are going to use these sticky flags on the bookmarks to code or mark our thinking spots as we read. I will use different codes in different parts of the book. As I read something, it might remind me of what I already know about this. If it does, I put the flag with the tick mark next to that part, right on the outside edge of the page. This way I can quickly find it to share. When I read the next part, I might have a question. I will put the flag with the question mark there.

Show Me

Introduce the book. Model how you code your thinking for different events or facts.

This book is about _____. I will read the first two pages and show my thinking with a code.

Example: *Sebastian Gets the Hiccups* by Jenny Feely (2001)

> *"Oh, no!" said Sebastian. "I have the hiccups, Mom. What should I do?"*
> *"Hold your breath and count to one hundred," said Mom.*

What am I thinking about when I read this part? Which code could I use to show my thinking? I am wondering if holding your breath and counting to one hundred will work. I will put my "I wonder" sticky flag next to this part.

> *"I tried holding my breath and counting to one hundred, but I still have the hiccups." "Drink from the wrong side of a glass," said Dad.*

Now I am thinking that doesn't make sense. How can you drink from the wrong side of a glass? I am confused about this. I will put my cents sign next to this part. Then I will try a fix-up tool; I will read on. Oh, I see in the picture that Sebastian has turned his head around to drink from the other side of the glass. That must be what his dad meant when he said the wrong side; it was the other side of the glass. I will put my lightbulb/stoplight flag here to show that I stopped and fixed it, and now I understand.

Guide Me

Students read the text and mark their thinking spots with a coded flag. Specify which flags and how many.

Read pages ___ to ___. Use the [number and type] *flags on your bookmark to show what you were thinking.*

Have students share a place where they coded their thinking. Record this on a chart with the code on the left of the chart and the student response written alongside in a shared writing format.

Comprehension in Action: *Sebastian Gets the Hiccups* by Jenny Feely (2001)

🙂	I tried blowing into a paper bag, too. It didn't work and the bag blew up.
?	How can you rub your tummy and pat your head at the same time?
🙂	If I stand on my head I get dizzy.
🧩 🧩	Is Isabella his sister or a friend? I am puzzled about who she is.
💡	I figured out that she is probably his sister, because everyone in the story so far is in his family.
🙂	I would feel angry too if someone came up to me and shouted "Boo" like that.

Coach Me

Students continue to read as you coach and support.

What are you thinking about when you read this part? Which code could you use to show that?

○ **Partner Think-Pinch-Share**

Students show their partner where they have coded the text and explain what they were thinking about and why this was an appropriate code.

What was their thinking for this part of the story? Can they explain to you why they used that code? How does the code show their thinking?

○ **Group Share**

Have partners share how they coded the rest of the story.

○ **Restate the Teaching Point**

We marked the text with a code that showed our thinking. Thinking about the story in different ways helps us to understand what we are reading and to grow as readers.

Reading-Writing Connection

● Students draw the codes in their notebook and record their thinking alongside, just like they did on the group chart.

Practice at the Comprehension Center

Provide independent practice with these activities from *Differentiated Literacy Centers* (Southall, 2007)

● Read, Relate, Respond
● Sticky Questions

I CAN UNDERSTAND WHAT I READ
Bookmark

I can understand what I read

- **I connect**

- **I predict**

- **I wonder**

- **I figure it out**

- **I stop and fix**

- **I retell**

- **I sum it up**

1 + 1 = 2

I CAN CONNECT
Bookmark

I can connect

- **I know**

- **This is like**

- **This reminds me of**

me

a book or story

the world

Differentiated Small Group Reading Lessons © 2009 by Margo Southall, Scholastic Teaching Resources page 151

I CAN PREDICT
Bookmark

I can predict

Predict

- I bet...
- I predict...
- I will find out...
- I think I will learn...
- I know what will happen...

Hold it

Read and check

- I will think back
- Does it match? Yes? No?
- Do I need to change it?

Predict again

- Now I know...
- I am thinking that...

I CAN FIGURE IT OUT
Bookmark

I can figure it out

Look for clues

in the picture

I see...

This tell me that...

in the words

The author says ...

This means that...

It could be that ...

Maybe ...Perhaps ...

Think about what I know

The author doesn't say...

but I know... because...

Make a picture in my mind

I can picture...

This helps me understand...

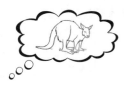

Differentiated Small Group Reading Lessons © 2009 by Margo Southall, Scholastic Teaching Resources page 152

I CAN WONDER
Literal Questions Bookmark

Seek and find

- **Who**

- **What**

- **Where**

- **When**

- **How**

I CAN WONDER
Inferential and Evaluative Questions Bookmark

Think and feel

- **I think**

- **I feel**

- **Why**

- **What if**

- **Should**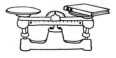

- **How might**

STOP AND FIX
Bookmark

I can stop and fix

 STOP

Look at pictures

Reread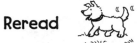

Read on

What do I know?

Use parts of words I know

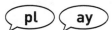 pl ay

Picture in my mind

 WAIT

Check it makes sense ¢

 GO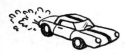

Keep reading

STOP AND FIX
Bookmark

I can stop and fix

STOP

Look at pictures

Reread

Read on

What do I know?

Use parts of words I know

 pl  ay

Picture in my mind

WAIT

Check it makes sense ¢

GO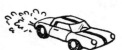

Keep reading

I CAN RETELL
Bookmark

I can retell

People

What they do and say

What they are like ___

Their goal

Places

What it looks like

How it feels there

Problems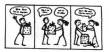

___ has a problem because ___

They try ___ and ___

They solve it by___

Ending

In the end...

I CAN SUM UP
Bookmark

I can sum it up

• **I know**

• **I learned**

• **An important word**

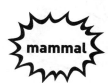
mammal

• **An important fact**

 kangaroos are...

• **This was about**

Retelling Cards

Places
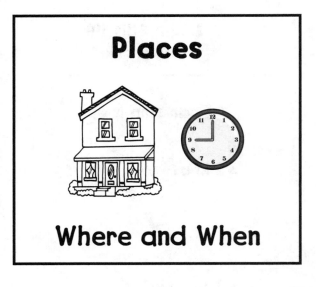
Where and When

People and Goals
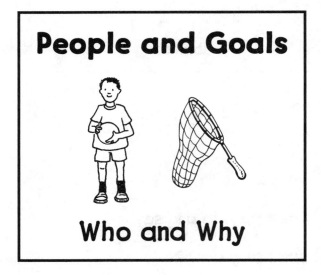
Who and Why

Problems
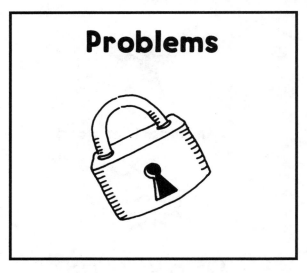

Main Events
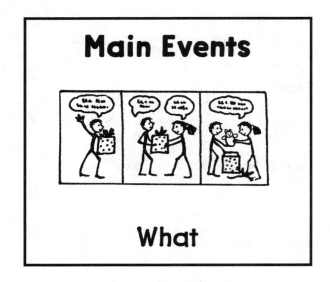
What

Solution
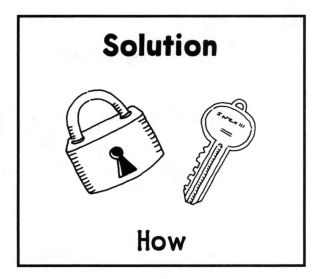
How

Ending
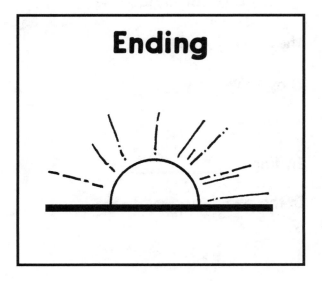

Summary Cards

I know	I wondered
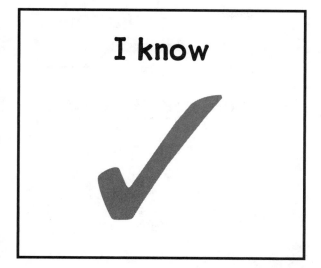	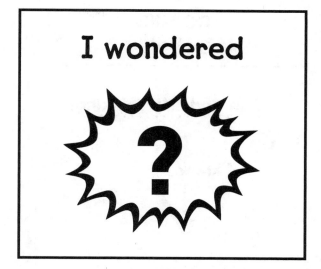

I learned	Some important words were
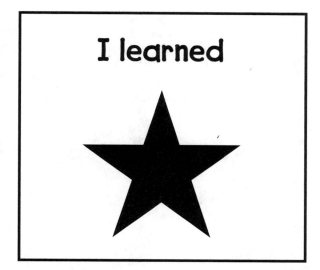	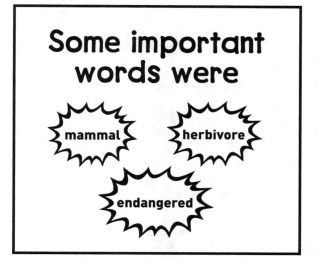

An important fact or event was	This was about...
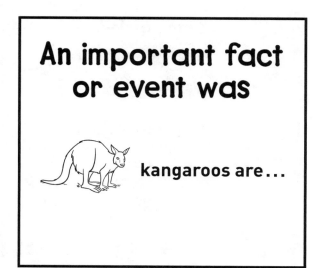	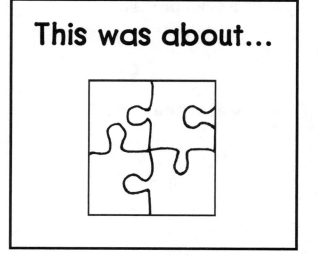

CODING
Bookmark

I Can Code My Thinking

- **I know**

- **This reminds me**

- **I wonder**

- **I learned**

- **I am puzzled**

- **Aha! Now I get it**

CODING
Bookmark

I Can Code My Thinking

- **I know**

- **This reminds me**

- **I wonder**

- **I learned**

- **I am puzzled**

- **Aha! Now I get it**

References

Allen, Mary Beth. (2007) *Current, best strategies for teaching reading comprehension: Resource handbook.* Bellevue, WA: Bureau of Education and Research.

Allington, Richard. (2005). *What really matters for struggling readers: Designing research-based programs.* (2nd ed). Boston: Pearson.

Applegate, Mary Dekonty, Quinn Kathleen Benson, & Applegate, Anthony J., (2006). Profiles in comprehension. *The Reading Teacher, Vol. 60, No. 1.*

Badian, N.A. (2000) It's not just phonological awareness! The importance of orthographic processing in reading. Paper presented at the 27th Annual Conference on Dyslexia and Related Reading Disorders, New York.

Bear, D. R. Invernizzi, M. Templeton, S. & Johnston, F. (2004) *Words their way: Word study for phonics, vocabulary, and spelling instruction.* (3rd ed.). Upper Saddle River, New Jersey: Pearson.

Beck, Isabel L. (2006). *Making sense of phonics: The hows and whys.* New York: Guilford Press.

Blevins, Wiley. (2006). *Phonics from A to Z.* New York: Scholastic.

Blevins, Wiley. (2002). *Building fluency: Lessons and strategies for reading success.* New York: Scholastic.

Blair, T.R., Rupley W.H., & Nichols, W. (2007). The effective teaching of reading: Considering the "what" and "how" of instruction. *The Reading Teacher Vol. 60, No. 5,* 442-438.

Boyles, Nancy. (2004). *Constructing meaning through kid-friendly strategy instruction.* FL: Maupin House.

Brown, Kathleen. (2003). What do you say when they get stuck on a word? Aligning teachers prompts with students development. *The Reading Teacher, Vol. 56. No. 8.*

Caldwell, JoAnne Schudt & Leslie Lauren. (2005). *Intervention strategies to follow informal reading inventory assessment.* Boston: Pearson Education Inc.

Clay, Marie. (2001). *Running records for classroom teachers.* Portsmouth, NH: Heinemann.

Clay, Marie. (1997). *Reading recovery: A guidebook for teachers in training.* Portsmouth, NH: Heinemann.

Clark, Kathleen. (2004). What can I say besides "sound it out"? Coaching word recognition in beginning reading. *The Reading Teacher, Vol. 57, No. 5.*

Cooper, J. David, Chard, David J., & Kiger, Nancy D. (2007). *The struggling reader: Interventions that work.* New York: Scholastic.

Duffy, Gerald, G. (2003). *Explaining reading: A resource for teaching concepts, skills, and strategies.* New York: The Guilford Press.

Dufresne, Michelle. (2002). *Word solvers.* Portsmouth, NH: Heinemann.

Fountas, I.C. & Pinnell, G.S. (1999). *Leveled books: Matching texts to readers.* Portsmouth, NH: Heinemann.

Ganske, Kathy. (2000). *Word journeys: Assessment-guided phonics, spelling and vocabulary instruction.* New York: Guilford.

Gaskins, I.L., Ehri, C. Cress, L., O'Hara C., & Donnelly, K. (1997). Procedures for word learning: Making discoveries about words. *The Reading Teacher, Vol. 50.*

Gibson, Vicki & Hasbrouck, Jan. (2007). *Differentiated instruction: Grouping for success.* New York: McGraw-Hill.

Gunning, Thomas G. (2002). *Assessing and correcting reading and writing difficulties.* Boston: Allyn and Bacon.

Harvey, S. & Goudvis, A. (2007). *Strategies that work: Teaching comprehension to enhance understanding.* (2nd ed). Portland, ME: Stenhouse.

Hasbrouck, Jan & Denton, Carolyn. (2005). *The reading coach: A how-to manual for success.* Boston: Sopris West.

Hoyt, Linda. (2002). Make it real: *Strategies for success with informational text.* Portsmouth, NH: Heinemann.

Juel, Connie & Minden-Cupp, Cecilia. (2000). One down and 80,000 to go: Word recognition instruction in the primary grades. *The Reading Teacher, Vol. 53, No. 4.*

Johnson, Pat. (2006). *One child at a time: making the most of your time with struggling readers K-6.* Portland, Maine: Stenhouse.

Klingner, Janette K., Vaughn, Sharon, & Boardman, Alison. (2007). *Teaching reading comprehension to students with learning difficulties.* New York: Guilford Press.

Kosanovich, Marcia, Ladinsky, Karen, Nelson, Luanne, & Torgesen, Joseph. (2006). Differentiated reading instruction: small group alternative lesson structures for all students. Florida Center for Reading Research. Retrieved from www.fcrr.org.

Lynch, Judy. (2002). *Word learning, word making, word sorting: 50 lessons for success.* New York: Scholastic.

Marcell, Barclay. (2007). Traffic light reading: Fostering the independent usage of comprehension strategies with informational text. *The Reading Teacher, Vol 60 (8),* 778-781.

McCandliss, B., Beck, I. L. , Sandak, R., & Perfetti, C. (2003) Focusing attention on decoding for children with poor reading skills: Design and preliminary tests of the word building intervention. *Scientific Studies in Reading,* 7 (1), 75-104.

McGregor, Tanny. (2007). *Comprehension connections: Bridges to strategic reading.* Portsmouth, NH: Heinemann.

Miller, Debbie. (2002) *Reading for meaning: Teaching comprehension in the primary grades.* Portland, ME: Stenhouse.

Morrison, Ian. (1994). *Keeping it together: Linking reading theory and practice.* Lower Hutt, New Zealand: Lands End Publishing.

Moss, Barbara. (2004). Teaching expository text structures through information trade books retellings. *The Reading Teacher, Vol. 57, No. 8.*

National Institute of Child Health and Human Development. (2000). *Report of the National Reading Panel. Teaching children to read: An evidence-based assessment of the scientific literature on reading and its implications for reading instruction.* (NIH – 00 – 4769). Washington, DC: Government Printing Office.

O'Connor, Rollanda E. (2007). *Teaching word recognition to students with learning difficulties.* New York: Guilford Press.

Pearson, P.D. & Gallagher, M.C. (1993). The instruction of reading comprehension. *Contemporary Educational Psychology 18,* 317-344.

Prescott-Griffin, Mary Lese & Witherell, Nancy L. (2004). *Fluency in focus.* Portsmouth, NH: Heinemann.

Raphael, Taffy E., Highfield, Kathy & Au., Kathryn H. (2006). *QAR now.* New York: Scholastic.

Rasinski, Timothy. (2003). *The fluent reader.* New York: Scholastic.

Richards, Janet C. & Anderson, Nancy A. (2003). How do you know? A strategy to help emergent readers make inferences. *The Reading Teacher Vol. 57, No. 3.*

Richek, Margaret. (2001). *Vocabulary strategies that boost your students' reading comprehension: Video resource guide.* Bureau of Education and Research, WA.

Robb, Laura. (2008). *Differentiating reading instruction.* New York: Scholastic.

Schwartz, Robert M. (1997). Self-monitoring in beginning reading. *The Reading Teacher, Vol. 51, No. 1.*

Shaywitz, Sally. (2003). *Overcoming dyslexia.* New York: Alfred Knopf.

Southall, Margo. (2007). *Differentiated literacy centers.* New York: Scholastic.

Taylor, Barbara M, & Pearson, P. David, Clark, Kathleen F., & Walpole, Sharon. (1999). Effective schools/accomplished teachers. *The Reading Teacher, Vol. 53, No. 2.*

Torgesen, Joseph. (2005). Preventing reading disabilities in young children: Requirements at the classroom and school level. University of Florida. Florida Center for Reading Research. Presentation for the International Dyslexia Association. Retrieved from www.fcrr.org.

Vogt, MaryEllen & Nagano, Patty. (2003). Turn it on with light bulb reading! Sound-switching strategies for struggling readers. *The Reading Teacher Vol. 57, No. 3.*

Wagstaff, Janiel. (1999). *Teaching reading and writing with word walls.* New York: Scholastic.

Walpole, Sharon & McKenna, Richard. (2007). *Differentiated instruction in the primary grades.* New York: Guilford Press.

Walpole, Sharon & McKenna, Richard. (2006). The role of informal reading inventories in assessing word recognition. *The Reading Teacher, 59, 592-594.*

Willner, Elizabeth Harden. (2003). Body parts reading: Giving your two cents, worth. *The Reading Teacher, Vol. 56, No. 6.*